Non-metallic biomaterials for tooth repair and replacement

Related titles:

Biomedical composites (ISBN 978-1-84569-436-4)

Materials science for dentistry: Ninth edition (ISBN 978-1-84569-529-3)

Dental biomaterials: imaging, testing and modelling (ISBN 978-1-84569-296-4)

Details of these books and a complete list of titles from Woodhead Publishing can be obtained by:

- visiting our web site at www.woodheadpublishing.com
- contacting Customer Services (e-mail: sales@woodheadpublishing.com; fax: +44 (0) 1223 832819; tel.: +44 (0) 1223 499140 ext. 130; address: Woodhead Publishing Limited, 80, High Street, Sawston, Cambridge CB22 3HJ, UK)
- in North America, contacting our US office (e-mail: usmarketing@woodheadpublishing.com; tel.: (215) 928 9112; address: Woodhead Publishing, 1518 Walnut Street, Suite 1100, Philadelphia, PA 19102-3406, USA

If you would like e-versions of our content, please visit our online platform: www.woodheadpublishingonline.com. Please recommend it to your librarian so that everyone in your institution can benefit from the wealth of content on the site.

We are always happy to receive suggestions for new books from potential editors. To enquire about contributing to our Biomaterials series, please send your name, contact address and details of the topic/s you are interested in to laura.overend@woodheadpublishing.com. We look forward to hearing from you.

The Woodhead team responsible for publishing this book:
Commissioning Editor: Laura Overend
Publications Co-ordinator: Lucy Beg
Project Editor: Cathryn Freear
Editorial and Production Manager: Mary Campbell
Production Editor: Richard Fairclough
Copyeditor: Marilyn J. Grant BSc
Proofreader: George Moore
Cover Designer: Terry Callanan

Woodhead Publishing Series in Biomaterials: Number 53

Non-metallic biomaterials for tooth repair and replacement

Edited by
Pekka Vallittu

WP
WOODHEAD PUBLISHING

Oxford Cambridge Philadelphia New Delhi

Published by Woodhead Publishing Limited,
80 High Street, Sawston, Cambridge CB22 3HJ, UK
www.woodheadpublishing.com
www.woodheadpublishingonline.com

Woodhead Publishing, 1518 Walnut Street, Suite 1100, Philadelphia,
PA 19102-3406, USA

Woodhead Publishing India Private Limited, G-2, Vardaan House, 7/28 Ansari Road,
Daryaganj, New Delhi – 110002, India
www.woodheadpublishingindia.com

First published 2013, Woodhead Publishing Limited

British Library Cataloguing in Publication Data
A catalogue record for this book is available from the British Library.

Library of Congress Control Number: 2012949692

ISBN 978-0-85709-244-1 (print)
ISBN 978-0-85709-643-2 (online)
ISSN 2049-9485 Woodhead Publishing Series in Biomaterials (print)
ISSN 2049-9493 Woodhead Publishing Series in Biomaterials (online)

Typeset by Toppan Best-set Premedia Limited, Hong Kong

Contents

Contributor contact details

(* = main contact)

Editor and Chapter 12

Professor Pekka K. Vallittu
Department of Biomaterials Science and Turku Clinical Biomaterials Centre (TCBC)
Institute of Dentistry
University of Turku
Lemminkäisenkatu 2
FI-20520 Turku
Finland

E-mail: pekka.vallittu@utu.fi

Chapter 1

Van P. Thompson
Biomaterials & Biomimetics
NYU College of Dentistry
345 East 24th Street
Room 838-S
New York 10010
USA

E-mail: van.thompson@nyu.edu

Nelson R. F. A Silva
Department of Restorative Dentistry
School of Dentistry (UFMG/FO)
Federal University of Minas Gerais
Alameda do ipe branco 520
Sao Luiz – Pampulha
Belo Horizonte 31275-080
Brazil

Chapter 2

Vuk Uskoković
Therapeutic Micro and Nanotechnology Laboratory
Department of Bioengineering and Therapeutic Sciences
University of California
San Francisco
CA, 94158-2330
USA

E-mail: vuk21@yahoo.com

Chapter 3

Jorge Perdigão*
University of Minnesota
Department of Restorative Sciences
Minneapolis, MN 55455
USA

E-mail: perdi001@umn.edu

Ana Sezinando
University Rey Juan Carlos
Alcorcón, Madrid
Spain

Chapter 4

Professor Nikolaos Donos*
UCL-Eastman Dental Institute
Periodontology Unit
Department of Clinical Research
UK

E-mail: n.donos@eastman.ucl.ac.uk

Dr Xanthippi Dereka
Department of Periodontology
School of Dentistry
National and Kapodistrian University of Athens
Greece

Dr Harsh D. Amin
Department of Bioengineering
Imperial College London
UK

Chapter 5

Dr Jukka P. Matinlinna
Associate Professor in Dental Materials Science
Faculty of Dentistry
Dental Materials Science
The University of Hong Kong
The Prince Philip Dental Hospital
34 Hospital Road
Sai Ying Pun
Hong Kong SAR
PR China

E-mail: jpmat@hku.hk; jumatin@utu.fi

Chapter 6

Professor Maged K. Etman
Division of Prosthodontics
College of Dentistry
University of Saskatchewan
105 Wiggins Road, Saskatoon
Saskatchewan
S7N 5E4
Canada

E-mail: maged.etman@usask.ca

Chapter 7

X. Chatzistavrou
Department of Orthodontics and Pediatric Dentistry
School of Dentistry
University of Michigan
1011 N University
Ann Arbor
MI 48109
USA

E. Kontonasaki and P. Koidis
Department of Fixed Prosthesis and Implant Prosthodontics
School of Dentistry
Aristotle University of Thessaloniki
54124 Thessaloniki
Greece

K. M. Paraskevopoulos
Department of Physics
Solid State Section
Aristotle University of Thessaloniki
54124 Thessaloniki
Greece

A. R. Boccaccini*
Institute of Biomaterials
University of Erlangen-Nuremberg
91058 Erlangen
Germany

E-mail: aldo.boccaccini@ww.uni-erlangen.de

Chapter 8

Dr Michael F. Burrow
Oral Diagnosis and Polyclinics
Faculty of Dentistry
The University of Hong Kong
Prince Philip Dental Hospital
34 Hospital Rd
Sai Ying Pun
Hong Kong (SAR)
PR China

E-mail: mfburr58@hku.hk

Chapter 9

Dr Idris Mohamed Mehdawi*
Department of Restorative Dentistry and Endodontics
Faculty of Dentistry
Benghazi University
Benghazi
Libya

E-mail: idr_meh@yahoo.com

Dr Anne Young
Department of Biomaterials and Tissue Engineering
UCL Eastman Dental Institute
256 Grays Inn Road
London
WC1X 8LD

E-mail: Anne.Young@ucl.ac.uk

Chapter 10

Dr Jack L. Ferracane*
Department of Restorative Dentistry
Division of Biomaterials and Biomechanics
Oregon Health & Science University
611 S.W. Campus Drive
Portland
Oregon 97239
USA

E-mail: ferracan@ohsu.edu

Dr William M. Palin
University of Birmingham
College of Medical and Dental Sciences
School of Dentistry, Biomaterials Unit
St Chads Queensway
Birmingham
B4 6NN
UK

E-mail: w.m.palin@bham.ac.uk

Chapter 11

Professor Timo O. Närhi*
Department of Prosthetic Dentistry
Institute of Dentistry
University of Turku
Turku
Finland

E-mail: timo.narhi@utu.fi

Dr Ahmed M. Ballo
Department of Biomaterials
Institute of Clinical Sciences
The Sahlgrenska Academy
Gothenburg University
Gothenburg
Sweden

and

Dental Implant and Osseointegration Research Chair
College of Dentistry
King Saud University
Riyadh
Saudi Arabia

Professor Pekka K. Vallittu
Department of Biomaterials Science
Institute of Dentistry
University of Turku
Lemminkäisenkatu 2
FI-20520 Turku
Finland

E-mail: pekka.vallittu@utu.fi

Chapter 13

Professor Mutlu Özcan
University of Zurich
Rämistrasse 71
CH-8006 Zurich
Switzerland

E-mail: mutlu.ozcan@zzmk.uzh.ch

Woodhead Publishing Series in Biomaterials

1 **Sterilisation of tissues using ionising radiations**
Edited by J. F. Kennedy, G. O. Phillips and P. A. Williams

2 **Surfaces and interfaces for biomaterials**
Edited by P. Vadgama

3 **Molecular interfacial phenomena of polymers and biopolymers**
Edited by C. Chen

4 **Biomaterials, artificial organs and tissue engineering**
Edited by L. Hench and J. Jones

5 **Medical modelling**
R. Bibb

6 **Artificial cells, cell engineering and therapy**
Edited by S. Prakash

7 **Biomedical polymers**
Edited by M. Jenkins

8 **Tissue engineering using ceramics and polymers**
Edited by A. R. Boccaccini and J. Gough

9 **Bioceramics and their clinical applications**
Edited by T. Kokubo

10 **Dental biomaterials**
Edited by R. V. Curtis and T. F. Watson

11 **Joint replacement technology**
Edited by P. A. Revell

12 **Natural-based polymers for biomedical applications**
Edited by R. L. Reiss et al

13 **Degradation rate of bioresorbable materials**
Edited by F. J. Buchanan

14 **Orthopaedic bone cements**
Edited by S. Deb

15 **Shape memory alloys for biomedical applications**
Edited by T. Yoneyama and S. Miyazaki

16 **Cellular response to biomaterials**
Edited by L. Di Silvio

17 **Biomaterials for treating skin loss**
Edited by D. P. Orgill and C. Blanco

18 **Biomaterials and tissue engineering in urology**
Edited by J. Denstedt and A. Atala

19 **Materials science for dentistry**
B. W. Darvell

20 **Bone repair biomaterials**
Edited by J. A. Planell et al.

21 **Biomedical composites**
Edited by L. Ambrosio

22 **Drug-device combination products**
Edited by A. Lewis

23 **Biomaterials and regenerative medicine in ophthalmology**
Edited by T. V. Chirila

24 **Regenerative medicine and biomaterials for the repair of connective tissues**
Edited by C. Archer and J. Ralphs

25 **Metals for biomedical devices**
Edited by M. Ninomi

26 **Biointegration of medical implant materials: science and design**
Edited by C. P. Sharma

27 **Biomaterials and devices for the circulatory system**
Edited by T. Gourlay and R. Black

28 **Surface modification of biomaterials: methods analysis and applications**
Edited by R. Williams

29 **Biomaterials for artificial organs**
Edited by M. Lysaght and T. Webster

30 **Injectable biomaterials: science and applications**
Edited by B. Vernon

31 **Biomedical hydrogels: biochemistry, manufacture and medical applications**
Edited by S. Rimmer

32 **Preprosthetic and maxillofacial surgery: biomaterials, bone grafting and tissue engineering**
Edited by J. Ferri and E. Hunziker

33 **Bioactive materials in medicine: design and applications**
Edited by X. Zhao, J. M. Courtney and H. Qian

34 **Advanced wound repair therapies**
Edited by D. Farrar

35 **Electrospinning for tissue regeneration**
Edited by L. Bosworth and S. Downes

36 **Bioactive glasses: materials, properties and applications**
Edited by H. O. Ylänen

37 **Coatings for biomedical applications**
Edited by M. Driver

38 **Progenitor and stem cell technologies and therapies**
Edited by A. Atala

39 **Biomaterials for spinal surgery**
Edited by L. Ambrosio and E. Tanner

40 **Minimized cardiopulmonary bypass techniques and technologies**
Edited by T. Gourlay and S. Gunaydin

41 **Wear of orthopaedic implants and artificial joints**
Edited by S. Affatato

42 **Biomaterials in plastic surgery: breast implants**
Edited by W. Peters, H. Brandon, K. L. Jerina, C. Wolf and V. L. Young

43 **MEMS for biomedical applications**
Edited by S. Bhansali and A. Vasudev

44 **Durability and reliability of medical polymers**
Edited by M. Jenkins and A. Stamboulis

45 **Biosensors for medical applications**
Edited by S. Higson

46 **Sterilisation of biomaterials**
Edited by S. Lerouge and A. Simmons

47 **The hip resurfacing handbook: a practical guide to the use and management of modern hip resurfacings**
Edited by K. De Smet, P. Campbell and C. Van Der Straeten

48 **Developments in tissue engineered and regenerative medicine products**
J. Basu and John W. Ludlow

49 **Nanomedicine: technologies and applications**
Edited by T. J. Webster

50 **Biocompatibility and performance of medical devices**
Edited by J-P. Boutrand

51 **Medical robotics**
Edited by P. Gomes

52 **Implantable sensor systems for medical applications**
Edited by A. Inmann and D. Hodgins

53 **Non-metallic biomaterials for tooth repair and replacement**
Edited by P. Vallittu

54 **Joining and assembly of medical materials and devices**
Edited by Y. N. Zhou and M. D. Breyen

55 **Diamond based materials for biomedical applications**
Edited by R. Narayan

56 **Nanomaterials in tissue engineering: characterization, fabrication and applications**
Edited by A. K. Gaharwar, S. Sant, M. J. Hancock and S. A. Hacking

57 **Biomimetic biomaterials: structure and applications**
Edited by A. Ruys

58 **Standardisation in cell and tissue engineering: methods and protocols**
Edited by V. Salih

59 **Inhaler devices: fundamentals, design and drug delivery**
Edited by P. Prokopovich

60 **Bio-tribocorrosion in biomaterials and medical implants**
Edited by Y. Yan

61 **Microfluidics for biomedical applications**
Edited by X. J. J. Li and Y. Zhou

62 **Decontamination in hospitals and healthcare**
Edited by J. T. Walker

63 **Biomedical imaging: applications and advances**
Edited by P. Morris

Foreword

The task of providing a reliable replacement for anatomic loss falls short of the original biology in both elegance and durability. Although prosthetic replacements are poor substitutes for healthy biology, disease and destruction leave clinicians few alternatives. Teeth and their prosthetic replacement typify this dilemma. The healthy tooth is a thing to be admired – strong, compliant, chemically resistant, and even beautiful. Despite the best efforts of clinicians and technicians, dental restorations have a long history characterized by failure, non-vitality, and a lack of true satisfaction. In the last 100 years, however, there has been success and beauty. These successes have provided important principles and the foundation from which current researchers and clinicians strive to improve the science of anatomic replacement.

Perhaps the greatest shift in restorative treatment ideology is the concept of minimal invasiveness. When preventative and regenerative therapies exist, they should be recommended and encouraged. The protection and regeneration of biological structures should be the goal of every clinician and researcher. Where resection and prosthetic reconstruction are the only possibility, however, the modern clinician should ask, what may remain? To this question, the modern answer emerges: retain all but the diseased state. Comparing the native biological structure with any restoration should affirm that answer, as should the relative lifespan of most restorations.

The increased usage of non-metallic materials has somewhat aided the principle of minimal resection and minimal invasiveness. The clinician and researcher are cautioned that if simply changing materials increases the need for biological resection, then the progress must be skeptically assessed. The materials described in the following chapters have great potential to create minimally invasive restorations. It is the methodology, however, of the preparation and fabrication that allows a minimally invasive result. With that understanding, the question may be posed, how may these modern materials be leveraged to create less invasive restorations for the patient? The definitive answer is yet unknown, but many results are very encouraging. These non-metallic materials provide clinicians with the possibility of imitating biological structures when restoration is the course of treatment. This biomimicry is a great opportunity to parallel the characteristics of teeth and other anatomic structures when resect and restore is the predominant course of action. While esthetic mimicry has long held the attention of clinician and patient, imitating other materials and biological properties will continue to gain in importance. Consequently, for this biomimicry to be more fully realized, current materials will need to be improved and skillfully employed.

Lastly, what is our obligation and responsibility as clinicians, researchers and readers? Perhaps it is to be inspired. Certainly, it is to encourage current and future generations of investigators. The editor asks us to bring our best science, to let us compare and learn. Either prove these concepts and ideas wrong, or push them forward. Regardless, consider that when our task is to restore prosthetically, we may create and use materials in a manner that preserves and parallels the natural biology.

'To read is to borrow; to create out of one's readings is paying off one's debts.' Charles Lilliard

Scott R. Dyer, DMD, MS, PhD
Portland, Oregon, USA

Part I

Structure, modification and repair of dental tissues

1

Structure and properties of enamel and dentin

V. P. THOMPSON, NYU College of Dentistry, USA and
N. R. F. A. SILVA, Federal University of Minas Gerais, Brazil

DOI: 10.1533/9780857096432.1.3

Abstract: This chapter addresses the mineralized tissues of teeth – enamel and dentin – and how they develop into structural components with unique physical properties. Tooth structure includes an epithelium-derived outer shell of enamel that is highly mineralized, hard, stiff and wear resistant. This is supported both mechanically and biochemically by a mesenchyme-derived dentin, which is vital, less mineralized, softer and more compliant. The dentin is maintained by the dental pulp, which is cellular and innervated, and has a vascular plexus.

Key words: dentin, enamel, mechanical properties of tooth structure, mineralized tissues.

1.1 Introduction

Much is known about teeth and their structure. Teeth have long been studied by paleontologists, since they degrade much more slowly than bone; in fact, they are the source of our primary knowledge of many ancient species. Nonetheless our understanding of their intriguing structure is still incomplete. Human teeth are generally representative, with an epithelium-derived outer shell of enamel that is highly mineralized, hard, stiff and wear resistant. The enamel is supported both mechanically and biochemically by a mesenchyme-derived dentin, which is vital, less mineralized, softer and more compliant. Dentin is maintained by the dental pulp, which is cellular and innervated, and has a vascular plexus. In this chapter we give details of each of the mineralized tissues and how they develop into structural components with unique physical properties.

1.2 Enamel

1.2.1 Development

Tooth enamel is the hardest tissue in the body, with a hardness comparable to that of window glass, and is highly fatigue- and wear-resistant. Human enamel is laid down by cells in a programmed temporal and spatial sequence to provide the overall shape of the tooth. The cells that make enamel develop from the invagination of epithelial tissue during fetal development. In what is known, because of its shape, as the 'bell stage' of tooth development (ca. 14th week of intrauterine life), the epithelial cells on the inside of the bell align with a concentration of mesenchyme cells in what appears to be a one-to-one relationship. More accurately the latter are 'ectomesenchyme' cells, as the first branchial arch, whose ectodermal cells migrates into the mesenchyme in the area of the developing jaws (Nanci, 2008). During this alignment an extracellular collagen network is created that extends from the epithelial cells to the mesenchyme cells. The epithelial cells begin to elongate and transform into ameloblasts, and the mesenchyme cells transform into odontoblasts (Nanci, 2008). The elongation of the ameloblasts when compared with the odontoblasts leads to pulling on the collagen network formed between the two, creating a local puckering of this structure that will become the dentin–enamel junction (DEJ). Seen in cross-section the DEJ appears as scalloped, but viewed in three dimensions (3-D), when the enamel has been dissolved, the circular ridges and pits of the DEJ structure become apparent. The gene expression controlling this process is not fully understood, but a large number of genes involved in tooth development have been identified (Nieminen, 2007).

1.2.2 Enamel prisms

The ameloblasts are arranged in a close, overlapping array. Each cell has a tail that extends between its neighbors (see Fig. 1.1), so that if observed from above the DEJ, they interdigitate.

Once aligned with their neighbors, the ameloblasts begin to mature and to lay down the enamel structure. The maturation of ameloblasts starts from what will become the cusp tip or the incisal edge of the tooth (but at this stage is the inner top of the bell) and proceeds apically. The last enamel to begin formation will be that closest to the cement–enamel junction (CEJ). The ameloblast at its terminal end (nearest to the DEJ) takes on a 'brush border' appearance and begins to excrete proteins, in particular amelogenins; these are the template molecules for the nucleation of calcium phosphate to form, with maturation, ribbons of dense hydroxyapatite (HA). In this process each ameloblast will create one enamel prism of approximately 5 μm in diameter, which is also referred to as an 'enamel rod' (Fig. 1.2). Individual prisms are currently thought to extend from the DEJ to the enamel surface through various paths and not to change diameter.

Prisms are joined to their neighbors by a thin organic layer referred to as a 'prism sheath'. When loaded to the point of cracking, the resultant cracks preferentially propagate through the protein sheath, going around and along the prism (Fig. 1.3).

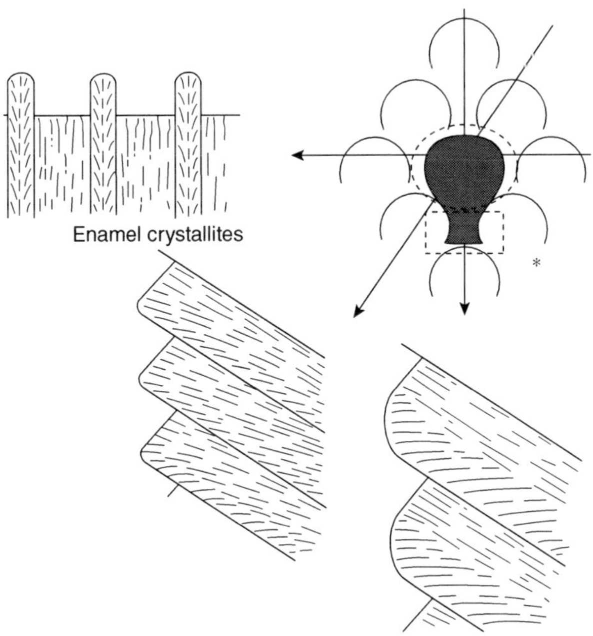

1.1 Ameloblasts arranged next to one another (upper right). Each cell has a head (dotted black oval) and a tail (dotted black box) that extends between its neighbors. Observe the discontinuity of the enamel crystallites. Asterisk shows secondary territories. Each arrow in the upper right denotes a sectioning plane through the enamel. Each arrow points to the diagram depicting the microscopic view of that sectioning plane in the enamel. Image modified from Boyde (1989).

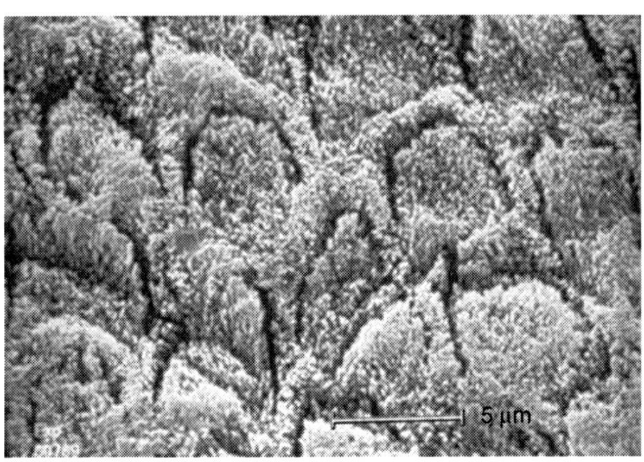

1.2 Scanning electron micrograph of enamel rods: alignment of enamel prisms observed when the enamel surface is etched by acid.

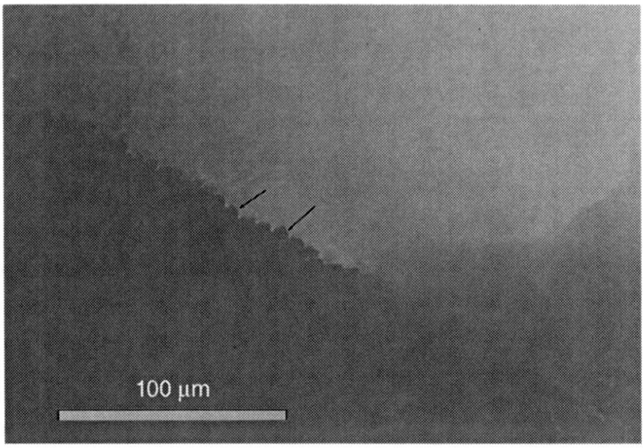

1.3 Cracks (crenellations) propagating through the protein sheath going around and along the prisms following Vickers indentation.

The tensile strength of enamel is lower when loaded perpendicular to the prism direction (11.4 ± 6.3 MPa) than when it is when loaded parallel (24.7 ± 9.6 MPa) (Carvalho *et al.*, 2000). When acid etched, the shear bond of adhesive applied end-on to the prism direction (enamel surface) is approximately 40% higher than when the adhesive is applied parallel to the enamel prism direction (Ikeda *et al.*, 2002). However, self-etch adhesives, which do not employ a separate etching step, do not result in a significant difference in bond strength relative to enamel prism orientation (Shimada and Tagami, 2003).

The laying down of enamel by the ameloblasts proceeds at a rate of about 4 μm per day (Dean, 1998). If an ameloblast were to migrate directly to the enamel surface, the fastest it could reach the outer dimension of a 1.2-mm-thick enamel cusp would be (1200/4 =) 300 days, but we note that ameloblasts do not proceed directly radially from the DEJ to the surface (as discussed below), so much more time is necessary to develop enamel for permanent teeth. Molar enamel thickness varies by cusp from 1.2–1.7 mm (Mahoney, 2008), increases from the first molar to the third (Grine, 2005) and is generally slightly thicker for females (Smith *et al.*, 2006). The enamel thickness on the facial or incisal of a central incisor is approximately 1.3 mm (Shillingburg Jr. and Grace, 1973). Once ameloblasts reach the outer extent of the enamel they transform to a more cuboidal shape and die. What signaling controls this process is not known. The calcification of the developing enamel prism occurs gradually and continues for a some time even after the tooth erupts into the mouth. This makes newly erupted teeth sensitive to decalcification and caries for more than a year.

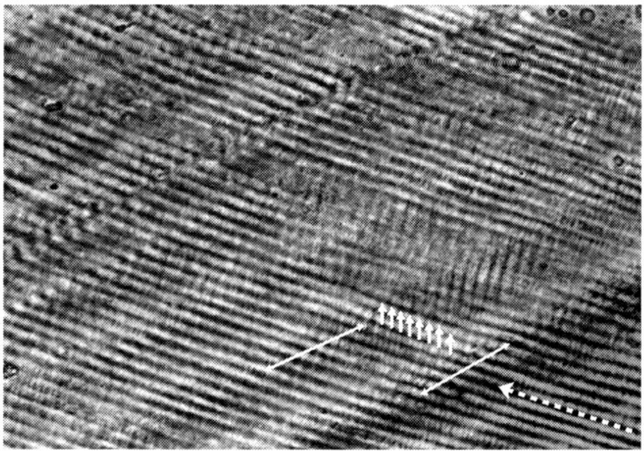

1.4 Variation in the width of the daily growth increment and in the density of calcification. Note striae of Retzius (double headed arrows) and the instantaneous forming front (white solid arrows) and enamel prism orientation and direction of growth (white dotted arrow).

Enamel growth periods are seen via structural features in the enamel. Ameloblasts mature in layers or fronts from the cusp toward the DEJ, resulting in layers called 'striae of Retzius'. These appear at the external surface of the tooth as 'perikymata', more pronounced layers in the cervical enamel surface. Between striae in humans, there are 8–9-day growth increments designated as the 'repeat interval' (Bromage *et al.*, 2011). Within the repeat interval of enamel there are 'rhythms', seen as variation in the width of the daily growth increment and in the density of calcification (Fig. 1.4). These same rhythms are seen in the lamellae of bone (Bromage *et al.*, 2011).

The properties of enamel prisms and how these properties change with prism orientation have been studied extensively since the advent of nano-indentation techniques (Carvalho *et al.*, 2000; He and Swain, 2007, 2009; Guidoni *et al.*, 2008). Enamel is hardest along the central axis of the enamel prism because of the alignment of the HA crystallites in this direction. The crystallite direction changes across the prism diameter (face) as well as in the transition between the tail and the body of the rod (Jeng *et al.*, 2011) (Fig. 1.5). Nanoindentation across the enamel allows the mapping of hardness and elastic modulus, with enamel shown to be both harder and of higher modulus at the outer surface of the tooth (Angker *et al.*, 2004; Xie *et al.*, 2009). Higher hardness and modulus are the basis for the wear resistance of the enamel surface. The higher hardness is likely to be related to the parallel alignment of the enamel prisms over large areas of the outer enamel surface, an alignment observed when the enamel surface is etched by acid (see Fig. 1.2). Enamel changes with age, becoming harder at the surface but not at the DEJ (Park *et al.*, 2008).

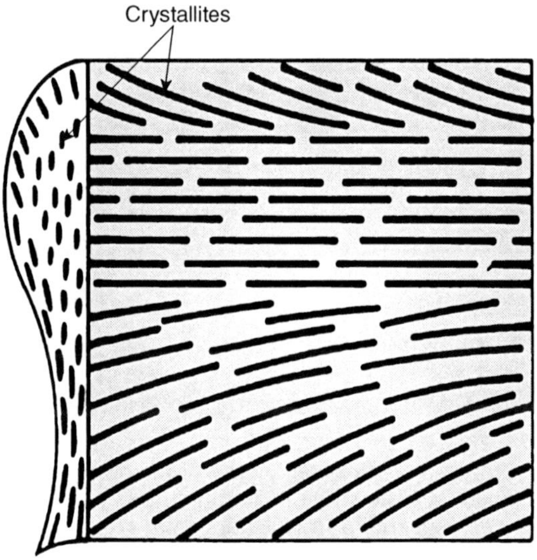

1.5 Crystallite direction changes across the prism diameter (face) as well as in the transition between the tail and the body of the rod (black arrows). Image modified from Avery and Chiego (2005).

The unique abilities of enamel, based upon its structure, to withstand cracking and resist fatigue are in part attributed to the complex pattern made by the ameloblasts as they traverse and fill the space between the dentin and enamel surface. A finite number of ameloblasts must each contribute to this process and groups of them seem to act in unison to create what is known as 'enamel prism decussation' (crossing of groups of rods). Decussation leads to the Hunter–Schreger bands (HSB) seen in sections of enamel viewed with the light microscope (Lynch *et al.*, 2011). In humans such decussation is derived from bundles of what are thought to be 50–100 prisms that follow a complex path from the DEJ to the surface in what is known as 'multiserial patterning'. These prism groups may be those associated with a scallop on the DEJ. They can be seen fanning out from the DEJ in incremental, stacked planes proceeding apically from the cusp tip or the incisal edge, each plane oriented approximately parallel to the occlusal plane of the tooth. In each plane the ameloblast groups grow outward at roughly a 40-degree angle to the radial direction, with one plane orienting left and the maturing plane below it orienting right. From incisal to gingival in each plane there are several prism groups. This thickness of the bands can be seen in a buccal to lingual vertical section of a molar cusp taken in polarized light (Fig. 1.6). Note that the decussation plane also changes direction occlusally and gingivally as it proceeds outward. Near the cusp tip or

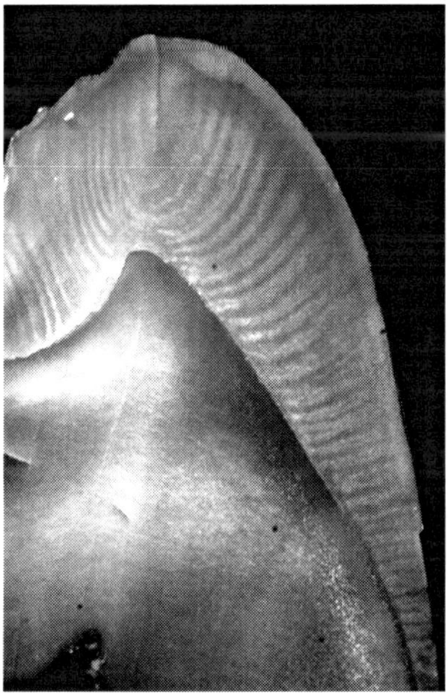

1.6 Enamel decussation plane changes direction occlusally and gingivally as it proceeds outwards.

incisal edge the decussation pattern becomes more complex as the ameloblast fronts proceed to fill the space. When sectioned this complex pattern beneath the cusp tip is referred to as 'gnarled enamel' (Dean, 1998).

The incisal or occlusal plane of decussation provides enamel with the ability to resist cracking in this overall direction, as a crack must run a very long distance to traverse the structure (Bajaj and Arola, 2009a; Myoung *et al.*, 2009; Bechtle *et al.*, 2010; Ivancik *et al.*, 2011). This is not the case in the incisal or occlusal to gingival direction. Teeth often show vertical cracks in enamel without consequence but rarely horizontal cracks, as the latter are quite detrimental (Lee *et al.*, 2011). Researchers have been investigating the 'fracture toughness' of enamel, that is, the energy necessary to propagate a crack (Bajaj *et al.*, 2008; Bajaj and Arola, 2009a; Ivancik *et al.*, 2011). Using very small sections of enamel to make compact tension and fracture toughness coupons, they have shown that the fracture toughness from surface inward or from the DEJ outward increases by an order of magnitude as the crack extends from either surface. They attribute this impressive behavior to enamel decussation (Bajaj and Arola, 2009b). Testing of whole teeth shows high resistance to cracking, with exceptional resistance in the occlusal as opposed to the vertical plane (Chai *et al.* 2009, 2011).

Although enamel is hard and wear resistant with its high HA content (> 95% by weight), it is still a hydrated tissue and chemicals can diffuse through the structure surprisingly rapidly. Once through the enamel the chemical species makes rapid access to the pulp via the dentinal tubules containing the odontoblastic process, making dentin highly permeable. In a cat canine model Lucifer Yellow dye can penetrate from the enamel surface to the odontoblasts in the pulp within 30 min (Ikeda and Suda, 2006). In extracted teeth subjected to bleaching agents, peroxide is present in the pulp within 30 min of external application (Gokay *et al.*, 2000). Given the ready permeability of enamel we can hypothesize that microscopic cracks on the surface and at the DEJ may be able to heal through remineralization from saliva or from dentin interstitial fluid, respectively.

1.3 Dentin–enamel junction (DEJ)

As noted earlier, the DEJ is the interphase between enamel and dentin, initially formed by the alignment of ameloblast and odontoblast during the bell stage of tooth development. It is approximately 60–100 μm in width and is a 'graded structure', in that the elastic modulus makes a nearly linear transition from the enamel (~70 GPa for inner enamel) to that of dentin (~15 GPa) (Marshall *et al.*, 2001; Chan *et al.*, 2011). The change in the calcium and phosphate content from the enamel to the dentin is thought to be responsible for this gradient in modulus. A graded structure serves to lower tensile stresses substantially at the interface of a brittle material with one of lower elastic modulus, resulting in increased strength and fatigue resistance (Zhang and Ma, 2009; Ren *et al.*, 2011). The DEJ gradient moves the highest tensile stresses into the bulk of the enamel during function and reduces those at the interface by nearly 50% (Huang *et al.*, 2007).

A graded interphase has also been identified between cementum and dentin (Ho *et al.*, 2004). Dentin mineral content changes from the DEJ toward the pulp, as noted by change in HA particle size (Marten *et al.*, 2010).

1.4 Dentin

The ectomesenchyme cells that become odontoblasts align with the ectodermal cap cells that become ameloblasts (Nanci, 2008). While the ameloblasts are elongating, the odontoblasts are already beginning to produce the collagen network that becomes the DEJ; they then make the transition to elaboration of the more complex collagen and proteoglycan structure of dentin. The elaboration of the dentin structure and its following calcification proceed inwards at an initial rate of ~2.8 μm per day. This rate slows as the odontoblasts approach the pulp space and slows further when

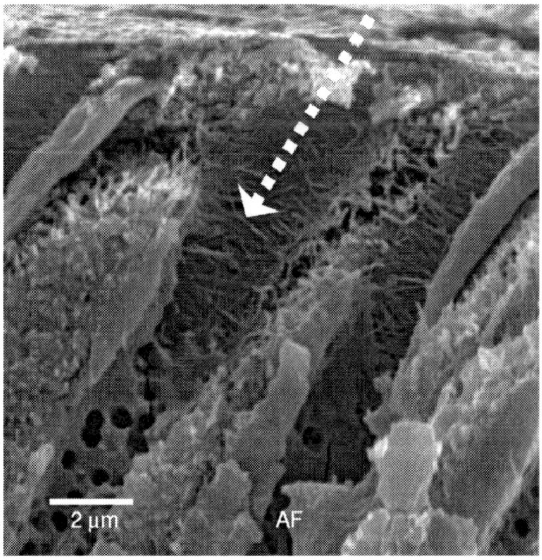

1.7 Lateral extension of dentinal tubule (white dotted arrow) of an etched dentin substrate.

root formation and tooth eruption are complete. Dentin continues to grow inwards for the life of the individual and leaves a record of growth-altering events. This is termed 'secondary dentin formation'. Dentin is also dynamic in that it can respond to insults to the enamel, such as caries or excessive wear, and lay down additional dentin, referred to as 'reactionary dentin' or 'tertiary dentin' (Bjorndal and Darvann, 1999; Bjorndal, 2001). Wear of root surfaces can also lead to laying down of reactionary dentin (Nanci, 2008).

Dentin has a structure with tubules that course from the DEJ to the pulp radially inwards, with a broad S shape when the tooth is sectioned axially. Within the tubules are cellular processes extending from the odontoblasts that line the pulp. The tubules have smaller lateral extensions along their length that communicate with neighboring tubules, creating a communication and interstitial fluid network that maintains the dentin. These lateral extensions can be seen in sections of etched dentin (Fig. 1.7).

The collagen structure of dentin is complex, with the collagen oriented in helical-like structures forming tubules but then changing to a more radial orientation in the plane perpendicular to the tubule direction. There are proteogylcans aligned along collagen fibers and these play a role in mineralization and physical properties (Chiu *et al.*, 2012). Calcification of dentin starts with nucleation in the gap space between collagen strands and proceeds outwards expanding in the direction of the fibers, forming elongated crystals of HA that are anisotropically oriented to withstand loading

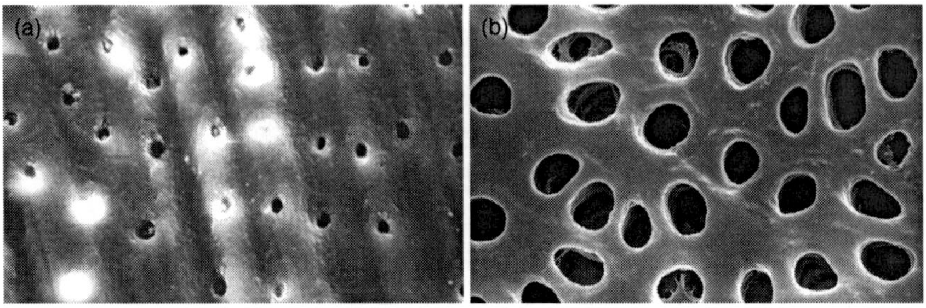

1.8 (a) Near DEJ dentin tubules that are widely spaced and about 0.8–1.2 μm in diameter, with a distance between tubules of nearly 10 μm. (b) Tubule density increases to approximately 40000 per mm^2 near the pulp.

(Marten *et al.*, 2010). The dentin around the tubules is more highly mineralized; this zone of mineralization, approximately the thickness of the tubule diameter, is called the 'peritubular dentin'. Outside this zone the mineral content is lower; these regions comprise the 'intertubular dentin'.

Near the DEJ, the dentin that forms has tubules that are widely spaced and about 0.8–1.2 μm in diameter, with a distance between tubules of nearly 10 μm (Fig. 1.8(a)). This gives a tubule density of 17000–20000 per mm^2. With the radial orientation of the tubules, tubule density increases to ~40 000 per mm^2 near the pulp (Pashley *et al.*, 1985) (Fig. 1.8(b)).

Inner dentin has a reduced amount of intertubular dentin, but this does not lead to an increase in hardness: the overall mineral content changes from the DEJ toward pulp as the HA particle size decreases with depth (Pashley *et al.*, 1985; Marten *et al.*, 2010). Note that dentin that has been etched and then dried has a collapsed collagen layer that appears as a gel (Fig. 1.9). Contrast this with the visible collagen seen in freeze-dried etched dentin (Fig. 1.10).

The properties of dentin have been studied to determine its strength with orientation as well as its fracture toughness. Using microtensile specimens Gianni and others (Giannini *et al.*, 2004) have shown that the tensile strength of dentin perpendicular to the tubule direction is 62 GPa near the DEJ and reduces to ~34 GPa near the pulp. This group also related the ability to bond adhesively to dentin to the area of the intertubular dentin (Giannini *et al.*, 2001) and, inversely, to the tubule density. The hardness of dentin on a macroscopic scale (Knoop or Vickers indentation) is isotropic perpendicular or parallel to the tubule direction at the same relative depth in the enamel (Pashley *et al.*, 1985). Hardness is reduced with depth in dentin (Hosoya and Marshall, 2004) and varies from buccal to lingual (Brauer *et al.*, 2011). Radicular intertubular dentin has a reduced elastic modulus and hardness compared to coronal intertubular dentin (Inoue *et al.*, 2009).

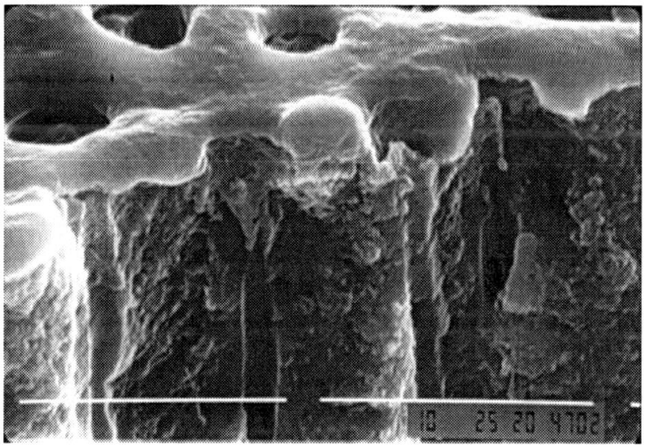

1.9 Scanning electron image of a dentin substrate that has been etched and then dried, showing a collapsed collagen layer that appears as a gel.

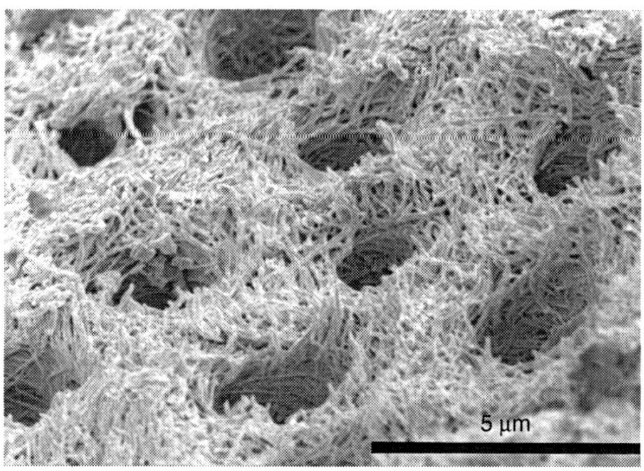

1.10 Scanning electron image of collagen seen in a freeze-dried etched dentin surface (courtesy of Dr Jorge Perdigão).

Dentin can also be considered to be a graded structure, given that it changes properties with location (Tesch *et al.*, 2001).

Dentin toughness has been studied to understand the mechanisms that limit crack extension (Imbeni *et al.*, 2003; Kruzic *et al.*, 2003; Nalla *et al.*, 2003). In their review, Nalla and others (Nalla, *et al.*, 2003) show that crack bridging and the formation of daughter cracks are significant mechanisms for the dissipation of crack energy, so that the process leading to the toughness of dentin is similar to that of fracture toughness in bone. Replacing the

Table 1.1 Physical properties of enamel and dentin compared to other dental materials

Tooth	Modulus (GPa)	Hardness (GPa)	Toughness (MPa m$^{1/2}$)
Enamel	94	3.2	0.8
Dentin	16	0.6	3.1
Resin cement	4–5	0.3	1.1
Composites (Z 100)	18	–	1.3
Glass-ceramic	67–96	3.4–6.3	100–420

water in dentin with less polar solvents, such as ethanol, increases the fracture toughness of dentin (Nalla *et al.*, 2005, 2006). However, dentin fracture toughness is reduced with age (Kinney *et al.* 2005; Nazari *et al.* 2009), which may help to explain the significant increase in cusp fracture of posterior teeth with age, in particular those that have been restored. Restoration often leads to volumes of dentin where the dentin tubules have been cut and thus can no longer supply interstitial fluid minerals to the dentin and associated DEJ and enamel. Table 1.1 presents physical properties of enamel and dentin compared to commonly use restorative materials.

Dentin is dynamic in that it reacts to the caries process with a low permeability zone and can remineralize caries-affected areas if the caries is sealed from the oral environment (ten Cate, 2001, 2008). Caries established in dentin is characterized as comprising a bacterial infected layer adjacent to the enamel and, beneath this, an acid-altered demineralized zone designated as 'affected dentin'. This demineralized zone, detected by dyes, is inaccurately perceived by clinicians to be 'infected dentin' (Boston and Liao, 2004). Within the affected dentin near the bacterial front the acid attack has dissolved most of the mineral, but beneath this is a zone where the acid attack is actively dissolving the HA. This dissolution yields a significant concentration of calcium and phosphate, leading to precipitation of an acid-resistant compound, whitlockite, in the dentinal tubules (Daculsi *et al.*, 1987). Histologically this is seen in thin section and identified as the 'transparent zone'. This tubule precipitate lowers the dentin permeability (Pashley *et al.*, 1991), allowing excavation of infected and overlaying affected dentin without anesthetic being required (Boston, 2003; Allen *et al.*, 2005).

Exposed dentin root surfaces of teeth may become worn through abrasion, erosion, or a combination of both, perhaps accelerated by occlusal stress (Gallien *et al.*, 1994; Terry *et al.*, 2003; Pecie *et al.*, 2011). Often such dentin has a smooth, hypermineralized surface called 'sclerotic dentin' (Aw *et al.*, 2002). The low-permeability zone in affected dentin is sometimes referred to as 'sclerotic dentin', but this is a misnomer: the calcification is in the tubules, whereas the surrounding dentin may be undergoing decalcification. Root surface sclerotic dentin in non-carious cervical lesions presents a challenge for dentin bonding agent procedures (Yoshiyama *et al.*, 1996; Marshall *et al.*, 2000), as most are evaluated on normal or caries-affected dentin.

Now well established but not appreciated clinically is the ability of caries to be arrested and undergo varying degrees of remineralization if sealed from the oral environment (Carvalho *et al.*, 1998; Thompson and Kaim, 2005; ten Cate, 2008; Alves *et al.*, 2010; Bjorndal, 2011). Quantification of this process has recently been observed with and without use of a calcification-promoting liner containing amorphous calcium phosphate compounds (Bresciani *et al.*, 2010; Peters *et al.*, 2010).

1.5 Conclusion

Teeth are unique biological structures that can last a lifetime in service. Nature, using a cellular approach, has constructed a fatigue- and damage-resistant structure, and to some extent a self-healing one, that is now only being approached in performance by ceramic and resin-based composite formulations. In studying the structure of enamel and dentin we may be provided with clues about the design and development of new materials with broad-ranging applications.

1.6 References

Allen K L, Salgado T L, Janal M N and Thompson V P (2005), 'Removing carious dentin using a polymer instrument without anesthesia versus a carbide bur with anesthesia', *J Am Dent Assoc*, **136**(5), 643–51.

Alves L S, Fontanella V, Damo A C, Ferreira de Oliveira E and Maltz M (2010), 'Qualitative and quantitative radiographic assessment of sealed carious dentin: a 10-year prospective study', *Oral Surg Oral Med Oral Pathol Oral Radiol Endod*, **109**(1), 135–41.

Angker L, Nockolds C, Swain M V and Kilpatrick N (2004), 'Correlating the mechanical properties to the mineral content of carious dentine – a comparative study using an ultra-micro indentation system (UMIS) and SEM–BSE signals', *Arch Oral Biol*, **49**(5), 369–78.

Avery J K and Chiego D J (2005), *Essentials of Oral Histology and Embryology: A Clinical Approach*, 3rd Edition, Elsevier Mosby, St Louis, p 99.

Aw T C, Lepe X, Johnson G H and Mancl L (2002), 'Characteristics of noncarious cervical lesions: a clinical investigation', *J Am Dent Assoc*, **133**(6), 725–33.

Bajaj D and Arola D (2009a), 'Role of prism decussation on fatigue crack growth and fracture of human enamel', *Acta Biomater*, **5**(8), 3045–56.

Bajaj D and Arola D D (2009b), 'On the R-curve behavior of human tooth enamel', *Biomaterials*, **30**(23–24), 4037–46.

Bajaj D, Nazari A, Eidelman N and Arola D D (2008), 'A comparison of fatigue crack growth in human enamel and hydroxyapatite', *Biomaterials*, **29**(36), 4847–54.

Bechtle S, Habelitz S, Klocke A, Fett T and Schneider G A (2010), 'The fracture behaviour of dental enamel', *Biomaterials*, **31**(2), 375–84.

Bjørndal L (2001), 'Presence or absence of tertiary dentinogenesis in relation to caries progression', *Adv Dent Res*, **15**, 80–3.

Bjørndal L (2011), 'In deep cavities stepwise excavation of caries can preserve the pulp', *Evid Based Dent*, **12**(3), 68.

Bjørndal L and Darvann T (1999), 'A light microscopic study of odontoblastic and non-odontoblastic cells involved in tertiary dentinogenesis in well-defined cavitated carious lesions', *Caries Res*, **33**(1), 50–60.

Boston D W (2003), 'New device for selective dentin caries removal', *Quintessence Int*, **34**(9), 678–85.

Boston D W and Liao J (2004), 'Staining of non-carious human coronal dentin by caries dyes', *Oper Dent*, **29**(3), 280–6.

Boyde A (1989), 'Enamel'. In *Handbook of Microscopic Anatomy, Volume 6: Teeth*, Oksche A and Vollarth L (eds), Springer-Verlag, New York.

Brauer D S, Hilton J F, Marshall G W and Marshall S J (2011), 'Nano- and micro-mechanical properties of dentine: investigation of differences with tooth side', *J Biomech*, **44**(8), 1626–9.

Bresciani E, Wagner W C, Navarro M F, Dickens S H and Peters M C (2010), '*In vivo* dentin microhardness beneath a calcium-phosphate cement', *J Dent Res*, **89**(8), 836–41.

Bromage T G, Juwayeyi Y M, Smolyar I, Hu B, Gomez S and Chisi J (2011), 'Enamel-calibrated lamellar bone reveals long period growth rate variability in humans', *Cells Tissues Organs*, **194**(2–4), 124–30.

Carvalho J C, Mestrinho H D, Bezerra A C and Maltz M (1998), 'Onset, development and arrest of dental caries in Brazilian pre-school children', *Clin Oral Investig*, **2**(2), 96–100.

Carvalho R M, Santiago S L, Fernandes C A, Suh B I and Pashley D H (2000), 'Effects of prism orientation on tensile strength of enamel', *J Adhes Dent*, **2**(4), 251–7.

Chai H, Lee J J, Constantino P J, Lucas P W and Lawn B R (2009), 'Remarkable resilience of teeth', *Proc Natl Acad Sci USA*, **106**(18), 7289–93.

Chai H, Lee J J and Lawn B R (2011), 'On the chipping and splitting of teeth', *J Mech Behav Biomed Mater*, **4**(3), 315–21.

Chan Y L, Ngan A H and King N M (2011), 'Nano-scale structure and mechanical properties of the human dentine–enamel junction', *J Mech Behav Biomed Mater*, **4**(5), 785–95.

Chiu R, Li W, Herber R P, Marshall S J, Young M and Ho S P (2012), 'Effects of biglycan on physico-chemical properties of ligament-mineralized tissue attachment sites', *Arch Oral Biol*, **57**(2), 177–87.

Daculsi G, LeGeros R Z, Jean A and Kerebel B (1987), 'Possible physico-chemical processes in human dentin caries', *J Dent Res*, **66**(8), 1356–9.

Dean M C (1998), 'A comparative study of cross striation spacings in cuspal enamel and of four methods of estimating the time taken to grow molar cuspal enamel in *Pan, Pongo* and *Homo*', *J Hum Evol*, **35**(4–5), 449–62.

Gallien G S, Kaplan I and Owens B M (1994), 'A review of noncarious dental cervical lesions', *Compendium*, **15**(11), 1366, 1368–72, 1374; quiz 1374.
Giannini M, Carvalho R M, Martins L R, Dias C T and Pashley D H (2001), 'The influence of tubule density and area of solid dentin on bond strength of two adhesive systems to dentin', *J Adhes Dent*, **3**(4), 315–24.
Giannini M, Soares C J and de Carvalho R M (2004), 'Ultimate tensile strength of tooth structures', *Dent Mater*, **20**(4), 322–9.
Gökay O, Tunçbilek M and Ertan R (2000), 'Penetration of the pulp chamber by carbamide peroxide bleaching agents on teeth restored with a composite resin', *J Oral Rehabil*, **27**(5), 428–31.
Grine F E (2005), 'Enamel thickness of deciduous and permanent molars in modern *Homo sapiens*', *Am J Phys Anthropol*, **126**(1), 14–31.
Guidoni G, Swain M and Jäger I (2008), 'Enamel: from brittle to ductile like tribological response', *J Dent*, **36**(10), 786–94.
He L H and Swain M V (2007), 'Enamel—a 'metallic-like', deformable biocomposite', *J Dent*, **35**(5), 431–7.
He L H and Swain M V (2009), 'Nanoindentation creep behavior of human enamel', *J Biomed Mater Res, Part A*, **91**(2), 352–9.
Ho S P, Balooch M, Marshall S J and Marshall G W (2004), 'Local properties of a functionally graded interphase between cementum and dentin', *J Biomed Mater Res, Part A*, **70**(3), 480–9.
Hosoya Y and Marshall G W Jr (2004), 'The nano-hardness and elastic modulus of carious and sound primary canine dentin', *Oper Dent*, **29**(2), 142–9.
Huang M, Wang R, Thompson V, Rekow D and Soboyejo W O (2007), 'Bioinspired design of dental multilayers', *J Mater Sci Mater Med*, **18**(1), 57–64.
Ikeda H and Suda H (2006), 'Rapid penetration of lucifer yellow into vital teeth and dye coupling between odontoblasts and neighbouring pulp cells in the cat', *Arch Oral Biol*, **51**(2), 123–8.
Ikeda T, Uno S, Tanaka T, Kawakami S, Komatsu H and Sano H (2002), 'Relation of enamel prism orientation to microtensile bond strength', *Am J Dent*, **15**(2), 109–13.
Imbeni V, Nalla R K, Bosi C, Kinney JH and Ritchie RO (2003), '*In vitro* fracture toughness of human dentin', *J Biomed Mater Res, Part A*, **66**(1), 1–9.
Inoue T, Saito M, Yamamoto M, Debari K, Kou K, Nishimura F and Miyazaki T (2009), 'Comparison of nanohardness between coronal and radicular intertubular dentin', *Dent Mater J*, **28**(3), 295–300.
Ivancik J, Neerchal N K, Romberg E and Arola D (2011), 'The reduction in fatigue crack growth resistance of dentin with depth', *J Dent Res*, **90**(8), 1031–6.
Jeng Y R, Lin T T, Hsu H M, Chang H J and Shieh D B (2011), 'Human enamel rod presents anisotropic nanotribological properties', *J Mech Behav Biomed Mater*, **4**(4), 515–22.
Kinney J H, Nalla R K, Pople J A, Breunig T M and Ritchie R O (2005), 'Age-related transparent root dentin: mineral concentration, crystallite size, and mechanical properties', *Biomaterials*, **26**(16), 3363–76.
Kruzic J J, Nalla R K, Kinney J H and Ritchie R O (2003), 'Crack blunting, crack bridging and resistance-curve fracture mechanics in dentin: effect of hydration', *Biomaterials*, **24**(28), 5209–21.

Lee J J, Constantino P J, Lucas PW and Lawn BR (2011), 'Fracture in teeth: a diagnostic for inferring bite force and tooth function', *Biol Rev Camb Philos Soc*, **86**(4), 959–74.

Lynch C D, O'Sullivan V R, Dockery P, McGillycuddy C T, Rees J S amd Sloan A J (2011), 'Hunter–Schreger Band patterns and their implications for clinical dentistry', *J Oral Rehabil*, **38**(5), 359–65.

Mahoney P (2008), 'Intraspecific variation in M1 enamel development in modern humans: implications for human evolution', *J Hum Evol*, **55**(1), 131–47.

Marshall G W Jr, Chang Y J, Saeki K, Gansky S A and Marshall S J (2000), 'Citric acid etching of cervical sclerotic dentin lesions: an AFM study', *J Biomed Mater Res*, **49**(3), 338–44.

Marshall G W Jr, Balooch M, Gallagher R R, Gansky S A and Marshall S J (2001), 'Mechanical properties of the dentinoenamel junction: AFM studies of nanohardness, elastic modulus, and fracture', *J Biomed Mater Res*, **54**(1), 87–95.

Märten A, Fratzl P, Paris O and Zaslansky P (2010), 'On the mineral in collagen of human crown dentine', *Biomaterials*, **31**(20), 5479–90.

Myoung S, Lee J, Constantino P, Lucas P, Chai H and Lawn B (2009), 'Morphology and fracture of enamel', *J Biomech*, **42**(12), 1947–51.

Nalla R K, Kinney J H and Ritchie R O (2003), 'Effect of orientation on the *in vitro* fracture toughness of dentin: the role of toughening mechanisms', *Biomaterials*, **24**(22), 3955–68.

Nalla R K, Balooch M, Ager J W III, Kruzic J J, Kinney J H and Ritchie R O (2005), 'Effects of polar solvents on the fracture resistance of dentin: role of water hydration', *Acta Biomater*, **1**(1), 31–43.

Nalla R K, Kinney J H, Tomsia A P and Ritchie R O (2006), 'Role of alcohol in the fracture resistance of teeth', *J Dent Res*, **85**(11), 1022–6.

Nanci A (2008), *Ten Cate's oral histology: development, structure, and function*, 7th edn, St Louis, Mosby Elsevier.

Nazari A, Bajaj D, Zhang D, Romberg E and Arola D (2009), 'Aging and the reduction in fracture toughness of human dentin', *J Mech Behav Biomed Mater*, **2**(5), 550–9.

Nieminen P (2007), *Gene expression in tooth*, Helsinki, University of Helsinki. Available from: http://bite-it.helsinki.fi/ [Accessed 08 05 12].

Park S, Wang D H, Zhang D, Romberg E and Arola D (2008), 'Mechanical properties of human enamel as a function of age and location in the tooth', *J Mater Sci Mater Med*, **19**(6), 2317–24.

Pashley D, Okabe A and Parham P (1985), 'The relationship between dentin microhardness and tubule density', *Endod Dent Traumatol*, **1**(5), 176–9.

Pashley E L, Talman R, Horner JA and Pashley D H (1991), 'Permeability of normal versus carious dentin', *Endod Dent Traumatol*, **7**(5), 207–11.

Pecie R, Krejci I, Garcia-Godoy F and Bortolotto T (2011), 'Noncarious cervical lesions—a clinical concept based on the literature review, Part 1: prevention', *Am J Dent*, **24**(1), 49–56.

Peters M C, Bresciani E, Barata T J, Fagundes T C, Navarro R L, Navarro M F and Dickens S H (2010), '*In vivo* dentin remineralization by calcium-phosphate cement', *J Dent Res*, **89**(3), 286–91.

Ren L, Janal M N and Zhang Y (2011), 'Sliding contact fatigue of graded zirconia with external esthetic glass', *J Dent Res*, **90**(9), 1116–21.

Shillingburg H T Jr and Grace C S (1973), 'Thickness of enamel and dentin', *J South Calif Dent Assoc*, **41**(1): 33–52.
Shimada Y and Tagami J (2003), 'Effects of regional enamel and prism orientation on resin bond strengths', *Oper Dent*, **28**(1), 20–27.
Smith T M, Olejniczak A J, Reid D J, Ferrell R J and Hublin J J (2006), 'Modern human molar enamel thickness and enamel–dentine junction shape', *Arch Oral Biol*, **51**(11), 974–95.
ten Cate J M (2001), 'Remineralization of caries lesions extending into dentin', *J Dent Res*, **80**(5), 1407–11.
ten Cate J M (2008), 'Remineralization of deep enamel dentine caries lesions', *Aust Dent J*, **53**(3), 281–5.
Terry D A, McGuire M K, McLaren E, Fulton R and Swift E J Jr (2003), 'Perio-esthetic approach to the diagnosis and treatment of carious and noncarious cervical lesions: Part II', *J Esthet Restor Dent*, **15**(5), 284–96.
Tesch W, Eidelman N, Roschger P, Goldenberg F, Klaushofer K and Fratzl P (2001), 'Graded microstructure and mechanical properties of human crown dentin', *Calcif Tissue Int*, **69**(3), 147–57.
Thompson V P and Kaim J M (2005), 'Nonsurgical treatment of incipient and hidden caries', *Dent Clin North Am*, **49**(4), 905–21, viii.
Xie Z H, Swain M V, Swadener G, Munroe P and Hoffman M (2009), 'Effect of microstructure upon elastic behaviour of human tooth enamel', *J Biomech*, **42**(8), 1075–80.
Yoshiyama M, Sano H, Ebisu S, Tagami J, Ciucchi B, Carvalho R M, Johnson M H and Pashley D H (1996), 'Regional strengths of bonding agents to cervical sclerotic root dentin', *J Dent Res*, **75**(6), 1404–13.
Zhang Y and Ma L (2009), 'Optimization of ceramic strength using elastic gradients', *Acta Mater*, **57**(9), 2721–9.

2
Biomineralization and biomimicry of tooth enamel

VUK USKOKOVIĆ, University of California, USA

DOI: 10.1533/9780857096432.1.20

Abstract: This critical review sommarizes the basics of biomineralization of tooth enamel and scrutinizes attempts to replicate this intricate biological process *in vitro*. Special emphasis is given to the author's results, obtained during studies on the formation of enamel by biomimetic means. Fundamental insights found regarding the latter process are presented. Some paradigmatically accepted aspects of the mechanism of amelogenesis, that is, biomineralization of enamel, are challenged. Amelogenin, the major protein of the developing enamel matrix, is thus claimed to be a mineralization inductor, rather than an inhibitor, presumably acting as a channel between the ionic growth units in the protein matrix and the uniaxially growing crystals of apatite. The role of water and other minor constituents of enamel is questioned, as well as the biologically active morphology of amelogenin aggregates and the reliability of recombinant proteins in studying amelogenesis *in vitro*. Appropriate crystal growth rates, the Ostwald–Lussac law, Tomes' process and mineralization of dentin present other aspects of amelogenesis discussed here. It is also claimed that three fundamental facets of amelogenesis ought to be coordinated in parallel for successful biomimetic replication of the given process in the laboratory: protein assembly, proteolytic digestion and crystal growth.

Key words: amelogenesis, biomimicry, biomineralization, enamel, self-assembly.

2.1 Introduction

Tooth enamel presents a prototype of a miniscule and yet extraordinarily intricate segment of the vertebrate body, research into which bears potential significance not only for dental science and orofacial therapies, but for understanding the essence of biomineralization processes *per se*. This explains why it attracts the attention of scientists from a wide array of fields. Not only is the complexity of the formation of this tissue such that its understanding and thorough investigation require knowledge of various materials science and life science fields, but insights obtained by research open trajectories for numerous other biomaterial- and biomedicine-related areas of knowledge. In addition to these fundamental merits, understanding biomineralization of tooth enamel carries an important medical significance. For, finding soft chemical ways to disinfect and remineralize the diseased enamel is the first step in ensuring less invasive and more biocompatible ways of treating enamel dissolution that occurs by attacks by cariogenic bacteria.

This chapter starts with a description of biomineralization of tooth enamel, followed by questions that touch upon some currently disputable or plainly unknown details about this biomineralization. In this way, important questions will be raised around which future research in this field will be based.

2.2 Structure of enamel

Tooth enamel is crowned in the realm of biominerals as the hardest of its members. Another of its peculiar attributes is that it is the only epithelium-derived mineralized tissue. It is also the only biomineral among vertebrates to be almost fully deprived of soft organic components, as 96–98 wt% is accounted for by mineral content only. Despite its almost purely mineral composition, tooth enamel is unlike typical ceramics, as it is typified by an exceptional toughness and only moderate brittleness, all owing to its extraordinarily complex microstructure. Namely, enamel is composed of apatite fibers, 40–60 nm wide and up to several hundred micrometers long, assembled in bundles, that is, rod-shaped aggregates 4–8 μm in width (Fig. 2.1). Having length-to-width aspect ratios of up to 3×10^4, apatite crystals in enamel are 1000 times longer than those found in bone ($50 \times 20 \times 3$ nm on average). This is made possible since the maintenance of this tissue does not depend on intrinsic cell proliferation and vascularization, as is the case with collagenous hard tissues that comprise bone.[1] Approximately 1000 apatite fibers are bundled within each enamel rod, 5–12 million of which are found on a single tooth crown, lined up parallel to each other. The long axis of the enamel rod is, within each row, generally perpendicular to the

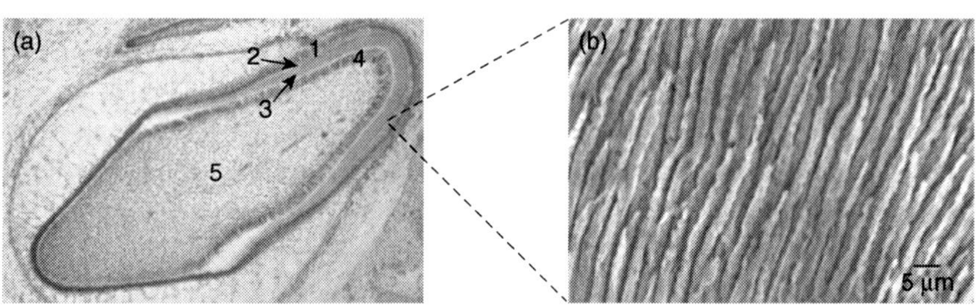

2.1 Histological section of the developing human tooth in the maturation stage (a) and a micrograph showing parallel arrangement of enamel rods (b). 1, ameloblasts; 2, enamel; 3, dentin; 4, odontoblasts; 5, pulp.

underlying dentin, the only exception being that enamel rods near the cement–enamel junction (CEJ) in permanent teeth tilt slightly toward the root of the tooth.

2.3 Amelogenesis at the molecular scale

The biological formation of enamel is known as amelogenesis, a process that lasts for about four years at an appositional crystal growth rate of about 4 μm per day in humans. The slow timescale of the process, making it lengthier than embryogenesis, implicitly speaks in favor of its extraordinary complexity. Besides specific cells, ameloblasts, the process engages numerous macromolecular species, divisible into families of proteins, proteases and protease inhibitors. Although the chronology of amelogenesis is typically divided into three stages – the secretory, the processing and the maturation stage – in view of the pronounced overlap of these stages at the molecular scale, the correctness of this classification can be questioned. For example, the key components involved in protein assembly are secreted during the processing stage, while no precise boundary has been established between the end of processing and the beginning of maturation. Also, although maturation stage can be thought of being the one during which the grown crystals are merely refined, concentration of the mineral phase in the developing enamel is estimated to increase in this stage from 15–20 % to its final percentage.[2] Two-thirds of the time spent in the process of amelogenesis thus belongs to the maturation stage rather than to the processing one. Therefore, the following three events, taking place in parallel during amelogenesis, may be said to describe this process more accurately at the nanoscale.

2.3.1 Protein expression, secretion and assembly

The process of amelogenesis can be said to begin with ameloblasts expressing and secreting proteins that make up the enamel matrix, 90% of which are composed of a single protein, amelogenin. The remaining 10% consists of other proteins: ameloblastin, enamelin, serum albumin (not expressed by ameloblasts and thought to arrive by diffusion through the extracellular matrix (ECM) from the adjacent soft tissues), amelotin and proteolytic enzymes. Together, they assemble into a scaffold that acts as a template for the growth of uniaxially oriented apatite crystals.

2.3.2 Nucleation and crystal growth

Proteins involved in amelogenesis are typically divided to predominantly hydrophilic and predominantly hydrophobic ones. The epithet 'predominantly' is attached here to both kinds of species because, strictly speaking, there are neither perfectly hydrophilic nor perfectly hydrophobic proteins. They are both hydrophobic and hydrophilic in their molecular nature; if this were not so, protein globules would either swiftly unfold had they been completely hydrophilic or wind down into dysfunctional clumps had they been fully hydrophobic. Still, some proteins involved in amelogenesis, including enamelin and ameloblastin, can be considered comparatively hydrophilic in nature; as such, they are supposed to act as nucleation sites for crystallization of apatite.[3,4] This hypothesis is supported by the fact that enamelin is expressed only in the secretory stage, whereas its expression is halted during the maturation stage.[5] Initial enamel crystals also nucleate along the dentin–enamel junction (DEJ) at an early time point when amelogenin is hardly present at all in the protein matrix, which is mainly composed of enamelin and ameloblastin. On the other hand, amelogenin, a low-molecular weight protein, the full-length isoform of which contains between 160 and 200 amino acids, depending on the species in question, is comparatively hydrophobic and has been assumed to inhibit apatite growth.[6] It contains only one phosphorylated site (^{16}Ser), which makes it different from the highly phosphorylated matrix macromolecules that control biomineralization in bone and dentin or the acidic glycoproteins of mollusk shells.[7] It also contains a short, 12-carboxyl-terminal residue sequence of hydrophilic amino acids at the C-terminal (Fig. 2.2), which makes its molecular structure arguably amphiphilic.

Of course, as shown in Fig. 2.2, although amelogenin, usually endowed with the epithet 'hydrophobic', is indeed more hydrophobic than most proteins, it is more hydrophilic than human hemoglobin alpha chain, for example. Still, owing to a large content of proline residues (25–30% of all the amino acids in the peptide chain of amelogenin) as well as those of histidine, glutamine and leucine, amelogenin is considerably hydrophobic, which explains its tendency to form aggregates in contact with a polar solvent even at extremely low concentrations (<0.01 mg ml^{-1}). For the very same reason, attempts to crystallize amelogenin molecules have failed owing to their resistance to standing at a periodic distance from each other, leaving their secondary structure still in the domain of the unknown. Nevertheless, the current model of crystal growth during enamel formation presupposes that amelogenin proteins self-assemble into polydisperse nanospheres ~20 nm in size (Fig. 2.3) (comprising about 40–60 molecules per spherical aggregate of this size), which then align into beaded strings and adhere onto the ($hk0$) faces of the apatite crystals, promoting their growth in the direction of the crystallographic [001] axis. As such, they are hypothesized to prevent the growth and fusion of crystals perpendicular thereto, while aligning them approximately parallel to each other.

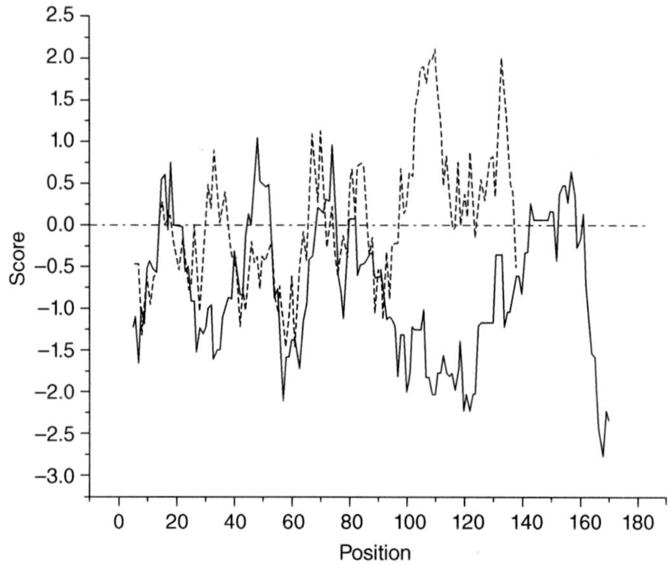

2.2 Hydrophobicity plots obtained using ExPASy ProtScale Kyte & Doolittle model (window size = 9; linear weight variation model) for human amelogenin (solid line) and human hemoglobin alpha chain (dashed line). The positive score on the diagram denotes hydrophobic sequences.

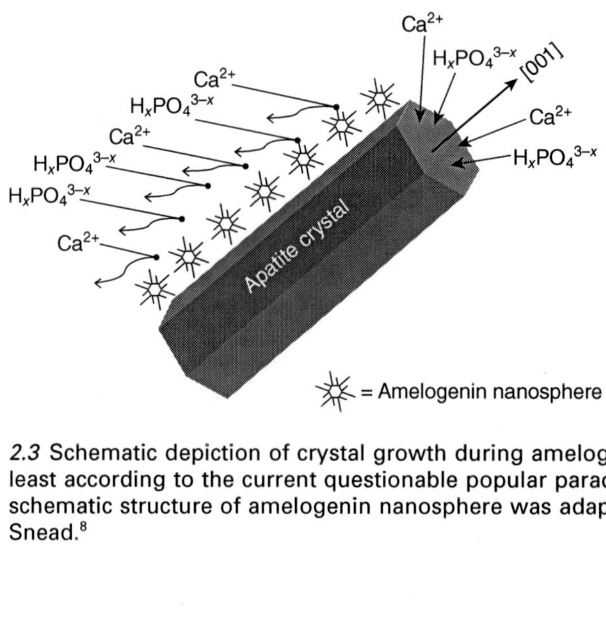

2.3 Schematic depiction of crystal growth during amelogenesis, at least according to the current questionable popular paradigm. The schematic structure of amelogenin nanosphere was adapted from Snead.[8]

2.3.3 Proteolysis

The action of proteases, including matrix metalloproteinase-20 (MMP-20, also known as enamelysin), enamel matrix serine protease 1 (EMSP1, also known as kallikrein-4), and cathepsin B, in hydrolysis of amelogenins and other ECM proteins presents a crucial segment of amelogenesis.[9] Owing to its high selectivity of the cleaved peptide bonds, MMP-20 is usually considered as the major protease in this process.[10] By controlling the modulation of full-length proteins, it is supposed to act as a regulator that controls the functionality of amelogenins. Since enamel is a 95 wt% mineralized tissue, it is clear that proteolytic degradation and removal of the protein matrix has to be orchestrated in synchrony with the lateral growth of apatite crystals.

Following proteolysis, amelogenins and ameloblastins are removed from mature enamel, leaving behind predominantly enamelins and tuftelin in trace amounts. Before the eruption of the tooth, but after the maturation stage, ameloblasts are also broken down and, consequently, enamel, unlike other tissue in the body (even dentin is able to partially remineralize itself, as the pulp cells form layers of reparative dentin whenever bacterial degradation of teeth reaches the pulp), has no way to regenerate itself 'from the inside'.

Finally, there is increasing evidence that these three aspects of amelogenesis – crystal growth, proteolysis and protein assembly – mutually affect each other, so that understanding any one of them individually is conditioned by the simultaneous understanding of the other two. Cooperative assembly of macromolecular species and crystal formation, probably first proposed by Eastoe in 1963,[11] rather than hierarchical and sequential conductance of crystal growth by a pre-assembled protein matrix is thus increasingly used as the hypothesis for describing amelogenesis at the molecular scale.[12–14] Henceforth, successive imitation of enamel growth *in vitro* can be imagined as a peak of a pyramid firmly based in the knowledge of all three given aspects of amelogenesis (Fig. 2.4).

2.4 Key issues in biomineralization and biomimicry of tooth enamel

2.4.1 Are the minor amounts of lipids, proteins and water accidentally remnant in enamel or structurally incorporated with a mechanical purpose?

The old school of thinking tends to consider the miniscule amounts of organic matter in enamel as mere non-functional impurities; however, some research groups are beginning to treat enamel as a composite ceramic

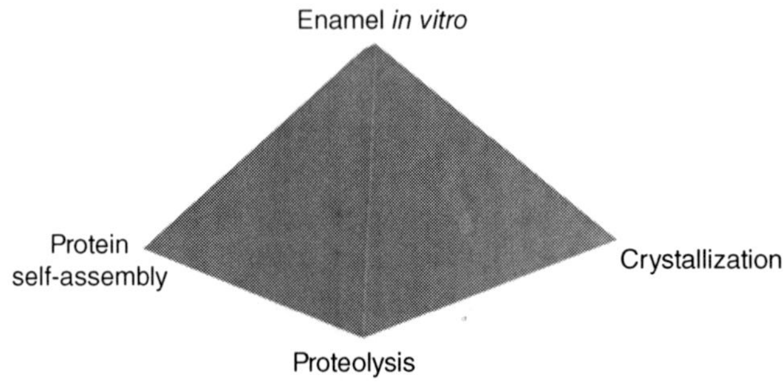

2.4 Biomimicry of amelogenesis is based on and utilizes three well understood and essential aspects of the process: protein self-assembly, proteolysis and crystallization.

material despite its low content of organic matter,[15] claiming that entrapment of such a small concentration of macromolecules increases the toughness and strength of what would be an otherwise brittle ceramic material enamel without them.[16] The biological material often referred to support this argument is the spine of sea urchin, which contains only 0.02 wt% of glycoprotein (~10 proteins per 10^6 unit cells). The amount is, however, large enough to absorb energy efficiently from propagating cracks and thus markedly enhances the resistance of the material to fracture.[17]

2.4.2 Is amelogenin acting as an inhibitor or promoter of nucleation, or both?

As shown in Fig. 2.5(a), recombinant human amelogenin is quite efficient in decreasing the nucleation lag time of metastable calcium phosphate solutions in direct proportion to its concentration. A set of biomimetic experiments based on slow titration of amelogenin sols with calcium and phosphate ions has also yielded conditions under which no crystal growth of apatite substrates was observed in the absence of amelogenin (Fig. 2.5(c),(d)), while the presence of amelogenin accelerated crystal formation in direct proportion to its concentration (Fig. 2.5(b)).[18] The results thus confirmed that the substrate-specific growth of apatite is conditioned by adsorption of amelogenin on the growing crystal surface.[19] Both of these insights have clearly suggested that amelogenins can act as effective nucleators for precipitation of calcium phosphates. In view of this, other recent reports on the ability of amelogenin to promote nucleation of apatite are not surprising.[14] Tarasevich *et al.* have shown that the nucleation promoting/inhibiting effect of amelogenin largely depends on its concentration,[20] confirming a well-known fact that additives may often exert diametrically opposite effects depending

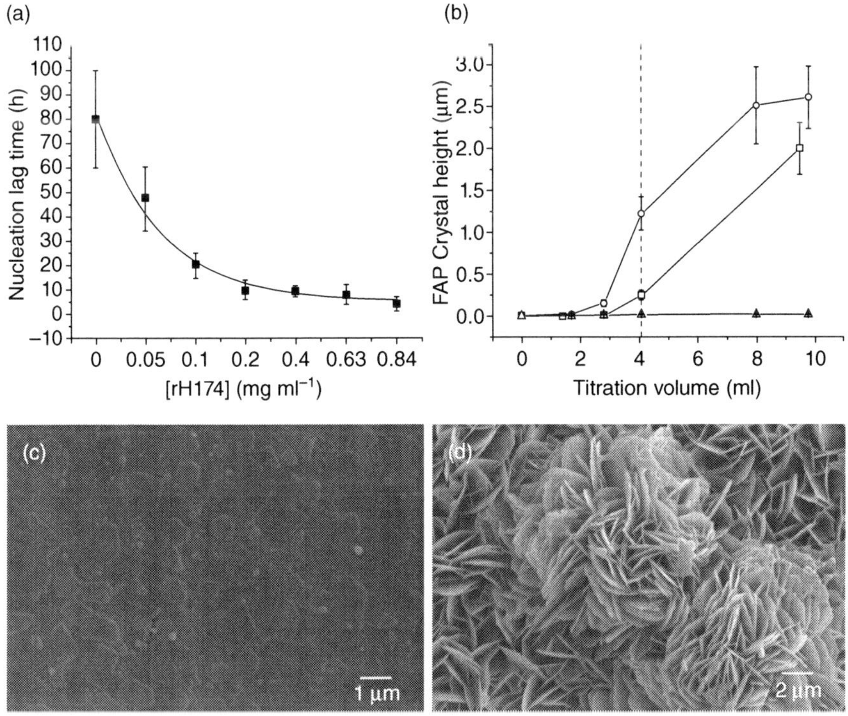

2.5 (a) Nucleation lag time decaying in proportion to the concentration of rH174, human recombinant amelogenin obtained from *Escherichia coli*, in the concentration range 0–0.84 mg ml^{-1}. (b) Crystal growth increasing in proportion to the concentration of rH174 as a function of titration volume. (c) Crystal formation absent from apatite/glass substrates at zero amelogenin concentration. (d) Plate-shaped calcium phosphate crystals obtained in the presence of amelogenin from metastable calcium phosphate solutions. Partially adapted from Uskoković *et al.*[18] and reprinted with permission from Elsevier.

on their concentration.[21] The crucial question today is no longer whether amelogenin can promote nucleation of calcium phosphates, but whether it can act both as a nucleator and inhibitor of nucleation depending on its conformation, morphology, concentration and cooperative assembly involving other protein species present in the developing enamel matrix.

By showing that adsorption of amelogenin is the first step in inducing controlled crystal growth we confirm the idea that evidence of adsorption does not necessarily imply protein–mineral interactions that hinder the crystal growth on the binding sites. For example, osteocalcin, one of the proteins involved in mineralization of bone, despite aligning with and binding to some of the growing crystal planes, does not constrain crystal

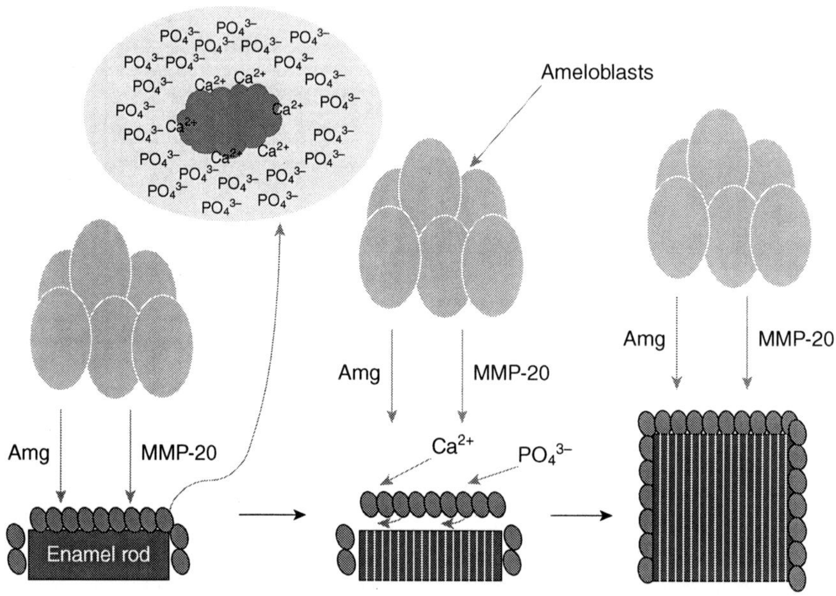

2.6 Scheme describing a model of the protein-controlled crystal growth in amelogenesis. Amelogenin assemblies, such as nanospheres or nanofibers, are adsorbed on the surface of apatite crystals where they channel their building blocks of either calcium and phosphate ions from the solution or amorphous calcium phosphate entities. These amorphous units may form by precise coordination of Ca^{2+} bound to the protein and phosphate ions diffusing in the hydrodynamic layer of the protein particles. Reprinted with permission from Uskokovic.[23]

growth along these directions.[22] Protein assemblies adsorbed on crystal surfaces were thus proposed to act as channels or bridges that transfer ions from the solution and promote their anchoring onto the growing faces. By reversing the old paradigm which has stated that the role of amelogenin assemblies is to block the approach of ions to the growing crystals, we have often joked that we have literally torn down the walls of the old way of thinking and transformed its steely gates into wonderful bridges, bringing forth a more inspiring picture of the way Nature crafts its materials (Fig. 2.6).

2.4.3 What is the biologically active morphology of amelogenin aggregates?

Unlike non-polar acetonitrile, where amelogenin can exist as a monomer within a certain concentration window,[24] in water, the medium of biological

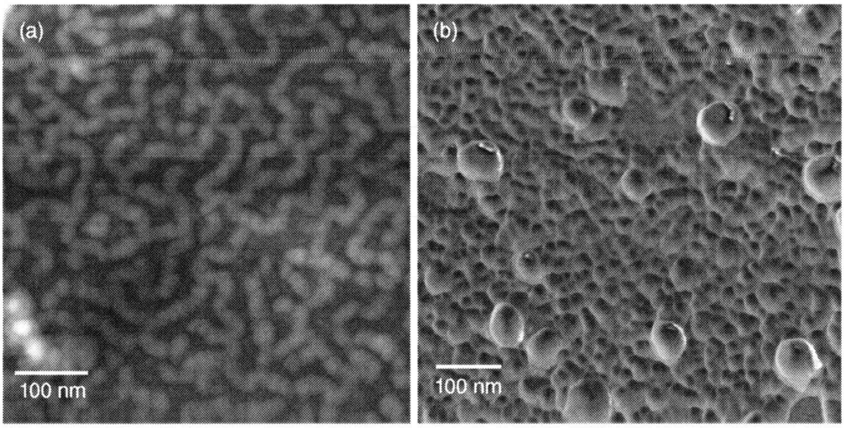

2.7 AFM images of recombinant full-length human amelogenin nanospheres 20–40 nm in size (right) and protofibrous nanostrings (left) formed by mixing amelogenin and water in the presence of calcium and phosphate ions.

importance, amelogenin readily aggregates and adopts one of two different morphologies: nanospheres or nanofibers of various length (Fig. 2.7). The latter have been shown to form owing to controlled aggregation of nanospheres as primary subunits.[25] However, observations of spherically shaped nanosized amelogenin aggregates *in vivo* have been far from convincing and questions regarding the biologically active morphology of amelogenin assemblies lie still unanswered. Biological molecules, especially the lengthy ones, such as proteins, comprise many active points on their surface which can engage in weak chemical interactions that are, in turn, responsible for their assembly into exciting morphological units.[26] However, without demonstrating the ability of these supramolecular symmetries to act in a biologically functional manner, their relevance within *in vivo* contexts is predestined to remain only a hypothesis.

2.4.4 Can recombinant proteins be reliable models for studying amelogenesis *in vitro*?

The first time amelogenin was expressed *in vitro* as a recombinant protein was in 1994.[27] Since then, most studies using this protein have been carried out with its recombinant versions rather than those isolated from animals, typically porcine, mouse or bovine. However, the structural difference between recombinant amelogenins and the nascent ones expressed by ameloblasts, although seemingly minor, may pose far greater limitations than routinely thought. For example, amelogenins expressed by ameloblasts are phosphorylated at one residue (^{16}Ser), whereas the recombinant proteins expressed by *E. coli* do not comprise any post-translational modifications. This causes concerns about the functional discrepancies that may occur owing to this slight structural variation, particularly in view of the fact that it is well known that phosphorylated groups are especially important in the formation of calcium phosphate minerals. The mineralization of dentin is, for example, directed by the phosphophoryn protein family typically with numerous repeats of the sequences Asp-Ser(P)-Ser(P)- and Ser(P)-Asp.[28] Studies have indicated that single-residue phosphorylation of amelogenins is absolutely crucial to ensure molecular conditions for the proper development of enamel.[29,30] Moreover, recombinant amelogenins dispossess the first residue at the N-terminal, which may also cause drastic differences in the mechanism of their folding.

Single-point mutations have been shown to lead to far greater implications, both *in vivo* and *in vitro*, than is insinuated by the magnitude of these structural perturbations. Aside from innumerable cases wherein single-point mutations disrupt the functionality of proteins (e.g. substitution of valine with glutamic acid in the β-chain of hemoglobin resulting in sickle cell anemia), single-point mutations have been shown to modify the peptide self-assembly too.[31] A single-point mutation in the amelogenin-coding gene thus resulted in a single amino acid substitution (Pro-41→Thr) in the primary structure of amelogenin and, hence, to a specific type of *amelogenesis imperfecta*, related to severe dental enamel malformation.[32,33] A similar single-point mutation (Pro-70→Thr) in recombinant full-length human amelogenin has been shown to result in significantly lower rates of apatite growth compared to that observed in the presence of the wild-type,[34] as demonstrated in Fig. 2.8. Moreover, mutations not only in amelogenin genes, but in those that encode MMP-20 cause *amelogenesis imperfecta*, a pathological state typified by abnormal and significantly weakened enamel.[35,36] The mutation g.2142G>A on the gene coding for this KLK-4 has also been shown to cause abnormal enzymatic activity, resulting in enamel crystals of normal length but insufficient thickness.[37]

2.4.5 What is the role of proteolysis in crystal formation?

While numerous studies have been carried out to assess the specificity of the proteolytic cleavage of amelogenins and other proteins in the enamel matrix and the morphogenetic effects of alterations in the native structures of these polypeptide reactants, the effects proteolysis exerts on crystal growth has not been tackled to a similar extent. As shown in Fig. 2.9, proteolytic digestion by means of MMP-20 can be suspected of playing an additional nucleation-promoting role compared to that played by amelogenin *per se*, as mentioned earlier. Proteolysis has been shown to cleave the

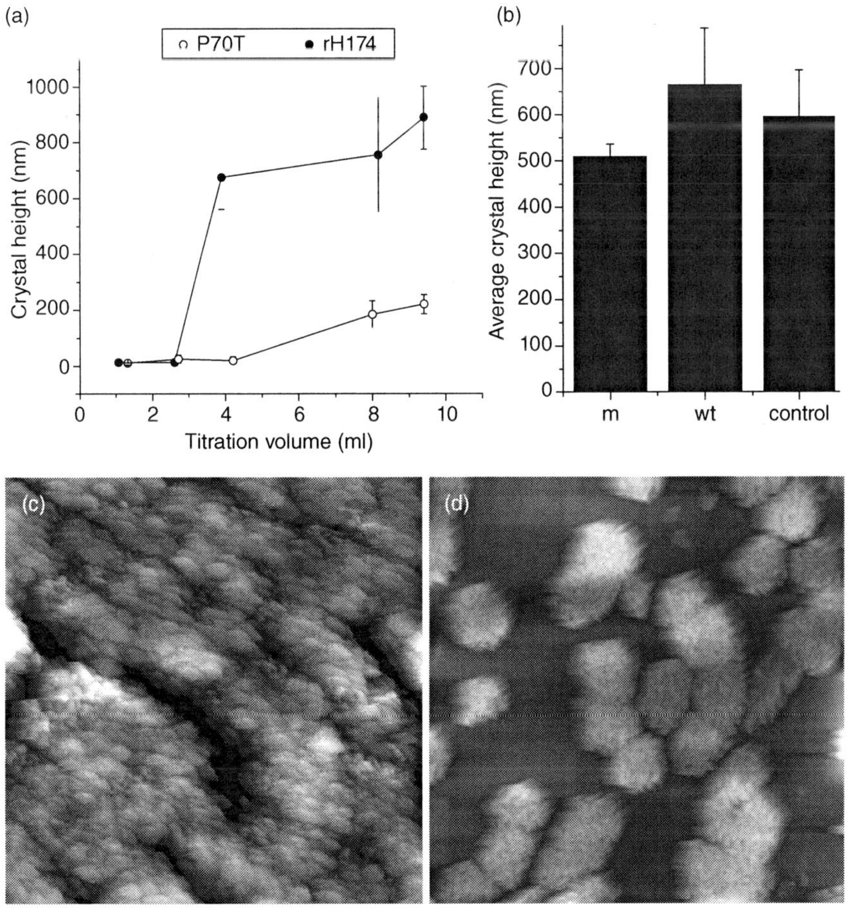

2.8 Significantly lower average calcium phosphate crystal height deposited on fluoroapatite substrates during titration of single-point Pro-70→Thr mutated human full-length recombinant amelogenin (P70T) in sol than that deposited in the presence of wild-type amelogenin (rH174), at different supersaturation ratios (a and b). Also, less specific crystal growth observed for mutated amelogenin (c) in comparison with the wild-type one (d). The size of both AMF micrographs is 10 × 10 mm. Partially adapted and reproduced with permission from Zhu *et al.*[34]

hydrophilic C-terminal of amelogenin and thus promote intensive aggregation and ripening of its nanospheres, detectable as an increase in the particle size during dynamic light scattering analysis. Consequently, the protein increasingly deposits onto the growing crystals and, since it supposedly acts as a bridge that facilitates the flow of ionic growing units from the solution to the crystalline faces, crystal growth becomes kinetically favored. In this

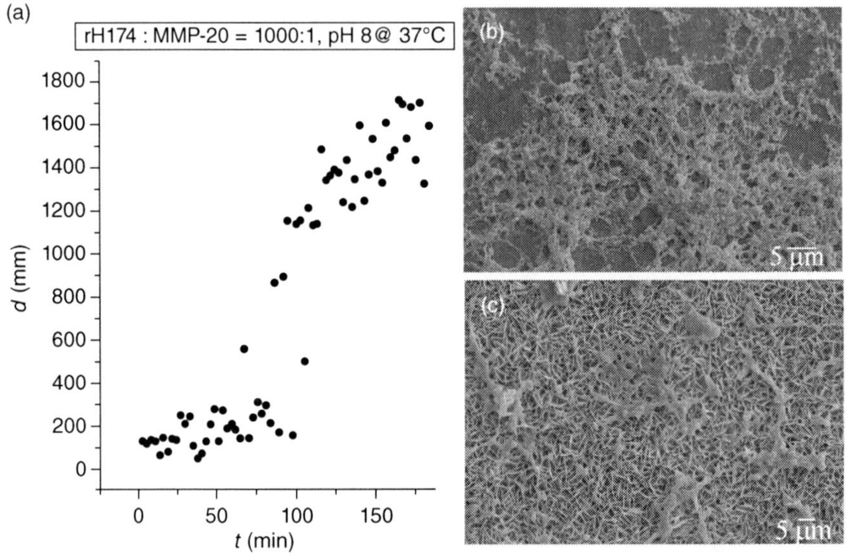

2.9 An increase in the average particle size of amelogenin following its proteolysis by MMP-20 (MMP-20/rH174 1:1000 weight ratio), starting at $t = 0$ (a). A moderate amount of crystal formation is observed during titration of amelogenin sols with calcium and phosphate ions (b) and a markedly greater amount of calcium phosphate precipitate forms under identical conditions when proteolytic reaction is coupled to the titration (c).

way, MMP-20 can be said to lower the energy of activation required for heterogeneous nucleation of calcium phosphate and serve as a potent kinetic factor that influences the thermodynamics of apatite growth.[38]

2.4.6 What is the role of micro-ions and less abundant protein species?

The role of many ions present in the enamel matrix in minor but controlled amounts are currently only the subject of hypotheses. For example, a steady, although probably carefully monitored and modulated inflow of zinc ions is known to exist owing to its role in regulating the activity of MMP-20. Fluoride is also present in natural enamel, where it has the effect of strengthening the apatite lattice. Still, in overly large amounts it leads to a counter-effect: increased porosity and weakening of the enamel structure.[39] It was also shown that increased levels of fluoride in developing enamel decrease the activity of MMP-20,[40] resulting in the condition known as fluorosis. The role of fluoride ions in promoting elongation of apatite crystals has, however, been well documented.[41,42] In a set of experiments, only a combination of amelogenin and fluoride led to formation of rod-like apatite crystals, while only octacalcium phosphate precipitated in the absence of fluoride.[43,44]

The role of other ions, including magnesium and sodium, known to be present in the natural enamel, should not be underestimated, especially in view of their inhibiting effect on apatite growth rates. Since crystal growth rates and the aspect ratio of grown crystals often stand in inverse proportion, it is possible that these growth-inhibiting ions may exert a pivotal influence on the overall process. Finally, variations in pH may also be crucial, particularly in view of the specificity of interaction between amelogenin and apatite, depending on the surface charge sign and magnitude.[45]

For example, as shown in Fig. 2.10, the fact the particle size measured by means of dynamic light scattering after mixing hydroxyapatite and amelogenin nanoparticles corresponds to that of their sum, while the resulting zeta potential is equal to the positive value of circa +5 mV, which amelogenin possesses at the given pH, clearly suggests that adsorption of the protein onto the mineral surface proceeds momentarily when their surface charges carry opposite signs.[45] The definitive role of pH changes is still not clear, although ameloblasts have been shown to modulate the pH of the enamel fluid rhythmically. Therefore, covering the micro-distance from smooth to ruffled endings of the cells is accompanied by a local pH change in the surrounding enamel fluid from nearly physiological (7.2 7.4) to slightly acidic (6.1–6.8) values.[46]

Reports on the role of enamel matrix proteins other than amelogenin in enamel formation have been relatively scarce to date.[47] Still, even simple requirements that entail proper crystal growth, such as controlling and modulating pH, are known to depend on a plethora of protein species secreted by ameloblasts and transitorily present in the enamel matrix.[48] The role of other protein species is still not even partially elucidated, especially not in synergy with other components of the developing enamel matrix. Studying these in parallel, however, introduces a lot more variables into the system than can be coped with on the timescale of a normal scientific project, especially considering the time-consuming kinetics required to replicate the naturally slow enamel-yielding reactions. However, signs still point to the essential role of these less abundant protein species in amelogenesis. For example, mutations on the enamelin-coding gene have been shown to result in severe phenotypic *amelogenesis imperfecta*.[12] This highly acidic glycoprotein is observed to form a sheath around the growing apatite crystals (their *c*-axes being perpendicular to the β sheets of the surrounding enamelin), which is in compliance with the current model of extracellular mineralization. According to this model, hydrophobic proteins, such as amelogenin, collagen or cellulose, are assumed to be involved in the buildup of the insoluble macromolecular matrix of the developing

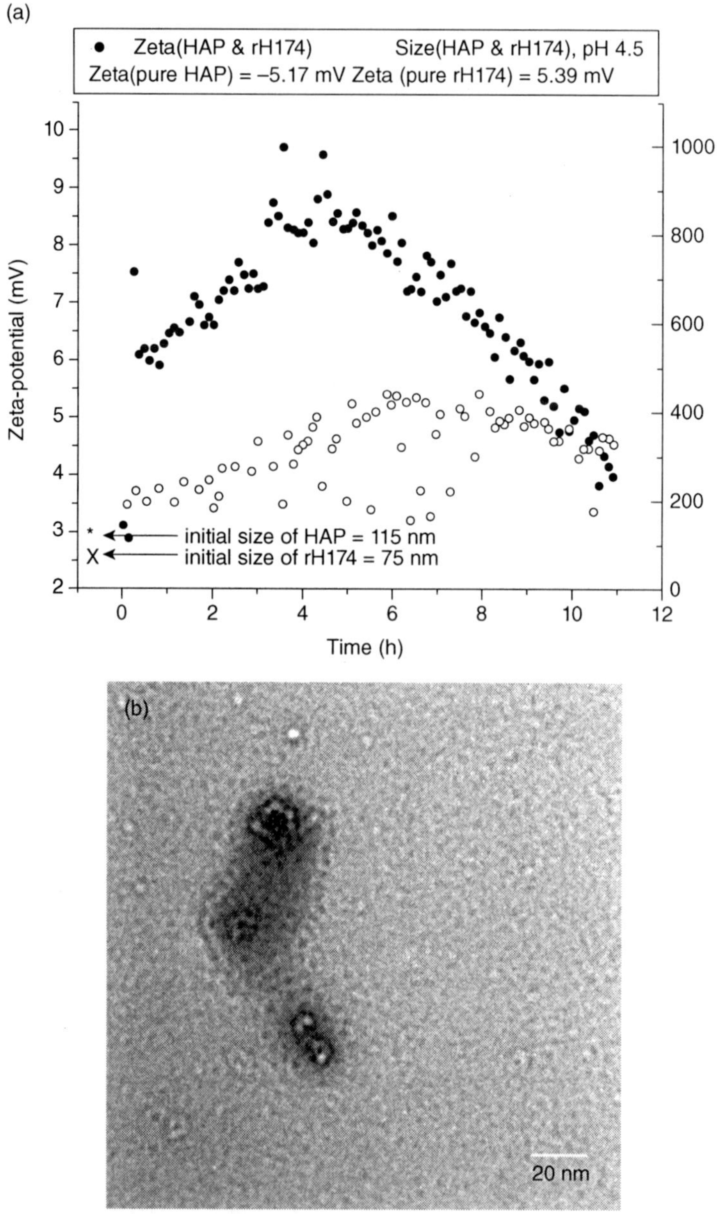

2.10 (a) Average hydrodynamic diameter and ζ-potential of the colloidal mixture of HAP and rH174 at [rH174] = 0.16 mM when rH174 was abruptly added to the HAP sol comprising 150 mM KCl, 20 mM Tris/HCl, at 25°C and pH 4.50 +–0.02, and continuously measured over 11 h aging time: (b) Transmission electron micrograph demonstrating the adsorption of amelogenin onto hydroxyapatite nanoparticles Partially adapted and reprinted with permission from Uskoković.[45]

hard tissue, whereas hydrophilic proteins are involved in attracting precursor ions and providing the nucleation surfaces.

Even though the low concentration of enamelin in the enamel matrix can be thought of as a sign of its low importance, that need not be necessarily so. For, there are many examples of macromolecular or amphiphilic additives that exhibit a cooperative effect on the assembly of the precipitated phase at low concentrations only.[6] The morphological specificity, such as preferential adsorption of the additive molecules along specific planes of the crystalline phase, in these cases rapidly diminishes at higher concentrations. Ameloblastin is also presumed to carry out a significant function, not only because of its localization at the secretory end of ameloblasts where the crystal growth is initiated, but because we know that both an elevated and hindered expression of ameloblastin results in *amelogenesis imperfecta*.[12] The roles of even less abundant components of the enamel matrix, such as KLK4, keratin K14, DLX3 or biglycan protein, the mutant expressions of which are also known to produce the conditions of *amelogenesis imperfecta*,[49] have also not been investigated thoroughly.

2.4.7 Can artificial enamel be synthesized at comparatively high growth rates?

Low metastable levels of supersaturation appear to be crucial for providing the right conditions for protein-guided crystal growth.[50] Low rates of nucleation and crystal growth naturally favor the formation of elongated crystals. In contrast, rapid mixing of reactants, yielding high initial concentrations of nuclei is a routine recipe for fabrication of ultrafine particles that are not to exceed a few nanometers in diameter. For example, when controlled degradation of urea is used slowly to increase alkalinity of the solution and provide conditions for precipitation, the apatite crystals formed turn out to be either plate-shaped or needle-shaped.[51] Single-crystal apatite fibers 20–60 μm in length and 100–300 nm in diameter were thus obtained by precipitation using decomposition of urea.[52] Attempts to initiate nucleation and crystal growth at a higher rate by increasing the supersaturation ratio would presumably deprive amelogenins of their ability to direct the crystallization events.[50]

Eventually, it is possible that an informal conclusion will be arrived at, stating that without slow growth comparable to the extraordinary slowness of amelogenesis, artificial replicas of enamel-like structures could not be synthesized. Even if a satisfactory degree of morphological semblance is reached, structural differences at the fine scale may possibly be large enough to render the given material mechanically inferior to natural enamel.

One thing is certain though. Namely, the elongated morphology and highly crystalline nature of apatite in enamel in comparison to smaller, nanosized and much less crystalline apatite particles formed in bone and dentin implies that different models of growth should be applicable in these two cases of biomineralization.[23] Indeed, a model involving template-based catalyzed nucleation and limited growth by hydrophilic proteins, such as osteocalcin, which is valid for bone and dentin, can thus be claimed not to be applicable to enamel. Instead, a model based on (a) slow crystal growth, (b) gradual increase of supersaturation levels and (c) the role of amelogenin in channeling the growth units onto the growing apatite surface, is given here as an alternative to the standard models of biomineralization that depict nucleation events as taking place on foreign organic surfaces, governed by their hydrophilic character and precisely matching lattice spacing, and crystal growth as proceeding while being inhibited by the adsorbing bioorganic particles.

2.4.8 To what extent does the Ostwald–Lussac rule apply to the mechanism of formation of apatite in enamel?

Crystallization of apatite under simple precipitation conditions in aqueous media is known to obey the Ostwald–Lussac rule, which dictates that precipitation of apatite as the most stable calcium phosphate phase has to be preceded by precipitation of the less soluble phases formable at low temperatures and in hydrated local environments (which excludes oxide phases: tricalcium phosphate polymorphs and tetracalcium phosphate). This is illustrated in Fig. 2.11: namely, a system undergoing a phase transition will tend

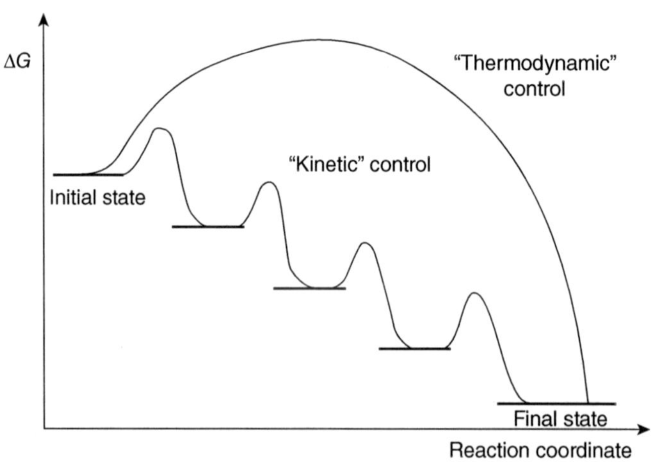

2.11 Free energy of a system undergoing phase transition through a multitude of transitory states.

to make multiple steps over transitory states separated from each other by a smaller energy barrier than the one posed between the initial and the final state.

Consequently, the precipitation of apatite at pH >7 should follow the following route in the absence of kinetic factors capable of inducing transcendence in some or all the stages in the process:

amorphous calcium phosphate → monocalcium phosphate → dicalcium phosphate → octacalcium phosphate → hydroxyapatite

In general, the higher the pH, the more rapid the transition from one stage to another and the less is the probability of halting the precipitation at an intermediate stage and detecting one of these transitory phases. At sufficiently high pH values, the solution will also be virtually undersaturated with respect to phases that dominate the low pH range, including monocalcium phosphate and dicalcium phosphates (brushite and monetite), which implies that they are missing in this stepwise progression of the precipitate toward the crystal structure of apatite. Still, opinion among biomineralization experts widely varies in terms of whether ECM proteins and other biointerfaces can provide sufficiently potent kinetic forces to enable transition of hydrated solutes directly to the most stable biomineral phase, apatite, following the onset of precipitation. Ever since a dark octacalcium phosphate line was found during a transmission election microscopy (TEM) analysis positioned in the center of enamel apatite fibers,[53] the belief that apatite is the phase that forms directly during amelogenesis has been intensively questioned. Since then, many studies have demonstrated that the amorphous calcium phosphate presents a transient phase in the course of amelogenesis.[54,55]

2.4.9 How crucial are the underlying Tomes' process and the mineralization of dentin for proper amelogenesis?

As can be seen from Fig. 2.1(a), the growing dentin and enamel are adjacent to each other. Although odontoblasts responsible for directing the growth of dentin, coming from mesenchymal tissue, and ameloblasts responsible for directing the growth of enamel, coming from epithelial tissue, are thoroughly separated after the mineral growth begins, these two types of cells are engaged in intensive communication prior to initiation of an almost simultaneous crystallization of dentin and enamel. Ameloblasts enter their first formative state after the first layer of dentin is formed, secreting the enamel matrix and at the same time retreating away from the DEJ, leaving the matrix to mineralize by itself.[56] The question that remains is to what extent does this initial dentin surface exert an effect on the nature of enamel

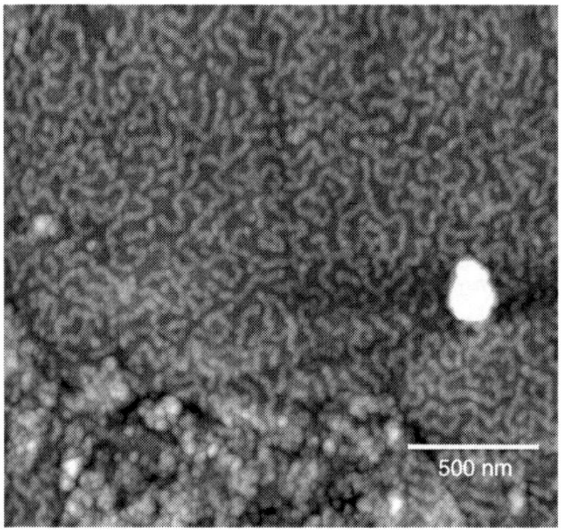

2.12 AFM image of fibrous amelogenin assemblies forming only on the flat glassy surface and not on the apatite crystal.

growth. For, just as in many other aspects of life, the first steps made during surface-specific growth greatly determine the direction which it will assume and, therefore, the nature and structure of the final product. After all, the smoothness and stiffness of the surface, as well as the nature and density of chemical groups residing on it, all crucially determine its activity and potential to be the starting point of growth of a new phase. This is nicely illustrated in Fig. 2.12, which shows how fibrous amelogenin assemblies form strictly on the flat silica glass surface and not on the rigged fluoroapatite crystals embedded in the glassy matrix. Furthermore, the underlying Tomes' process, during which ameloblasts retreat from the growing fibers and toward the epithelium, may be crucial in aligning the apatite fibers, bundling them up within prisms composed of rod and inter-rod enamel and preventing their random tilting in space.

2.4.10 Do biomimetic studies present a reliable approximation of the biological process?

Having been played around with, DNA molecules were assembled into an array of attractive morphologies, from cubes to triangles to pentagons to hexagons and octahedrons.[57] Yet, none of those probably have any significance for the biological domain, at least not in the evolutionary terms. Similarly, macrophage peptides have been intensively utilized to produce exciting material structures;[58,59] still, this also cannot be taken as a sign that somewhere in Nature they indeed act along these lines. As already pointed out, a high potential for molecular recognition predisposes organic molecules and particularly polypeptides to assemble into an endless variety of morphologies depending on the environmental conditions to which they are naturally structurally sensitive.[60] This versatility of interactions is responsible for a variety of mutually contradictory conclusions, that abound in literature reports on attempts to replicate amelogenesis *in vitro*. For, insights derived under one set of conditions may easily turn out to be at odds with those inferred from another seemingly similar, but in reality drastically different set of conditions. If we add an immense sensitivity to the slightest changes in boundary conditions on the evolution of these systems in time, we come to an awareness of a yet deeper gap that should prevent experimentalists from coming up with omnipotent conclusions from their studies. Strictly speaking, what is observed in a simplified biomimetic set of conditions may present only an indication that similar structures and mechanisms may occur *in vivo* as well.

Just as the absence of evidence is in no way equal to evidence of absence, so the evidence of an interesting effect in the laboratory setting does not imply that this effect is evidence of the principle investigated by laboratory mimicry. Whatever the insights obtained from biomimetic studies, precautionary measures ought to be taken against deriving premature and grandiose conclusions from them. For, what appears to be immanent in one context need not be as naturally derived from another. Some of the greatest blunders in science came not from cleverly framed propositions, but from pretentious broadening of their validity far beyond the scope proposed by their originators. A most striking example comes from Darwin's theory of evolution and the concept of 'survival of the fittest' which he proposed in his Origins. Namely, even though he mentioned that it ought to be grasped in a 'broad and metaphorical sense, so that it implies an interdependence of one creature on others, including not only individual lives, but the entire progeny',[61] the followers of his teaching should be blamed for irrational exaggeration and overly literal interpretation of this phrase, which nowadays holds a quite different casual connotation from that of which Darwin conceived.[62,63] Although this example may seem remote from the realm of dental science, it may not be so. For, whenever an intriguing discovery is glimpsed, it takes considerable modesty to keep on claiming its validity only under the experimental settings replicated in the laboratory rather than in the biological circumstances mimicked.

This leads to another important question, on which the research fate of many biomimeticians depends. It is whether *in vitro* remineralization of enamel, the precursor of soft and non-invasive clinical therapy, can be accomplished in a cell-deprived manner. Or, as Sherlock Holmes would have phrased it, 'We cannot imitate Nature, we can only recreate it as a whole'. Future insights in this field of research will certainly depend on how biomimeticians come to terms with this holistic saying of one of the world's dearest detectives.

2.5 Conclusion

The general feeling is that only a tip of an iceberg has been glimpsed in our understanding of the fascinating biomineralization process called amelogenesis. Despite the sense of confidence in what has already been verified or merely theorized as certain in the circle of 'enamel growers', digging deeper into the nature of their findings gives a sense that much more has been hypothesized than truly confirmed. Hypotheses are certainly not lacking in this field since almost every idea that can occur can be traced back to a hypothesis already proposed. However, inventiveness in designing experimental methods that would contribute to validation of these assumptions in reality are what this field needs in the foreseeable future.

Another trait of vital importance, on which the accomplishment of the aforementioned aims will depend, is the openness of the dental community to cross-disciplinary fertilization of ideas. Dental science has greatly benefited in the past from the constructive intrusion of physicists and physical chemists into its realm and although many may be skeptical, in view of the risks such interdisciplinary encounters bear, or may feel insecure about putting their research into hands of someone who will shape it into a different and often barely intelligible language, these will be challenges that need to be overcome with intellectual courage by members of the dental community.

Finally, insights into the mechanism by which the protein matrix guides the growth of apatite crystals in enamel, such as those presented here based in part on previously published results,[18,23,64,65] are not only relevant to dental researchers, educators and clinicians interested in amelogenesis. They are valuable for understanding the protein–mineral interactions that govern many other types of biomineralization. The broad relevance of findings obtained with a focus on enamel growth may remind us once again that small is beautiful, that each field of research hides universal meanings and that focusing on small things and details of physical reality may lead us to grasp answers to much greater secrets of the universe. Such an awareness of greatly potent findings awaiting in seemingly small research fields can motivate scientists from a plethora of other fields to peek into the world of dentistry and find either a temporary solace for their wonder therein or a safe academic nest.

2.6 Acknowledgments

The author acknowledges the NIH grants K99-DE021416, R01-DE17529 and R01-DE015821 for support.

2.7 References

1. Cai, Y., Liu, Y., Yan, W., Hu, Q., Tao, J., Zhang, M., Shi, Z. and Tang, R., 'Role of hydroxyapatite nanoparticle size in bone cell proliferation'. *J Mater Chem*, 2007, **17**, 3780.
2. Robinson, C., Kirkham, J. and Hallsworth, A.S., 'Volume distribution and concentration of protein, mineral and water in developing bovine enamel'. *Arch Oral Bio*, 1988, **33**, 159–62.
3. Bouropoulos, N. and Moradian-Oldak, J., 'Induction of apatite by the cooperative effect of amelogenin and the 32-kda enamelin'. *J Dent Res*, 2004, **83**, 278–82.
4. Bartlett J.D., Ganss B., Goldberg M., Moradian-Oldak J., Paine M.L., Snead M.L., Wen X., White S.N. and Zhou Y.L., 'Protein-protein interactions of the developing enamel matrix'. *Curr Top Dev Biol*, 2006, **74**, 57–115.
5. Smith, C.E., 'Enamel agenesis and aberrant mineralizations occur in enamelin null mice'. Presented at the *International Association of Dental Researchers Conference*, Toronto, July 2008.
6. Mann, S., *Biomineralization: Principles and Concepts in Bioinorganic Materials Chemistry*, Oxford University Press, Oxford, 2001.
7. Levi-Kalisman, Y., Falini, G., Addadi, L. and Weiner, S., 'Structure of the nacreous organic matrix of a bivalve mollusk shell examined in the hydrated state using cryo-TEM'. *J Struct Biol*, 2001, **135**, 8–17.
8. Snead, M.L., 'Amelogenin protein exhibits a modular design: implications for form and function'. *Connect Tissue Res*, 2003, **44**, 47–51.
9. Robinson, C., Brookes, S.J., Bonass, W.A., Shore and R.C., Kirkham, J. 'Enamel maturation'. *Ciba Foundation Symposium 205 – Dental Enamel*, D.J. Chadwick and G. Cardew (eds), John Wiley & Sons, Chichester, UK, 2007, 156–74.
10. Lu, Y., Papagerakis, P., Yamakoshi, Y., Hu, J.C., Bartlett, J.D. and Simmer, J.P., 'Functions of KLK4 and MMP-20 in dental enamel formation'. *Biol Chem*, 2008, **389**, 695–700.
11. Eastoe, J.E., 'The amino acid composition of proteins from the oral tissues – II The matrix proteins in dentine and enamel from developing human deciduous teeth. *Arch Oral Biol*, 1963, **8**, 633–52.
12. Margolis, H.C., Beniash, E. and Fowler, C.E., 'Role of macromolecular assembly of enamel matrix proteins in enamel formation'. *J Dent Res*, 2006, **85**, 775–93.
13. Cölfen, H. and Mann, S., 'Higher-order organization by mesoscale self-assembly and transformation of hybrid nanostructures'. *Angew Chem Int Ed*, 2003, **42**, 2350–65.
14. Wang, L., Guan, X., Du, C., Moradian-Oldak, J. and Nancollas, G.H., 'Amelogenin promotes the formation of elongated apatite microstructures in a controlled crystallization system'. *J Phys Chem C*, 2007, **111**, 6398–404.
15. White, S.N., Luo, W., Paine, M.L., Fong, H., Sarikaya, M. and Snead, M.L., 'Biological organization of hydroxyapatite crystallites into a fibrous continuum toughens and controls anisotropy in human enamel'. *J Dent Res*, 2001, **80**, 321–6.

16. He, L.H. and Swain, M.V., 'Understanding the mechanical behaviour of human enamel from its structural and compositional characteristics'. *J Mech Beha Biomed Mater*, 2008, **1**, 18–29.
17. Stupp, S.I., 'Molecular manipulation of microstructures: biomaterials, ceramics, and semiconductors'. *Science*, 1997, **277**, 1242–48.
18. Uskoković, V., Li, W. and Habelitz, S., 'Amelogenin as a promoter of nucleation and crystal growth of apatite'. *J Crystal Growth*, 2011, **316**, 106–17.
19. Habelitz, S., Kullar, A., Marshall, S.J., DenBesten, P.K., Balooch, M., Marshall, G.W. and Li, W., 'Amelogenin-guided crystal growth on fluoroapatite glass-ceramics'. *J Dent Res*, 2004, **83**, 698–702.
20. Tarasevich, B., Howard, C.J., Larson, J.L., Snead, M.L., Simmer, J.P., Paine, M. and Shaw, W.J., 'The nucleation and growth of calcium phosphate by amelogenin'. *J Cryst Growth*, 2007, **304**, 407–15.
21. Gower, L.B., 'Biomimetic model systems for investigating the amorphous precursor pathway and its role in biomineralization'. *Chem Rev*, 2008, **108**, 4551–627.
22. Robinson, C., 'Amelogenin assembly and function'. *Eur J Oral Sci*, 2006, **114**, 327–9.
23. Uskoković, V., 'Prospects and pits on the path of biomimetics: The case of tooth enamel'. *J Biomimetics, Biomate, Tissue Eng*, 2010, **8**, 45–78.
24. Moradian-Oldak, J. *et al.*, 'Detection of monodisperse aggregates of a recombinant amelogenin by dynamic light scattering'. *Biopolymers*, 1994, **34**, 1339–47.
25. He, X., Wu, S., Martinez-Avila, O., Cheng, Y. and Habelitz, S., 'Self-aligning amelogenin nanoribbons in oil–water system'. *J Struct Biol*, 2011, **174**, 203–12.
26. Uskokovic, V., 'Theoretical and practical aspects of colloid science and self-assembly phenomena revisited'. *Rev Chem Eng*, 2007, **23**, 301–72.
27. Simmer, J.P., Lau, E.C., Hu, C.C., Aoba, T., Lacey, M., Nelson, D., Zaichner-David, M., Snead, M.L., Slavkin, H.C. and Fincham, A.G., 'Isolation and characterization of a mouse amelogenin expressed in *Escherichia coli*'. *Calcif Tissue Int*, 1994, **54**, 312–19.
28. Hartgerink, J.D., 'Self-assembly and mineralization of peptide–amphiphile nanofibers'. *Science*, 2001, **294**, 1684–88.
29. Kwak, S.-Y., Wiedemann-Bidlack, F.B., Beniash, E. Yamakoshi, Y., Simmer, J.P., Litman, A. and Margolis, H.C., 'Role of 20-kDa amelogenin (P148) phosphorylation in calcium phosphate formation *in vitro*. *J Biol Chem*, 2009, **284**, 18972–79.
30. Wiedemann-Bidlack, F.B., Kwak, S.-Y., Beniash, E. Yamakoshi, Y., Simmer, J.P. and Margolis, H.C., 'Effects of phosphorylation on the self-assembly of native full-length porcine amelogenin and its regulation of calcium phosphate formation *in vitro*'. *J Struct Biol*, 2011, **173**, 250–60.
31. Dai, Q., Castellino, F.J. and Prorok, M., 'A single amino acid replacement results in the ca^{2+} -induced self-assembly of a helical conantokin-based peptide'. *Biochemistry*, 2004, **43**, 13225–32.
32. Collier, P., Sauk, J., Rosenbloom, J., Yuan, Z. and Gibson, C., 'An amelogenin gene defect associated with human X-linked amelogenesis imperfecta'. *Arch Oral Biol*, 1997, **42**, 235–42.
33. Tanimoto, K. *et al.*, 'Reduced amelogenin-MMP20 interactions in amelogenesis imperfecta'. *J Dent Res*, 2008, **87**, 451–5.

34. Zhu, L., Uskoković, V., Le, T., DenBesten, P., Huang, Y., Habelitz, S. and Li, W., 'Altered self-assembly and apatite binding of amelogenin induced by N-terminal proline mutation'. *Arch Oral Biol*, 2011, **56**, 331–6.
35. Bartlett, J.D., Skobe, Z., Lee, D.H., Wright, J.T., Li, Y., Kulkarni, A.B. and Gibson, C.W., 'A developmental comparison of matrix metalloproteinase-20 and amelogenin null mouse enamel'. *Eur J Oral Sci*, 2006, **114**, 18–23.
36. Caterina, J.J., Skobe, Z., Shi, J., Ding, Y., Simmer, J.P., Birkedal-Hansen, H. and Bartlett, J.D., 'Enamelysin (matrix metalloproteinase 20)-deficient mice display an *amelogenesis imperfecta* phenotype'. *J Biol Chem*, 2002, **277**, 49598–604.
37. Hart, P.S., Hart, T.C., Michalec, M.D., Ryu. O.H., Simmons, D., Hong, S. and Wright, J.T., 'Mutation in kallikrein 4 causes autosomal recessive hypomaturation amelogenesis imperfecta'. *J Med Genet*, 2004, **41**, 545–9.
38. Uskoković, V., Khan, F., Liu, H., Witkowska, H.E., Zhu, L., Li, W. and Habelitz S., 'Proteolytic hydrolysis of amelogenin by means of matrix metalloprotease-20 accelerates mineralization *in vitro*'. *Archives of Oral Biology*, 2011, **56**, 1548–59.
39. Garant, P.R., *Oral Cells and Tissues*, Quintessence, Carol Stream, IL, 2003.
40. Zhang, Y., Yan, Q., Li, W. and DenBesten, P.K., 'Fluoride down-regulates the expression of matrix metalloproteinase-20 in human fetal tooth ameloblast-lineage cells *in vitro*'. *Eur J Oral Sci*, 2006, **114**, 105–10.
41. Ma, G., Liu, X.Y. and Wang, M., 'Growth and mechanisms of enamel-like hierarchical nanostructures on single crystalline hydroxyapatite micro-ribbons'. *J Nanosci Nanotechnol*, 2011, **11**, 5199–206.
42. Fan, Y., Sun, Z. and Moradian-Oldak, J., 'Effect of fluoride on the morphology of calcium phosphate crystals grown on acid-etched human enamel'. *Caries Res*, 2009, **43**, 132–6.
43. Iijima, M., Du, C., Abbott, C., Doi, Y. and Moradian-Oldak, J., 'Control of apatite crystal growth by the co-operative effect of a recombinant porcine amelogenin and fluoride'. *Eur J Oral Sci*, 2006, **114**, 304–7.
44. Iijima, M. and Moradian-Oldak, J., 'Control of apatite crystal growth in a fluoride containing amelogenin-rich matrix'. *Biomaterials*, 2005, **26**, 1595–603.
45. Uskoković, V., Odsinada, R., Djordjevic, S. and Habelitz, S., 'Dynamic light scattering and zeta potential of colloidal mixtures of amelogenin and hydroxyapatite in calcium and phosphate rich ionic milieus'. *Arch Oral Biol*, 2011, **56**, 521–32.
46. Smith, C.E., 'Cellular and chemical events during enamel maturation'. *Crit Rev Oral Biol Med*, 1998, **9**, 128–61.
47. Wang, H., Tannukit, S., Zhu, D., Snead, M.L. and Paine, M.L., 'Enamel matrix protein interactions'. *J Bone Miner Res*, 2005, **20**, 1032–40.
48. Lacruz, R.S., Smith, C.E., Moffatt, P., Chang, E.H., Bromage, T.G., Bringas, P. Jr, Nanci, A., Baniwal, S.K., Zabner, J., Welsh, M.J., Kurtz, I. and Paine, M.L., 'Requirements for ion and solute transport, and pH regulation, during enamel maturation'. *J Cell Physiol*, 2011, **227**(4), 1776–85.
49. Stephanopoulos, G., Garefalaki, M.-E. and Lyroudia, K., 'Genes and related proteins involved in *amelogenesis imperfecta*'. *J Dent Res*, 2005, **84**, 1117–26.
50. Habelitz, S., DenBesten, P., Marshall, S., Marshall, G. and Li, W., 'Amelogenin control over apatite crystal growth is affected by the pH and degree of ionic saturation'. *Orthod Craniofacial Res*, 2005, **8**, 232–8.

51. Jevtić, M. and Uskoković, D., 'Influence of urea as homogeneous precipitation agent on sonochemical hydroxyapatite synthesis'. *Mater Sci Forum*, 2007, **555**, 285–90.
52. Aizawa, M., Porter, A., Best, S. and Bonfield, W., 'Ultrastructural observation of single-crystal apatite fibres'. *Biomaterials*, 2005, **26**, 3427–33.
53. Reyes-Gasga, J. and Alcantara-Rodriguez, C.M., 'Structural analysis of the human tooth enamel by transmission electron microscopy'. *Hydroxyapatite and Related Materials*, Paul W. Brown and Brent Constanz (eds), 1994, 295–304.
54. Beniash, E., Metzler, R.A., Lam, R.S.K. and Gilbert, P.U.P.A., 'Transient amorphous calcium phosphate in forming enamel'. *J Struct Biol*, 2009, **166**, 133–43.
55. Le Norcy, E., Kwak, S.-Y., Wiedemann-Bidlack, F.B., Beniash, E. Yamakoshi, Y., Simmer, J.P. and Margolis, H.C., 'Leucine-rich amelogenin peptides regulate mineralization *in vitro*. *J Dent Res*, 2011, **90**, 1091–7.
56. Simmer, J. and Hu, J., 'Expression, structure, and function of enamel proteinases'. *Connect Tissue Res*, 2002, **43**, 441–9.
57. Aldaye, F.A., Palmer, A.L. and Sleiman, H.F., 'Assembling materials with DNA as the guide'. *Science*, 2008, **321**, 1795–9.
58. Ahmad, G., Dickerson, M.B., Church, B.C., Cai. Y., Jones, S.E., Naik, R.R., King, J.S., Summers, C.J., Kroger, N. and Sandhage, K.H., 'Rapid, room-temperature formation of crystalline calcium molybdate phosphor microparticles via peptide-induced precipitation'. *Adv Mater*, 2006, **18**, 1759–63.
59. Dickerson, M.B., Naik, R.R., Stone, M.O., Cai, Y. and Sandhage, K.H., 'Identification of peptides that promote the rapid precipitation of germania nanoparticle networks via use of a peptide display library'. *Chem Commun*, 2004, 1776–7. Electronic Supplementary Information (ESI) is available describing the biopanning, germania precipitation assay, and molybdenum blue assay procedures. See http://www.rsc.org/suppdata/cc/b4/b402480j/.
60. Channon, K. and MacPhee, C.E., 'Possibilities for 'smart' materials exploiting the self-assembly of polypeptides into fibrils'. *Soft Matter*, 2008, **4**, 647.
61. Darwin, C., *On the Origin of Species by Means of Natural Selection, or the Preservation of Favoured Races in the Struggle for Life*. ElecBook, London, UK, 1859.
62. Whitehead, A.N., *Science and the Modern World*. The Free Press, New York, NY, 1925.
63. Loye, D., *Darwin's Second Revolution*. Benjamin Franklin Press, Pacific Grove, CA, 2010.
64. Uskokovic, V., Li, W. and Habelitz, S., 'Biomimetic precipitation of uniaxially grown calcium phosphate crystals from full-length human amelogenin sols'. *J Bionic Eng*, 2011, **8**, 114–21.
65. Uskoković, V., Kim, M.-K., Li, W. and Habelitz, S., 'Enzymatic processing of amelogenin during continuous crystallization of apatite'. *J Mater Res*, 2008, **23**, 3184–95.

3
Enamel and dentin bonding for adhesive restorations

JORGE PERDIGÃO, University of Minnesota, USA
and ANA SEZINANDO, University Rey Juan Carlos, Spain

DOI: 10.1533/9780857096432.1.45

Abstract: Since the introduction of the acid-etch technique many researchers have pursued methods for reliable and durable adhesion between resins and tooth structure. Numerous simplified adhesives have been introduced to the dental market within the last few years, without comprehensive clinical testing to validate the performance supported by *in vitro* tests. Because of the high hydrophilic nature of the monomers and the high water concentration required for ionization of the acidic monomers in self-etch solutions, it is likely that these materials have their bonding ability compromised over time. While *in vitro* tests are useful as a triage step, clinical studies are the ultimate test for any biomaterial. This chapter discusses recent developments in dental adhesives, their benefits, limitations, indications and contraindications.

Key words: chlorhexidine, dental bonding, dentin-bonding agents, hybrid layer, self-etch adhesive.

3.1 New trends in restorative dentistry

3.1.1 Introduction

The increasing demand for esthetic dentistry and the introduction of fluorides have revolutionized the practice of dentistry over the last two decades. The conventional concepts of tooth preparation introduced at the beginning of the 20th century (Black, 1917) have been challenged as a result of the more conservative approach prompted by the adhesion of resin-based restorative materials to tooth structure.

In 1955 Buonocore used 85% phosphoric acid to make enamel surfaces more susceptible to adhesion (Buonocore, 1955). Dr Buonocore applied a concept used in the paint industry to facilitate adhesion of paints and resins to metallic surfaces. Buonocore later foresaw the use of acids to etch enamel for sealing pits and fissures. The finding that caries incidence can be reduced in the pits and fissures of permanent teeth by as much as 86.3%, by sealing them with an adhesive at six-month intervals, pioneered the potential of this procedure in preventive dentistry (Cueto and Buonocore, 1967).

Since Buonocore's introduction of the acid-etch technique many researchers have pursued methods for reliable and durable adhesion between resins

Table 3.1 Indications and contraindications of dental adhesives

Indications	Contraindications
Direct anterior composite restorations	Patients with known allergies to resin-based materials and other components
Direct posterior composite restorations	Direct application in deep preparations of vital teeth (<0.5 mm from the pulp) (Costa *et al.*, 2003)
Indirect composite restorations	Contamination of the operating field – use of rubber dam may optimize the outcome
All-porcelain inlays/onlays, crowns and bridges	
Bonding of orthodontic brackets and bands	
Pit-and-fissure sealants	
Porcelain veneers	
Fiber-reinforced resin posts	
Improve retention for porcelain-metal or metallic crowns	
Periodontal splints and conservative tooth replacement prostheses	
Root desensitization	
Reattachment of fractured tooth fragments	
Repair of existing restorations	
Surface sealant for composite restorations	
Endodontic sealer	
Bond fractured fragments of anterior teeth	

and tooth structure. First, bonded resin-based restorations were used to replace missing or carious tooth structure. Then, indications moved gradually from anterior to posterior teeth. The acid-etch technique is now used in a wide variety of clinical situations in dentistry (Table 3.1).

Over the last decades there has been an enormous progress in dental materials research. Additionally, caries is now considered a complex or multi-factorial disease, in the same category as cardiovascular diseases and diabetes, in which many genetic, environmental and behavioral risk factors interact (Fejerskov, 2004). The relationship between *Streptococcus mutans* and dental caries is not linear. Relatively high proportions of this bacterium are found on tooth surfaces without caries progression (Fejerskov, 2004). The biofilm is now deemed to be the crucial factor responsible for caries lesions that develop where biofilms remain for extended periods of time (Fejerskov, 2004).

Another change occurred in dentistry. It involved a shift from methods that rely on visual–tactile inspection of the tooth surface and mechanical removal of carious tissues. More emphasis is now given to early diagnosis and conservative treatment of the diseased tissue (Hudson, 2004; Mount, 2007). Dentin caries lesions are difficult to detect under a macroscopically intact occlusal surface. Several studies (Rock and Kidd, 1988; Lussi, 1991) have demonstrated the inability of dentists to diagnose carious lesions within pit-and-fissure defects using the traditional dental explorer. The use of a dental explorer, as still taught in dental schools (visual–tactile inspection), has the potential to transfer cariogenic bacteria from one fissure to another (Loesche *et al.*, 1979) and damage sound fissures, facilitating the development of caries lesions (van Dorp *et al.*, 1988; Yassin, 1995). Additionally, the explorer does not improve accuracy of caries detection on non-cavitated occlusal surfaces (Lussi and Francescut, 2003).

3.1.2 Minimally invasive dentistry concept

The concept of minimally invasive dentistry (MID) has evolved as a consequence of an increased understanding of the caries process and the development of adhesive restorative materials. In 1896, Dr G.V. Black, a visionary for his time, stated that 'The day is surely coming . . .. when we will be engaged in practicing preventive, rather than reparative, dentistry' (Wolf *et al.*, 2007). A few years later, Dr Black compiled a great amount of knowledge on the caries process and clearly described the parameters of tooth preparation currently still taught in operative dentistry. Dr Black's classical operative dentistry concepts were based on:

- A wide 'surgical' approach to repair the caries lesion – extension for prevention;
- Material-driven geometrical preparation design – the need to retain a metal filling inside a box.

The traditional approach to the restoration of caries lesions leads to a retreatment cycle: excessive tooth reduction for a small caries lesion, subsequent replacement of the restoration and additional loss of tooth structure. This cycle is irreversible and results in progressive loss of tooth structure and tooth loss in some cases (Wendt *et al.*, 1998; Roberts *et al.*, 2001). It is now recognized that demineralized, but non-cavitated enamel and dentin, can be healed (Tyas *et al.*, 2000). Therefore, current concepts involve maximum preservation of the tooth structure (Fig. 3.1):

- No geometrically shaped preparation – no need to extend for prevention, but prevention of extension;

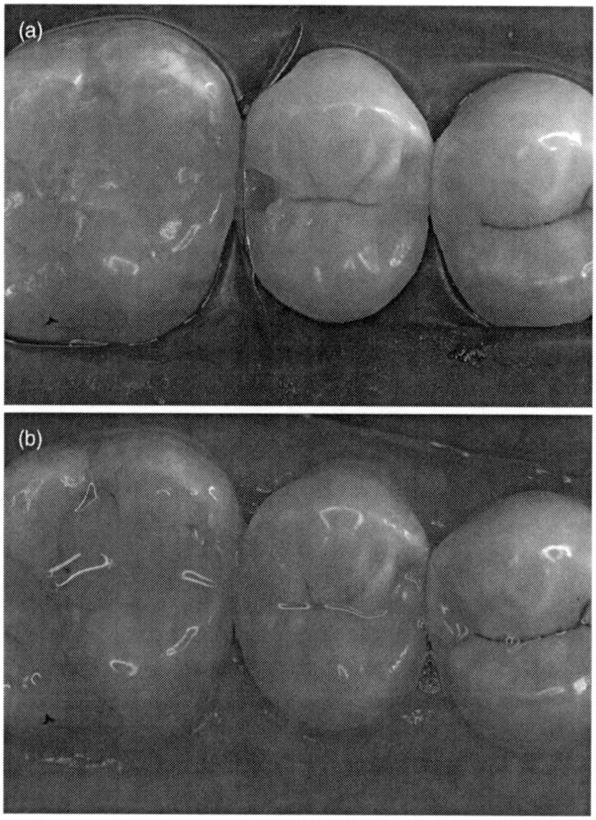

3.1 Class II caries lesion restored using MID concepts. The preparation involved removal of carious tissues without any extension. (a) Conservative preparation of a class II caries lesion using a lesion-specific approach; (b) tooth was restored with a 2-step etch-and-rinse adhesive and a resin composite. Courtesy of Dr George Gomes.

- A conservative approach, only removing the actual damaged area (lesion-specific).
- The classical philosophy of complete and invasive carious tissue removal has been challenged (Kidd, 2004).

As stated by Ericson, MID is the application of a systematic respect for the original tissue; MID goes beyond inserting small fillings to restore incipient lesions (Ericson, 2004). The development of adhesive dentistry and scientific progress in understanding the nature of caries as a systemic disease has enabled dentists to overcome the purely mechanical process of removing and replacing diseased tissue. ‘Extension for prevention’ has given way to the new paradigm of minimally invasive dentistry, as described by Tyas *et al.* (2000), and includes the following concepts:

- early caries diagnosis;
- assessment of each individual's caries risk;
- reduction of cariogenic bacteria;
- arresting active carious lesions and further remineralizing them;
- placement of restorations in teeth with cavitated lesions using lesion-specific designs;
- whenever feasible, repair rather than replace defective restorations;
- assessing disease management outcomes at pre-established intervals.

3.2 Dental adhesion

3.2.1 Basic concepts of adhesion

The word 'adhesion' comes from the latin *adhaerere* (to stick to). *Adhaerere* itself is composed of *ad* (to) and *haerere* (to stick) (Packham, 1992). An adherend is the surface to which an adhesive adheres. An adhesive is a material, generally a liquid that joins two substrates together and transfers a load from one adherend to the other. Adhesion or adhesive strength is the measure of the load-bearing capability of an adhesive joint. The American Society for Testing and Materials defines adhesion as 'the state in which two surfaces are held together by interfacial forces which may consist of valence forces or interlocking forces or both' (Packham, 1992). Theoretically, major criteria must be observed for adhesion to occur in the mouth (Eick *et al.*, 1972):

- An intimate contact must exist between the liquid adhesive and the solid adherend to allow structural interaction. This means that wetting of the solid by the liquid must occur.
- The stress concentration at the interface must be reduced.
- The interface must be protected from the oral environment.

Generally speaking, the liquid surface tension of the adhesive should be less than the critical wetting tension of the surface of the solid substrate (dentin and enamel) (Baier, 1992), promoting a contact angle as close as possible to zero. Dental enamel is composed of hydroxyapatite, a hard solid crystalline structure, with strong intermolecular forces and a high-energy surface; conversely, dentin is composed of hydroxyapatite and collagen. Dentin is intrinsically humid and less hard than enamel, with low intermolecular forces and a low-energy surface (Baier, 1992). Salivary films and composite resins also have a low-energy surface. Moreover, the instrumentation of tooth structure releases polar substances that form a low-energy smeared layer (Eick *et al.*, 1970).

Etching dentin and enamel with acids removes the surface contaminants and increases roughness by creating pits and microgrooves. These factors increase wettability and disrupt the adsorption of the organic layers. If the bonding adhesive wets the dental substrate poorly, air bubbles may form, which may result in reduced adhesion associated with local stress concentration (Eick *et al.*, 1972). Even with good wettability, local stresses depend on the polymerization shrinkage of the resins, the mechanical properties of both the adhesive and the adherend, and the coefficient of thermal expansion of the adhesive and the adherend (Eick *et al.*, 1972).

Dental adhesives are composed of monomers with either hydrophilic groups, which enhance the wettablity to the dental hard tissues, or hydrophobic groups, which allow interaction and copolymerization with the restorative material. A list of advantages and disadvantages of dental adhesives is displayed in Table 3.2.

Table 3.2 Advantages and disadvantages of dental adhesives

Dental adhesives	
Advantages	**Disadvantages**
Wide range of clinical applications Increased resistance to caries when dental tissues are impregnated with the adhesive More conservative procedures – lesion-specific preparations Reinforcement of residual tooth structure May minimize microleakage	Dentists may rely solely on adhesion, as the source of primary retention, even in clinical situations in which there is not enough residual tooth structure. Other forms of mechanical retention, such as slots, coves and retention locks, may be needed when more than half of the coronal tooth structure has been compromised. Degradation of the adhesive interface is common when margins are located in dentin/cementum, regardless of the type of adhesive material used. Dental adhesives may be the only biomaterials in health sciences that can be launched without proof of clinical efficacy. Clinical studies for some dental adhesives are published when that specific dental adhesive is not available any longer and has been replaced by a new version. Potential consequences of an inadequate adhesion are: bacterial leakage; pulpal inflammation; recurrent caries; fractured restorations; dental sensitivity; compromised esthetics; compromised function

During polymerization of methacrylate monomers in resin-based composites, shrinkage occurs and one of two phenomena can take place. (i) If the bonded interface resists the composite polymerization shrinkage, cuspal deflection may occur and enamel may fracture when stress is transferred to the bonded interface. (ii) If the composite polymerization shrinkage is higher than the adhesive bond strength, the margin will open and the resin tags will be pulled out from the tubules. The unsealed tubules will be susceptible to contamination. The gap formed may allow the penetration of bacteria and their products, fluids, molecules and ions (Asmussen, 1985).

3.3 Bonding substrates

3.3.1 Enamel as a bonding substrate

One of the major problems in operative dentistry is that dental materials do not adhere spontaneously to dental tissues. Therefore, marginal leakage may occur at the restorative interface, resulting in secondary caries, sensitivity to temperature changes, pulpal damage and marginal staining (Asmussen, 1985). After Buonocore introduced phosphoric acid etching of enamel (Buonocore, 1955), further research suggested that micromechanical entanglement of resins within enamel microporosities was the principal mechanism of bonding of resin to phosphoric acid-etched enamel. Several studies reported the formation of tag-like resin extensions into the enamel microporosities (Gwinnett and Matsui, 1967; Buonocore *et al.*, 1968). The 'acid-etch technique' has, therefore, transformed the way restorative dentistry is practiced (Swift *et al.*, 1995).

Phosphoric acid demineralizes enamel and dentin by removing calcium, creating microporosities. A classical study found that a concentration of 30% phosphoric acid created an enamel retentive surface (Silvestone, 1974). Barkmeier and co-workers measured identical enamel shear bond strengths after conditioning with 37% phosphoric acid for 15 s and compared them with those conditioned for 60 s (Barkmeier *et al.*, 1986). These *in vitro* results were corroborated by scanning election microscopy (SEM) observations of the conditioned enamel surfaces.

Phosphoric acid is now used in concentrations between 30% and 40%. The application of phosphoric acid to enamel transforms the smooth enamel into an irregular surface (Fig. 3.2(a) and (b)) and increases its surface-free energy. The enamel etching pattern is characterized by selective hydroxyapatite dissolution, creating microporosities that will be infiltrated by resins monomers through capillary attraction. Once the resin monomers polymerize, the resin becomes interlocked within the numerous porosities of the enamel surface (Fig. 3.3(a) and (b)) forming resin tags (Gwinnett and Matsui, 1967; Buonocore *et al.*, 1968; Shinchi *et al.*, 2000; Van Meerbeek

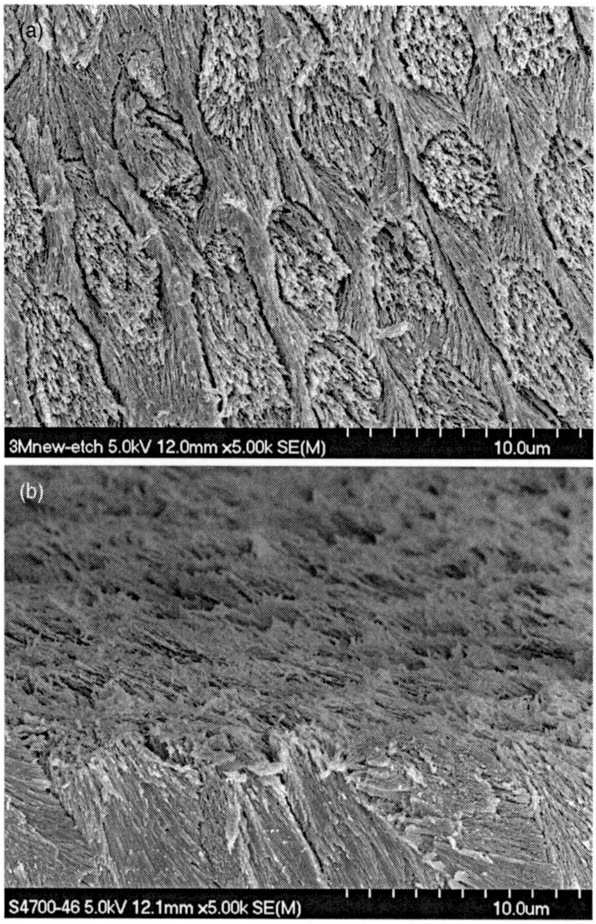

3.2 (a) Field emission scanning election microscopy (FESEM) micrograph of enamel etching pattern (occlusal view) of human enamel etched with 35% phosphoric acid (3M ESPE) for 15 seconds. Original magnification = ×5000. (b) FESEM micrograph of enamel etching pattern (lateral view) of human enamel etched with 34% phosphoric acid (Dentsply Caulk) for 15 seconds. Original magnification = ×5000.

et al., 2003a). These tags can be classified as macrotags if the resin surrounds the enamel prisms, or microtags if the resin infiltrates the very small porosities within the etched enamel prism core. Microtags are thought to be fundamental in resin-enamel retention (Van Meerbeek *et al.*, 2003a).

In vitro microtensile bond strengths of resin composite to phosphoric acid-etched enamel are usually above 40 MPa (Inoue *et al.*, 2003). Such bond strengths usually provide excellent retention. Clinically, enamel

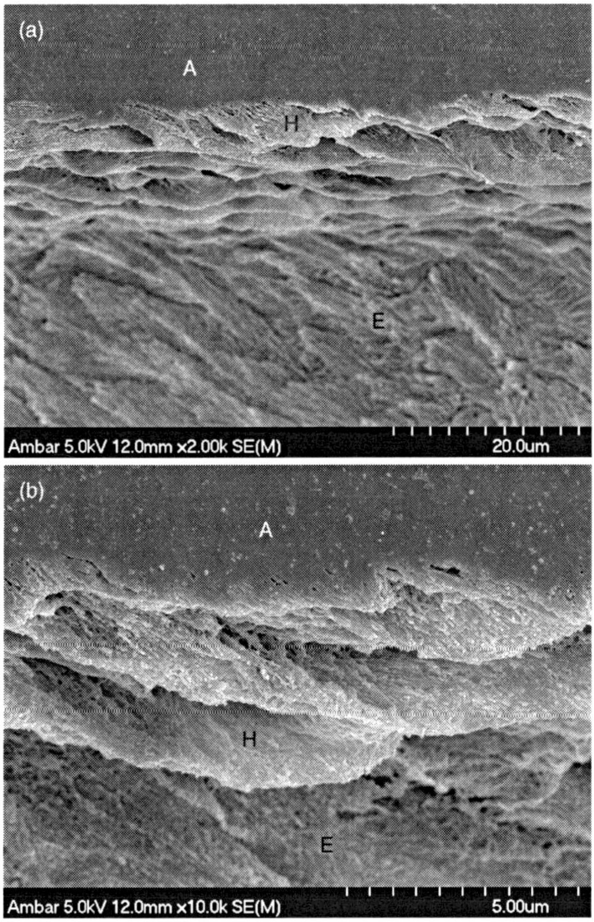

3.3 (a) FESEM micrograph of resin–enamel interface formed with Ambar two-step etch-and-rinse adhesive (FGM) after treatment with 6N HCL for 30 seconds. Original magnification = ×2000. (b) FESEM micrograph of resin–enamel interface formed with Ambar (FGM) after treatment with 6N HCL for 30 seconds. Original magnification = ×10 000. A = adhesive; E = enamel; H = enamel hybrid layer formed by enamel crystallites that were enveloped by the adhesive, therefore resisting dissolution in HCl.

etching also reduces leakage and improves marginal integrity around restorations with margins in enamel (Loguercio *et al.*, 2007; Perdigão *et al.*, 2009).

Resin-based restorations applied to etched enamel provide reinforcement of the residual tooth structure. When a cavity preparation is cut, the potential for cuspal fracture increases because the overall structure becomes

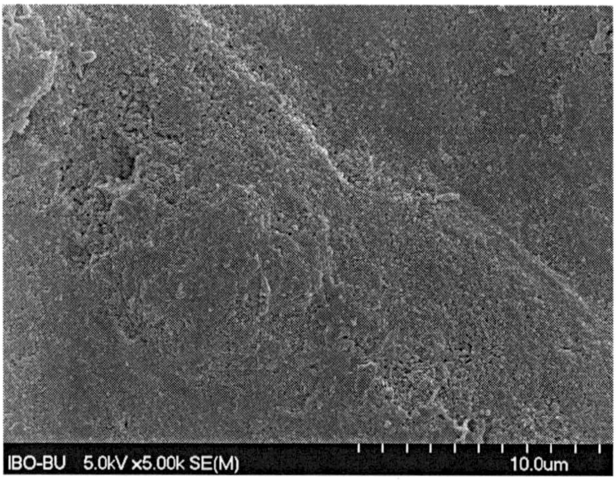

3.4 FESEM micrograph of enamel etching pattern (occlusal view) of beveled human enamel treated with the self-etch adhesive iBond one-step self-etch adhesive (Heraeus Kulzer), followed by resin dissolution in acetone for 2 h. Original magnification = ×5000.

weaker. Classic restorative materials, such as amalgam, do not bond to tooth structure, so they provide no reinforcement of the weakened tooth structure. Conversely, bonded resin composite restorations reinforce the remaining cusps (Morin *et al.*, 1984; McCullock and Smith, 1986).

Recently, acidic non-rinsing primers, which are solutions containing an organic solvent, water and acidic resin monomers, have been used in lieu of phosphoric acid to treat enamel. The enamel bond strengths of these self-etch adhesives are lower than the enamel bond strengths associated with their etch-and-rinse counterparts (those that rely on a separate etching step) (Pashley and Tay, 2001). Because of their higher pH, self-etch adhesives result in a shallow featureless enamel demineralization compared to that of phosphoric acid (Fig. 3.4) (Pashley and Tay, 2001; Perdigão and Geraldeli, 2003; Grégoire and Ahmed, 2007). However, roughening enamel to remove prismless enamel improves the enamel bonding ability of self-etch adhesives (Kanemura *et al.*, 1999). A separate phosphoric acid enamel-etching step also enhances the efficacy of self-etch adhesives (Van Meerbeek *et al.*, 2003b). As their etching pattern approaches that obtained with phosphoric acid (Grégoire and Ahmed, 2007), aggressive self-etch adhesives (Fig. 3.5) may be used for pit-and-fissure sealants in pediatric patients to shorten treatment time and reduce the procedure complexity (Feigal and Quelhas, 2003; Perdigão *et al.*, 2005a).

In spite of containing a mildly acidic primer, and, therefore, not being able to etch enamel to the same depth as phosphoric acid (Perdigão and

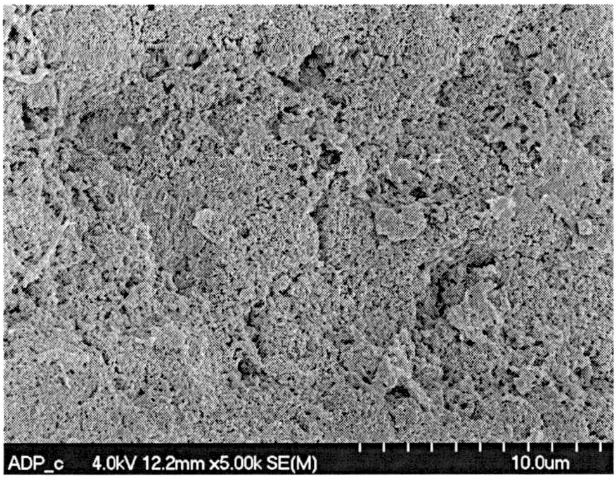

3.5 FESEM micrograph of enamel etching pattern (occlusal view) of beveled human enamel treated with the self-etch adhesive Adper Prompt L-Pop one-step self-etch adhesive (3M ESPE), followed by resin dissolution in acetone for 2 hours. Original magnification = ×5000.

Geraldeli, 2003), Clearfil SE Bond (Kuraray) has demonstrated very good clinical behavior in non-carious cervical lesions (Peumans *et al.*, 2010). However, enamel marginal staining is still a problem when enamel is not etched with phosphoric acid (Peumans *et al.*, 2010). In spite of marginal deficiencies in enamel, this adhesive resulted in a 97% retention rate after eight years with or without separate enamel etching (Peumans *et al.*, 2010). Another study reported a better retention rate for Clearfil SE Bond than for PQ1 (Ultradent) (a two-step etch-and-rinse adhesive) on a yearly basis up to 8 years (van Dijken, 2010). These findings challenge the need for a separate enamel acid-etching step. Clinical studies, nevertheless, have suggested that microleakage occurs around enamel margins after 1 year when phosphoric acid is not used. Therefore, enamel etching is still the recommended clinical protocol (Opdam *et al.*, 1998; Perdigão *et al.*, 2009).

3.3.2 Dentin as a bonding substrate

Dentin tubules run continuously from the dentin–enamel junction (DEJ) to the pulp in coronal dentin, and from the cementum–dentin junction (CEJ) to the pulp canal in the root. Pashley (1996) described dentin as a porous biological composite made up of apatite crystal filler particles in a collagen matrix.

During the development of the human tooth, dentin that is secreted until the completion of root formation is identified as primary dentin, which consists of the circumpulpal dentin matrix. Physiological secondary dentin is secreted after completion of root formation. While secondary dentin may be less tubular, it has the same morphological features as primary dentin.

Sclerotic dentin in non-carious cervical lesions (NCCL)

Sclerotic dentin is common in areas where dentin is exposed to the oral environment, such as in NCCL (Fig. 3.6(a)), being a complex substrate attributed to different ultrastructural layers (Tay and Pashley, 2004). The matrix of the 10–20 μm thick surface hypermineralized layer in sclerotic dentin of NCCL is composed of denatured collagen with bacteria (Tay and Pashley, 2004). Large hydroxyapatite crystallites are observed in the hypermineralized surface layer. Crystalline deposits obliterate the tubules and etch more slowly than the other dentin components (Fig. 3.6(b) and (c)). The fact that intertubular sclerotic dentin from NCCL etches differently from normal root dentin may explain the difficulties in restoring such lesions using current bonding procedures (Marshall *et al.*, 2000). Acid conditioning with 50% phosphoric acid for 60 seconds opens up some tubules occluded by intratubular deposits in NCCL dentin. The penetration of resin monomers is, however, limited by the presence of these deposits following acid conditioning (Gwinnett and Jendresen, 1978).

Bonding to sclerotic dentin in NCCL has resulted in compromised bonding (Yoshiyama *et al.*, 1996; Kwong *et al.*, 2002). Regardless of the dentin treatment, bond strengths to unaffected dentin were consistently higher than those made to sclerotic dentin (Kwong *et al.*, 2002). Because of their challenging nature, NCCL are recommended as the bonding substrate for dental adhesion clinical studies (ADA, 2001).

In spite of the lower bond strengths obtained when the substrate is sclerotic dentin from NCCL, other clinical studies have not totally corroborated the *in vitro* findings. van Dijken (2004, 2005) found that the differences in retention rates between the sclerotic and non-sclerotic dentin are not significant for some adhesive materials.

Caries-affected dentin

Carious dentin consists of a superficial first layer of highly decalcified and physiologically unrecalcifiable dentin and a deeper second layer which is intermediately decalcified, physiologically recalcifiable, with sound collagen fibers and apatite crystals bound to the fibers (Fusayama and Terachima, 1972; Ohgushi and Fusayama, 1975; Kuboki *et al.*, 1977).

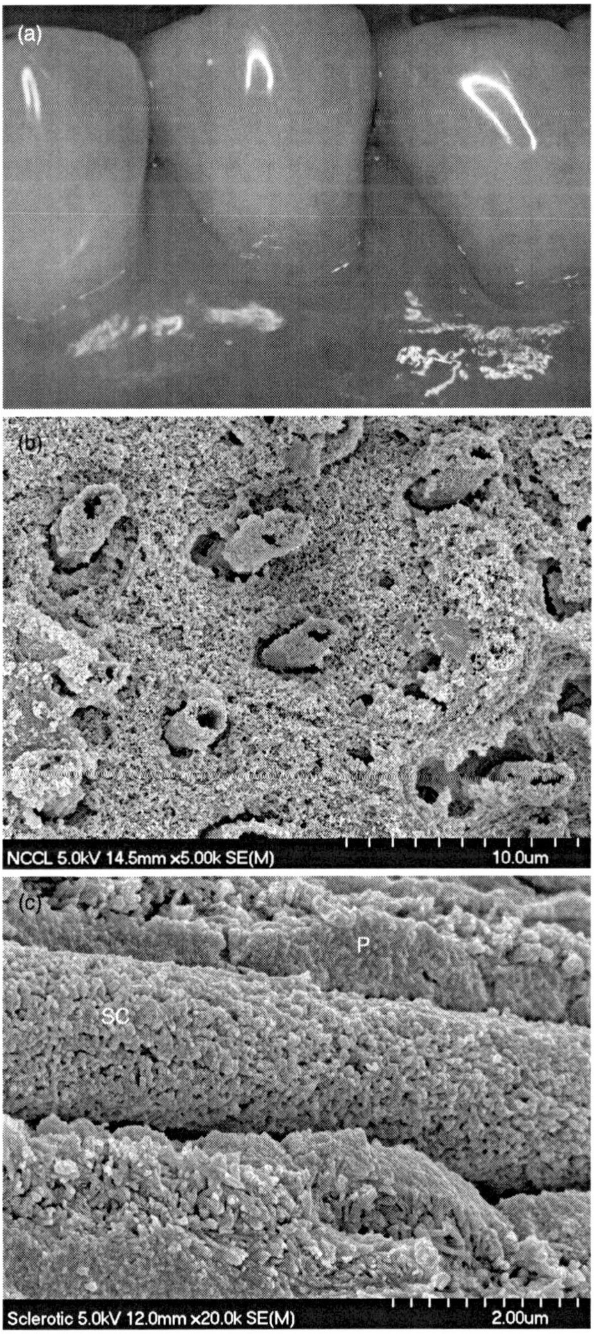

3.6 (a) Clinical aspect of a NCCL. Dark dentin is associated with higher sclerosis scale. (b) FESEM micrograph of etched NCCL with sclerotic cast partially obliterating the dentinal tubules. Original magnification = ×5000. (c) FESEM micrograph of sclerotic cast obliterating the dentinal tubule underneath an area of sclerotic dentin in an NCCL (20 μm below the surface). Original magnification = ×20 000. SC = sclerotic cast; P = peritubular dentin.

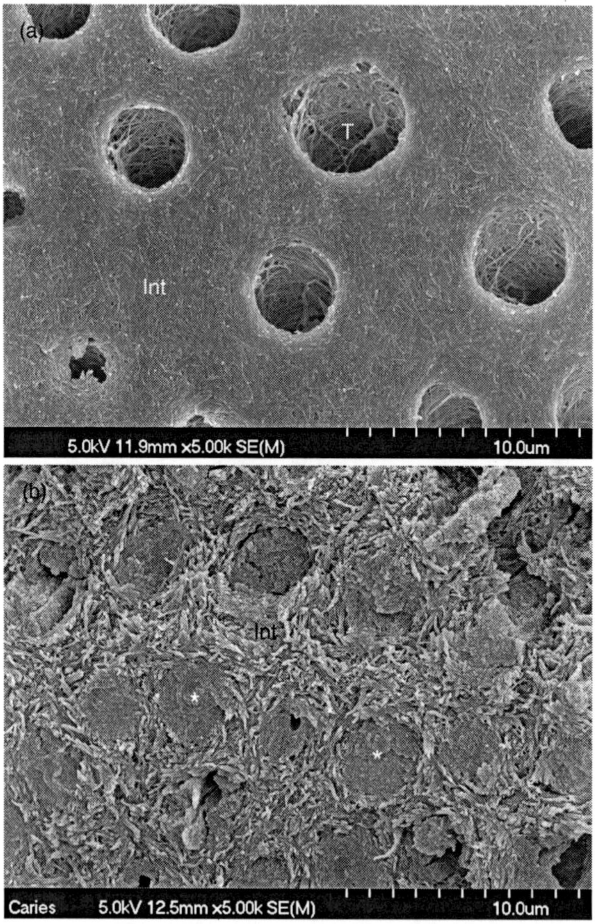

3.7 (a) FESEM micrograph: Occlusal view of unaffected dentin. Original magnification = ×5000. (b) FESEM micrograph: Occlusal view of dentin underneath a caries lesion showing tubules obliterated by mineral deposits (asterisks). Original magnification = ×5000. Int = intertubular dentin; P = peritubular dentin.

The pulp responds to the carious process either by completely blocking the lumen of the dentinal tubule (compare Fig. 3.7(a) with Fig. 3.7(b)), or by decreasing the tubule diameter through deposition of mineral, to assist in the prevention of further permeation of bacteria and toxic materials toward the pulp. Stanley *et al.* in 1983 found that the pulpo–dentinal complex responds to external injuries with dentin sclerosis, dead tracts or reparative dentin.

As a result of the deposition of mineral in the lumina of the tubules, resin infiltration into dentinal tubules of caries-affected dentin is also

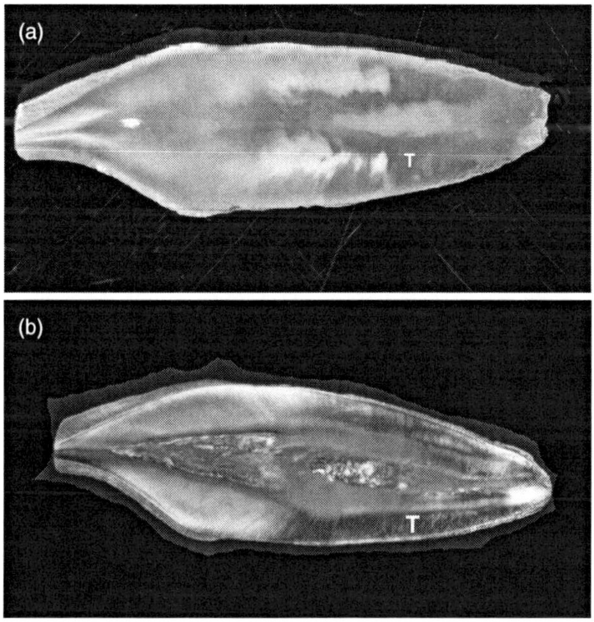

3.8 (a) Longitudinal section of extracted lower human incisor showing transparent dentin (T) in the radicular part of the tooth. (b) Polarized photograph of lower incisor showing the changes in light refraction caused by hypermineralization of transparent dentin.

hampered by the presence of mineral (Say *et al.*, 2005). The interface with caries-affected dentin is poorly mineralized and readily permeated by the acid etchant (Say *et al.*, 2005). The degree of conversion of the adhesive that penetrated the demineralized dentin in the caries-affected dentin specimens is lower than in the normal dentin specimens (Say *et al.*, 2005). Bond strengths to caries-affected dentin are typically lower than those obtained in normal unaffected dentin, regardless of the type of adhesive used (Yoshiyama *et al.*, 2002; Ceballos *et al.*, 2003; Say *et al.*, 2005; Wei *et al.*, 2008).

Substrate changes with aging

Secondary dentin is deposited over the entire inner circumpulpal surface throughout the life of the individual. Physiological transparent dentin forms as a natural part of ageing, without trauma or caries lesions being associated with it. The tubule lumina become filled with mineral from chemical precipitation (Vasiliadis *et al.*, 1983; Kinney *et al.*, 2005) decreasing the amount of light scatter and therefore being called transparent dentin (Fig. 3.8(a) (b)). As tubules become filled with mineral, the fracture toughness of dentin decreases (Kinney *et al.*, 2005). The fatigue strength of young dentin (17–30 years) is greater than that of older dentin (50–80 years) (Arola and Reprogel, 2005).

As a result of the reduction in tubule diameter there is also a decrease in dentin permeability. Teeth of subjects over 50 years old are more brittle and contain less water than teeth of subjects 10–20 years of age. With increasing age, dentinal thickness increases, while the density of odontoblasts and pulp fibroblasts decreases (Murray *et al.*, 2002).

Adhesion studies have not shown a direct correlation between dentin age and dentin bonding (Mixson *et al.*, 1993; Burrow *et al.*, 1994; Brackett *et al.*, 2008). A more recent study used Single Bond (3M ESPE) in dentin from 18 to 22-year old or 55 to 60-year-old patients (Lopes *et al.*, 2011). Bonding to older dentin after 30 seconds of etching time resulted in higher bond strength than when dentin was etched for 15 seconds. However, no statistical differences were found between young and older dentin for the same etching time (Lopes *et al.*, 2011).

Perdigão *et al.* (2012) used teeth from three age groups, less than 21 years old, between 21 and 40 and over 40. The substrate age was not a determinant factor when microtensile bond strengths were measured, except for a classical three-step etch-and-rinse adhesive Adper Scotchbond Multi-Purpose (3M ESPE), which resulted in higher bond strengths in the age group over 40 years old.

Tooth region and remaining dentin thickness (RDT)

The water content of dentin near the DEJ is about 1% by volume (area occupied by the tubule lumina), while that of dentin near the pulp is about 22% (Garberoglio and Brännström, 1976; Pashley, 1996). This difference in intrinsic moisture may result in differences in bond strengths between superficial and deep dentin. Superficial dentin normally results in higher composite–dentin bond strengths than deep dentin (Nakamichi *et al.*, 1983; Causton, 1984; Stanford *et al.*, 1985; Mitchem and Gronas, 1986; Suzuki and Finger, 1988). These differences tend to diminish when the smear layer is left intact, but lower bond strengths occur in deep dentin when the smear layer is removed (Tao and Pashley, 1988). As bonding systems become more hydrophilic, the sensitivity of bond strengths to dentin depth decreases (Prati and Pashley, 1992).

3.4 Current bonding strategies

The ultimate goal of a bonded restoration is to attain an intimate adaptation of the restorative material to the dental substrate. This task is difficult to

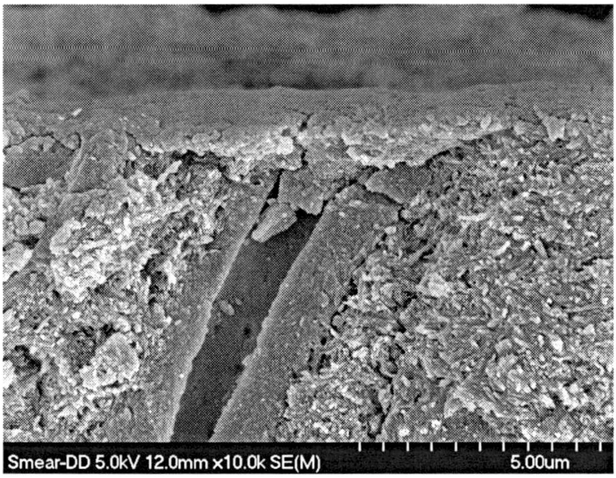

3.9 FESEM micrograph of human dentin (lateral view) showing the smear layer covering the occlusal aspect, and a smear plug obliterating the dentinal tubule. This smear layer was created with a carbide bur with water refrigeration. Original magnification = ×10 000.

achieve as the bonding process is different for enamel and for dentin; dentin is more humid and more organic than enamel (Pashley, 1992). While enamel is composed of 96 weight% hydroxyapatite (mineral), dentin contains a significant amount of water and organic material, mainly type I collagen (Asmussen and Uno, 1992). The humid and organic nature of dentin makes this hard tissue extremely difficult to bond to.

When tooth structure is prepared with a cutting instrument, the residual components form a 'smear layer' of debris on the surface (Bowen *et al.*, 1984) (Fig. 3.9). The basic composition of the smear layer is hydroxyapatite and altered collagen with an external surface formed by gel-like denatured collagen (Eick *et al.*, 1991). The morphology of the smear layer is determined by the type of instrument that creates it and by the site of dentin where it is formed (Gwinnett, 1984; Suzuki and Finger, 1988). These deposits form a uniform coating on enamel and dentin that plugs the entrance of the dentinal tubules reducing the permeability of dentin. The smear layer is porous and permeable as a result of submicrometer channels (Pashley, 1992).

As the smear layer constitutes a true physical barrier, it must be dissolved or made permeable so the monomers in dental adhesives are able to contact the dentin surface directly to provide adhesion. The current adhesion strategies depend exclusively on how dental adhesives interact with this smear layer:

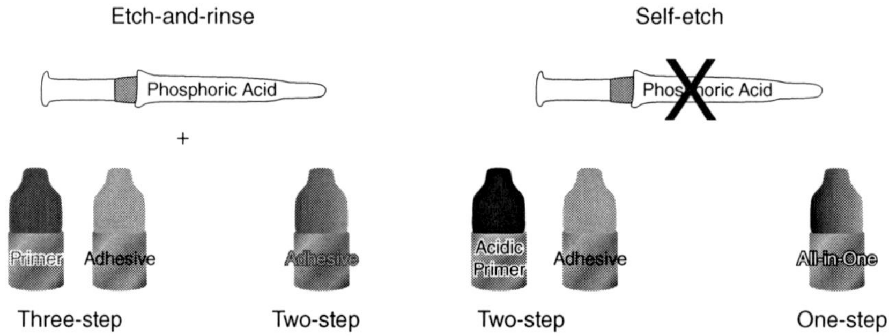

3.10 Current dental adhesion strategies are based on how the adhesives interact with the smear layer and secondly on the number of application steps.

Table 3.3 Advantages and disadvantages of etch-and-rinse adhesives

Advantages	Disadvantages
Universal use – ability to bond to composite, porcelain, fiber posts, etched or sandblasted metals.	Some acetone-based adhesives need more applications than those recommended by the manufacturer (Platt *et al.*, 2001).
Enamel and dentin are etched simultaneously for 15 seconds.	Over-etching decreases dentin bond strengths (Hashimoto *et al.*, 2002).
High dentin and enamel bond strengths in laboratory studies.	Most etch-and-rinse adhesives require moist dentin *in vitro* – bond strengths vary with the degree of moisture.
Clinical studies over 4 years have shown good results (Peumans *et al.*, 2005).	Hydrolytic degradation of the bonds when margins are in dentin (De Munck *et al.*, 2003).
As these adhesives contain organic solvents such as ethanol or acetone, minor contamination with oil and saliva does not decrease *in vitro* bond strengths.	
Still the standard for other dental adhesives (Peumans *et al.*, 2005).	

1. Etch-and-rinse (or total-etch) adhesives remove the smear layer and superficial hydroxyapatite through etching with a separate acid gel.
2. Self-etch adhesives make the smear layer permeable without removing it completely.

Figure 3.10 summarizes the current bonding strategies. The advantages and disadvantages of each strategy are summarized in Table 3.3 and Table 3.4.

Table 3.4 Advantages and disadvantages of self-etch adhesives

Advantages	Disadvantages
Extremely easy to apply, no etch, no rinsing.	Acidity pH = 1.0–2.5, therefore they do not etch enamel to the same depth as H_3PO_4 (Tay and Pashley, 2001; Grégoire and Ahmed, 2007).
Most are available in unidose to help the dental professional comply with infection control guidelines.	Self-etch adhesives may result in clinical signs of enamel leakage at 1 year (Perdigão *et al.*, 2009).
Some two-bottle self-etch adhesives (for example, Clearfil SE Bond, Kuraray) result in high dentin bond strengths *in vitro* and good clinical results. In fact, Clearfil SE Bond is still the reference against which all other self-etch adhesives are compared (Perdigão *et al.*, 2005b; Peumans *et al.*, 2010).	Long-term thermal cycling decreases already low enamel bond strengths (Miyazaki *et al.*, 2000; De Munck *et al.*, 2005a).
May cause lower incidence of post-operative sensitivity (clinical research reports have not been conclusive).	The acidity of 'all-in-one' (or 1-step) self-etch adhesives inhibits polymerization of chemically cured composites; this is especially important when dentists use chemically cured composite buildup materials and chemically cured luting cements with all-in-one adhesives (Swift *et al.*, 2001; Sanares *et al.*, 2001; Tay *et al.*, 2003a, 2003b).
	Self-etch adhesives result in the degradation of the resin–dentin interface by hydrolysis (Tay and Pashley, 2003).
	All-in-one self-etch adhesives behave as permeable membranes after polymerization, allowing permeation of fluids through the adhesive layer to the surface (Tay *et al.*, 2002a; Tay *et al.*, 2002b).
	On enamel, all-in-one self-etch adhesives result in the formation of water blisters on the surface of the adhesive, which may compromise the durability of enamel bonding (Tay *et al.*, 2004a).
	All-in-one self-etch adhesives undergo phase separation very rapidly (Van Landuyt *et al.*, 2005).
	Water in their composition may become entrapped, if not properly evaporated, which results in dentin leakage (Spreafico *et al.*, 2006; Furuse *et al.*, 2008).

3.4.1 Etch-and-rinse strategy

Dentin and enamel are treated with phosphoric acid (other acids have been used in the past, however phosphoric acid is now the most prevalent) to remove the smear layer and demineralize the most superficial dentin removing hydroxyapatite crystals (Fig. 3.11(a)(b)).

Following this chemical etching, a mixture of resin monomers (primer/adhesive) dissolved in an organic solvent is applied to infiltrate etched dentin (Perdigão, 2002). The resin monomers permeate the water-filled spaces between adjacent dentin collagen fibers and replace hydroxyapatite crystals that used to occupy those spaces. This infiltration results in a hybrid tissue composed of collagen, resin, residual hydroxyapatite and traces of water known as the resin–dentin interdiffusion zone, or hybrid layer (Fig. 3.12) (Nakabayashi *et al.*, 1982; Van Meerbeek *et al.*, 1992).

In 1952 it was reported that a resin containing glycerol phosphate dimethacrylate or GPDM stained the 'altered' dentin immediately below the filling material. This was the first historical report of changes in dentin promoted by an acidic monomer and may be considered to be the precursor of the hybrid layer concept (McLean and Kramer, 1952; Kramer, 1952). This intimate micromechanical entanglement of resin monomers with etched dentin may result in decreased post-operative sensitivity, better marginal fit, and may even act as an elastic buffer that compensates for the polymerization shrinkage stress during contraction of the restorative composite (Brännström and Nordenvall, 1977; Davidson *et al.*, 1984; Perdigão *et al.*, 1996).

Three-step etch-and-rinse adhesives have resulted in better laboratory and clinical performance than two-step etch-and-rinse adhesives (Armstrong *et al.*, 2003; Peumans *et al.*, 2005). The simplification from three- to two-step etch-and-rinse adhesives has resulted in some drawbacks, as some two-step etch-and-rinse adhesives may need more than one application to achieve micromechanical interlocking of monomers into the collagen-rich etched dentin (Platt *et al.*, 2001). Additionally, the lack of a hydrophobic resin coating in two-step etch-and-rinse adhesives may result in degradation of the bonded interface by hydrolysis from fluid transudation through the hybrid layer, which may be visualized as water trees (Fig. 3.13) (Tay *et al.*, 2004b).

3.4.2 Self-etch strategy

This strategy is based on simplification and reduced application time. These self-etch (non-rinsing) adhesives do not require a separate acid-etch step, as they condition and prime enamel and dentin simultaneously by infiltrating and partially dissolving the smear layer and hydroxyapatite, forming a hybrid zone with minerals mixed with residual smear layer and resin (Van

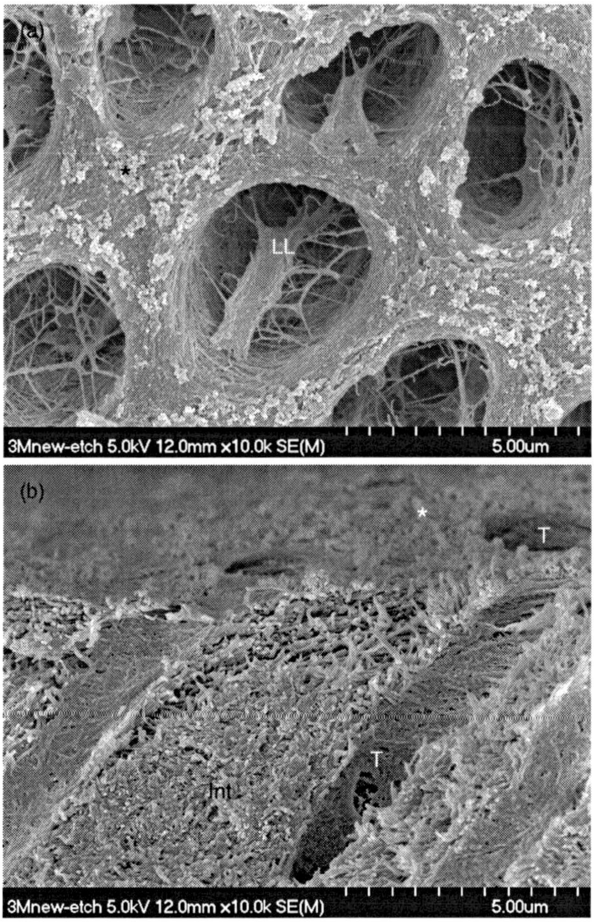

3.11 (a) FESEM micrograph: Occlusal view of dentin etched with 34% phosphoric acid (Scotchbond Universal Etchant, 3M ESPE) for 15 seconds. Most phosphoric acid gels are thickened with silica that is not removed even with vigorous water rinsing (asterisks). Original magnification = ×10 000. (b) FESEM micrograph: Lateral view of dentin etched with 34% phosphoric acid (Scotchbond Universal Etchant, 3M ESPE) for 15 seconds. The acidic gel demineralized 2.0–2.5 μm of the surface intertubular dentin, leaving only collagen fibers. The adhesive will infiltrate these spaces, formed by contiguous collagen fibers, to form a hybrid layer. Original magnification = ×10 000. P = peritubular dentin; T = tubule; LL = *lamina limitans.*

Meerbeek *et al.*, 2003a). The elimination of separate etching and rinsing steps simplified the bonding technique and has been responsible for the increased popularity of these systems in a daily practice (Van Meerbeek *et al.*, 1998).

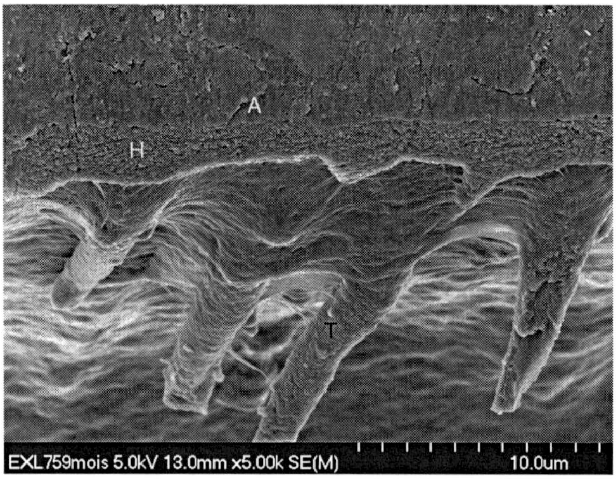

3.12 FESEM micrograph of resin–dentin interface after laboratory demineralization in 6N HCl followed by deproteinization in 2.5% NaOCl for 2.5 minutes. This interface was formed with Scotchbond Universal Adhesive (3M ESPE) applied as an etch-and-rinse adhesive, using the moist dentin technique. Original magnification = ×5000. A = adhesive; H = hybrid layer; T = resin tag.

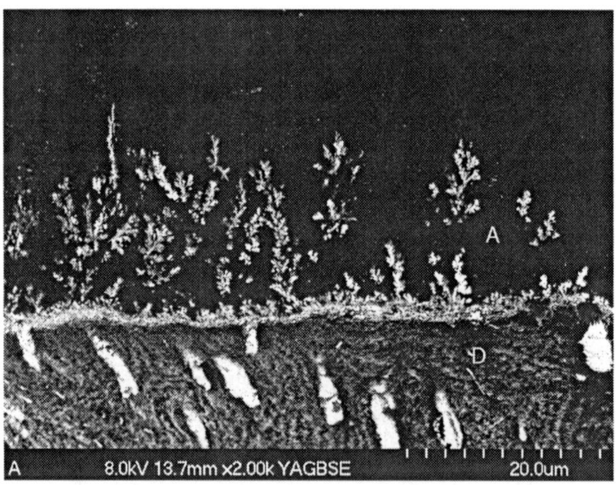

3.13 FESEM micrograph (with backscattered detector) of resin–dentin interface after an ammoniacal silver nitrate challenge, showing water trees inside the adhesive layer. This interface was formed with an Adper Easy Bond one-step self-etch adhesive (3M ESPE). Original magnification = ×2000. A = adhesive; D = dentin.

The first self-etch adhesives were composed of two solutions, a non-rinsing acidic primer and a bonding resin, and are currently known as two-step self-etch adhesives. More recently, the trend has shifted to one-step self-etch systems (also known as all-in-one adhesives) in which manufacturers have attempted to incorporate all the original components of an adhesive system (etchant, primer and bonding resin) into a single solution. All-in-one adhesives are user-friendly in that the number of steps required for the bonding protocol is reduced, although it has been shown that some all-in-one adhesives require multiple applications (Ito *et al.*, 2005). Both the acidic primers for two-step self-etch adhesives and the one-step self-etch adhesive solution are composed of aqueous mixtures of acidic functional monomers, generally phosphoric acid- or carboxylic acid-esters, with a pH higher than that of phosphoric acid gels (Pashley and Tay, 2001). Water is an essential component of self-etch adhesives as it participates in the ionization of the acidic moieties.

Because self-etch adhesives are not as aggressive as the phosphoric acid gel in etch-and-rinse adhesives, most self-etch adhesives do not remove the smear layer completely. The aggressiveness of self-etch adhesives (i.e. their ability to demineralize dentin and enamel) depends on their pH – mild, moderate or aggressive (Pashley and Tay, 2001; Tay and Pashley, 2001). Nevertheless, their pH is always greater than that of the phosphoric acid gel used in dentistry. Currently most self-etch adhesives available on the market are considered to be mild or moderate (pH >1.5) (Carvalho *et al.*, 2005; Van Landuyt *et al.*, 2005; Perdigão *et al.*, 2006; Nishitani *et al.*, 2006; Van Meerbeek *et al.*, 2011).

Self-etch adhesives have the potential to form a hybrid layer and seal dentin (Tay and Pashley, 2001). In contrast to etch-and-rinse adhesives, the hybrid layer formed by self-etch adhesives is not completely deprived of hydroxyapatite (Tay and Pashley, 2001). While mild self-etch (pH ~ 2) adhesives form a very thin submicrometer hybrid layer with less pronounced resin tag formation, strong self-etch adhesives (pH ~ 1) hybridize dentin resembling the hybridization formed by etch-and-rinse adhesives (Fig. 3.14) with the formation of abundant resin tags (Perdigão, 2002).

3.4.3 Moist versus dried dentin

Vital dentin is inherently wet, which means that it is quite difficult to dry dentin completely in a clinical situation. Consequently, manufacturers have developed dentin adhesives that are compatible with humid environments. Many adhesives combine hydrophilic and hydrophobic monomers in the same bottle. The 'moist bonding' technique (Kanca, 1992a) prevents the spatial alterations, that is collagen collapse, that occurs upon drying demineralized dentin. Such alterations might prevent the monomers from

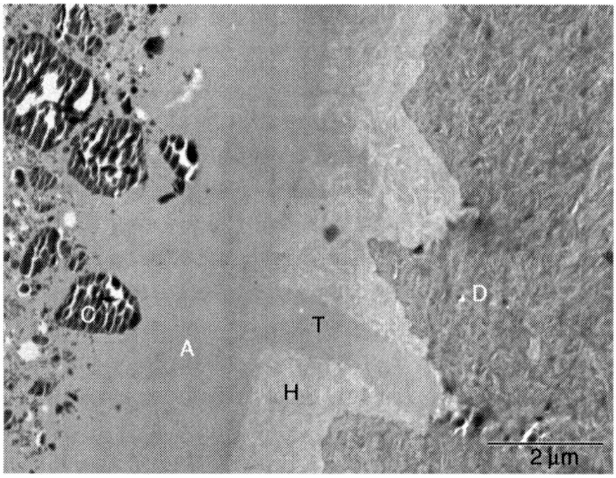

3.14 TEM micrograph of resin–dentin interface after laboratory decalcification in EDTA to facilitate ultramicrotomy. This interface was formed using Adper Prompt-L-Pop (3M ESPE). A = adhesive; C = composite resin; D = dentin; H = hybrid layer; T = resin tag.

penetrating the labyrinth of nanochannels formed by dissolution of hydroxyapatite crystals between collagen fibers. The use of adhesive systems on moist dentin is made possible by incorporation of the organic solvents acetone or ethanol into the primers or adhesives. Because the solvent can displace water from both the dentin surface and the moist collagen network, it promotes the infiltration of resin monomers throughout the nanospaces of the dense collagen web. The 'moist bonding' technique has been shown repeatedly to enhance bond strengths, as water preserves the porosity of collagen network that is available for monomer interdiffusion (Kanca, 1992a; Perdigão, 2002).

If the dentin surface is dried with air, the collagen collapses and prevents resin monomers from penetrating (Carvalho *et al.*, 1996). Many clinicians still dry the tooth preparation after rinsing away the etching gel to check for the etched enamel aspect. Because it is clinically impossible to dry enamel without simultaneously drying dentin, the collagen fibers collapse easily on air drying, closing the spaces between contiguous fibers (Tay *et al.*, 1996, 1997). These alterations in the collagen fiber network result in decreased *in vitro* bond strengths, especially for acetone-based dentin adhesive systems (Kanca, 1992b; Tay *et al.*, 1996).

The mechanism of collagen collapse with air-drying relies on changes in the molecular arrangement. When the dentin is air dried, the collagen molecules are arranged more compactly, as the interfibrillar spaces are not filled with water. Rewetting the dried dentin restores bond strengths and raises the collapsed collagen network to a level similar to a 'moist bonding' technique (Van der Graaf and ten Bosch 1993; Gwinnett, 1994; Maciel *et al.*, 1996; Perdigão *et al.*, 1999).

Despite numerous articles focused on the low *in vitro* bond strengths associated with air-dried dentin, it is difficult clinically to standardize the amount of moisture that should be left on the dentin surface before application of the adhesive system. Ideally, the dentin surface should have a shiny aspect. A study showed that excess water after rinsing the etching gel can be removed with a damp cotton pellet, disposable brush, or tissue paper without adversely affecting bond strengths (De Goes *et al.*, 1997). More recently, it has been shown that dentin moisture may not be crucial for the retention of etch-and-rinse adhesives as long as the adhesives are rubbed vigorously onto the dentin surface (Zander-Grande *et al.*, 2011).

All research focused on adhesion to moist dentin compared with dried dentin has been carried out in extracted teeth. Most *in vitro* bond strength studies use intact dentin from extracted sound molars or bovine teeth. Clinically, dentists rarely place adhesive restorations on sound dentin, but rather on caries-affected dentin, hypermineralized dentin in NCCL, or areas of dentin that had been underneath a base/liner. A clinical study in NCCL demonstrated that the 18-month retention rate was similar for dried and moist dentin using both an acetone- and an ethanol-based adhesive (Perdigão *et al.*, 2005b).

Recently, *in vitro* research has tested the replacement of water with ethanol in etched dentin, a technique known as 'ethanol wet-bonding' (Pashley *et al.*, 2007; Tay *et al.*, 2007; Hosaka *et al.*, 2009). When acid-etched dentin is saturated with 100% ethanol instead of water, the bond strengths of both hydrophilic and hydrophobic resins increase significantly. Although ethanol wet-bonding appears promising, it involves an extra step of replacing rinsing water with 100% ethanol. The time needed to replace water with ethanol in etched dentin would make the technique difficult to implement in a clinical environment.

3.4.4 Pretreatment of the substrate

One study suggested that the benefits of chlorhexidine in the treatment of periodontitis were a result of the inhibition of matrix metalloproteinases (MMPs) activity by chlorhexidine (Gendron *et al.*, 1999). MMPs are endopeptidases capable of degrading the extracellular matrix components (Martin-De Las Heras *et al.*, 2000; Sulkala *et al.*, 2002; Mazzoni *et al.*, 2006). Before being tested as a potential inhibitor of MMPs in dentin adhesion, chlorhexidine was first used as a dentin disinfectant prior to the application of dental adhesives. Under SEM, chlorhexidine residues were attached to the etched dentin surface after rinsing, but chlorhexidine did not influence dentin shear bond strengths (Perdigão *et al.*, 1994).

Chlorhexidine has been recently studied as a protease inhibitor to preserve the hybrid layer through the inhibition of MMPs (Pashley *et al.*, 2004). Dentinal collagen fibrils may undergo degradation by MMPs if they are not fully enveloped by resin (Mazzoni *et al.*, 2006). Human dentin contains gelatinases (MMP-2 and -9), collagenase (MMP-8) and enamelysin MMP-20 (Martin-De Las Heras *et al.*, 2000; Sulkala *et al.*, 2002; Mazzoni *et al.*, 2006). These enzymes are trapped within the mineralized dentin matrix during the development of the tooth (Martin-De Las Heras *et al.*, 2000; Sulkala *et al.*, 2002).

The use of chlorhexidine results in the preservation of dentin bond strengths and the integrity of the hybrid layer with time (Hebling *et al.*, 2005; Carrilho *et al.*, 2007; Ricci *et al.*, 2010). When phosphoric acid with 2% digluconate chlorhexidine was used, no significant reduction in bond strengths was observed for Adper Single Bond Plus (3M ESPE) and Prime&Bond NT (Dentsply) at six months. On the other hand, when chlorhexidine was not included in the etchant, a significant reduction in bond strengths is observed for both adhesives at six months and two years (Stanislawczuk *et al.*, 2009, 2011). Nanoleakage is more pronounced when the phosphoric acid gel is used without chlorhexidine.

The use of chlorhexidine as an MMP inhibitor results in an intact hybrid layer after 12 months of *in vivo* aging. However, preservation of the hybrid layer may occur in the absence of MMP inhibitors (Sadek *et al.*, 2010). Additionally, the use of chlorhexidine does not eliminate water from the bonding interface and does not prevent hydrolysis from the layer of adhesive on the top of the water-rich surface of the hybrid layer (Brackett *et al.*, 2011).

3.5 Dental adhesion mechanisms

3.5.1 Mechanical interlocking

Mechanical interlocking is a primary mechanism of resin adhesion to dental tissues, which is believed to be a prerequisite for durable adhesion, especially for etch-and-rinse adhesives (Van Meerbeek *et al.*, 2003a). Adhesive monomers diffuse into etched dentin, permeate into the collagen mesh and displace water. A mixed tissue of collagen and resin is then formed upon polymerization of the monomers – the interdiffusion zone or hybrid layer (Nakabayashi *et al.*, 1982; Van Meerbeek *et al.*, 1992).

Dentinal tubules and concomitant intertubular resin infiltration or hybridization represent an important contribution to the resin bond (Gwinnett, 1993) as lower bond strengths were reported when the bonding agent does not form a hybrid layer (Gwinnett and Kanca, 1992). Also gap-free areas, *in vivo*, are coincident with a hybrid layer with tags of different lengths. Debonding areas are associated with incomplete resin infiltration and no hybrid layer formation (Walshaw and McComb, 1994).

The role of resin tags in bonding is debatable, as tags have to be firmly bonded to tubules wall to provide retention. An SEM study with Scotchbond 2 (3M Company) showed resin tags withdrawal from the demineralized dentin tubules, sometimes in dense clusters, in areas where the resin bonding layer failed to adhere to the primed dentin surface (Walshaw and McComb, 1994). This represents the inability of resin tags to maintain adhesion to dentin on their own. The morphology, length and adaptation of resin tags are indicative of the wetting ability of the respective hydrophilic primers (Tay *et al.*, 1995). Even conventional hydrophobic enamel adhesive agents can form long resin tags in etched dentin, but resin does not wet or bond to tubule walls (Brännström and Nordenvall, 1977). Theoretically, when dentin is acid-etched, the bond strengths obtained are the sum of the strengths of the resin tags, hybrid layer and surface adhesion all together (Pashley *et al.*, 1995).

For the self-etch approach, the smear layer is preserved and infiltrated by hydrophilic monomers with affinity for the organic and inorganic components of the underlying dentin (Van Meerbeek *et al.*, 1992; Tay and Pashley, 2001). The degree of interaction with the smear layer and underlying dentin is dependent on the adhesive aggressiveness, that is pH and chemical composition (Tay and Pashley, 2001; Perdigão *et al.*, 2008). In general, self-etch adhesives demineralize dentin more superficially than etch-and rinse adhesives.

For self-etch adhesives, the hybrid layer is thicker when aggressive (acidic) self-etch adhesives are applied (Kenshima *et al.*, 2006), but also presents areas of irregular tag remnants with different sizes and shapes. For example Adper Prompt L-Pop (3M ESPE) (pH = 0.9–1.0) forms a hybrid layer 1.7–2.9 μm thick (Perdigão *et al.*, 2008), which approaches the thickness of that formed with etch-and-rinse adhesive, but with areas of debonding.

As described above, some self-etch adhesives slightly decalcify dentin to a nanometric extent, without exposing collagen fibers. Koshiro *et al.* proposed a new designation for this interface, the nanointeraction zone (NIZ) (Koshiro *et al.*, 2006), as opposed to the traditional and thicker hybrid layer.

3.5.2 Chemical bonding

The interaction of acids or acidic monomers with hydroxyapatite is a fundamental factor in the adhesion process. Acids demineralize dental hard tissues (Yoshioka *et al.*, 2002), opening a pathway for the infiltration of resin monomers into the microporosities previously occupied by hydroxyapatite crystals (Van Meerbeek *et al.*, 2003a). While micromechanical dentin–resin entanglement is essential for immediate dentin bond strengths, chemical adhesion is desirable to improve bonding stability (Van Meerbeek *et al.*, 2003a).

Glass ionomer cements (GIC) are the only direct restorative material to bond chemically to hard dental tissues owing to the formation of ionic bonds between carboxylate groups and calcium (Lin *et al.*, 1992; Yoshida *et al.*, 2001). The chemical adhesion provided by GIC has led some manufacturers to introduce carboxylate-based polymers into the composition of dental adhesives. The polyalkenoic acid copolymer first used in Vitrebond (3M ESPE) is now known as the 'Vitrebond copolymer' (VCP) (Mitra *et al.*, 2009). This specific copolymer bonds chemically to calcium in hydroxyapatite (Mitra *et al.*, 2009).

Mine *et al.* (2009) suggested that the chemical interaction between the carboxylate groups in mild self-etch adhesives and the hydroxyapatite crystals in slightly decalcified dentin might be responsible for chemical bonding. Polycarboxylates used in classical GIC-based materials do not demineralize dentin as deeply as phosphoric acid, however there is a stable chemical adhesion between COO^- groups in GIC materials and Ca^{2+} groups in hydroxyapatite (Lin *et al.*, 1992; Yoshida *et al.*, 2000; Mitra *et al.*, 2009). Carboxylic groups replace phosphate ions in the substrate and bond ionically with the calcium of hydroxyapatite (Yoshida *et al.*, 2000). This chemical bonding mechanism is explained by the adhesion–decalcification concept (Yoshioka *et al.*, 2002; Yoshihara *et al.*, 2010). A different reaction occurs with resin-modified GIC. The self-adhesive bonding mechanism of these materials is two-fold. First, there is ionic bonding to hydroxyapatite around collagen as in conventional GICs. Second, there is micromechanical interlocking for those resin-modified GIC (RMGIC) that additionally hybridize dentin (Fig. 3.15) (Tay *et al.*, 2004c; Coutinho *et al.*, 2007).

For Vitrebond, there is no evidence of the second mechanism, that is, hybridization or gel phase deposition (Coutinho *et al.*, 2007). Since the bonding associated with Vitrebond and Ketac Nano (3M ESPE) may be stable and there is an intimate relationship between these materials and dentin, chemical interaction may be their primary bonding mechanism (Coutinho *et al.*, 2007, 2009). Nevertheless, it is difficult to explain how resin-modified GIC is able to interact chemically with dentin when a light-cured resinous primer is cured prior to the application of the resin-modified GIC material (Fig. 3.16(a) and (b)).

A 5-year clinical study with a VCP-containing RMGIC material (like in Vitrebond) reported excellent retention rates (Franco *et al.*, 2006). The VCP bonds chemically to calcium in hydroxyapatite (Mitra *et al.*, 2009), which supports the idea that the VCP in dentin adhesives may also bond

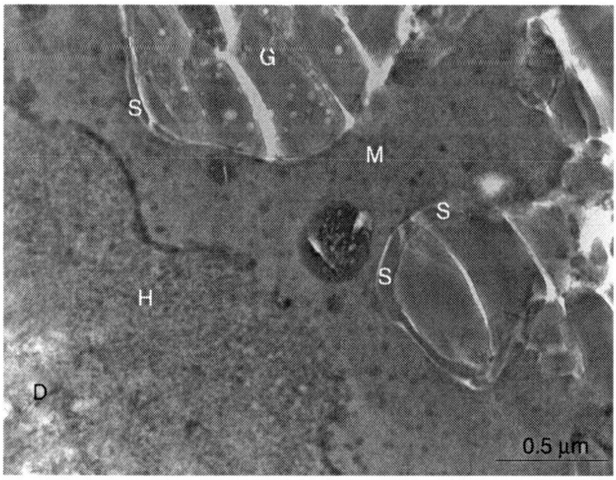

3.15 TEM micrograph of RMGIC–dentin interface formed using Fuji II LC RMGIC (GC Co.). Original magnification = ×50 000. D = dentin; H = hybrid layer; M = polycarboxylate matrix; G = glass particle; S = silica gel involving the glass particles as a result of the acid–base reaction.

chemically to hydroxyapatite. The percentage threshold of VCP for effective bonding effectiveness remains to be determined, as it may vary depending on the solvents and other components of each adhesive system. Nevertheless, this chemical adhesion may have somehow contributed to the good clinical performance of etch-and-rinse VCP-containing materials (Dalton Bittencourt *et al.*, 2005; Perdigão *et al.*, 2005c; Kubo *et al.*, 2006).

The clinical success of Clearfil SE Bond (Kuraray) at eight years (Peumans *et al.*, 2010) might be the result of its potential for chemical adhesion through the monomer 10-MDP. This monomer bonds chemically to hydroxyapatite by forming stable calcium phosphate salts without causing strong decalcification (Yoshihara *et al.*, 2010). The chemical bonding formed by 10-MDP is more stable in water than that of other monomers used in the composition of self-etch adhesives, such as 4-META and phenyl-P (Van Meerbeek *et al.*, 2011). The bonding ability of 10-MDP is a result, in part, of the Ca-10-MDP salt being one of the most hydrolytically stable salts (Van Landuyt *et al.*, 2008). According to the adhesion–decalcification concept (Yoshihara *et al.*, 2010), the less soluble the calcium salt of the acidic molecule is, the more intense and stable is the molecular adhesion to a hydroxyapatite-based substrate. MDP is adsorbed onto hydroxyapatite in a regularly layered structure at the hydroxyapatite surface (nano-interaction) (Yoshihara *et al.*, 2010) and at the same time decalcifies hydroxyapatite (Fukegawa *et al.*, 2006).

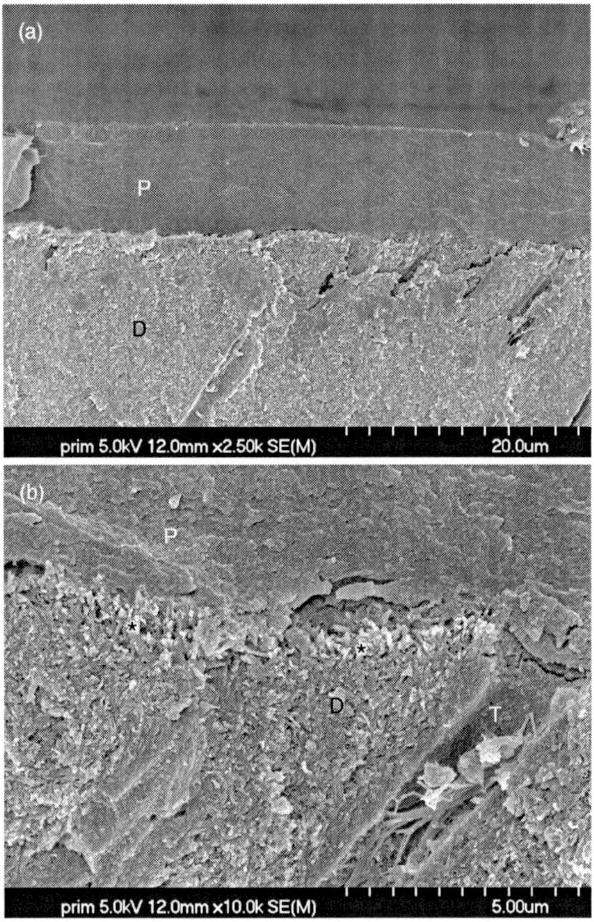

3.16 FESEM micrograph of resin–dentin interface (lateral view) formed by a resin-modified glass-ionomer cement that contains a resin-based primer. (a) Original magnification = ×2500. (b) Asterisks denote a zone of mild dentin decalcification. Original magnification = ×10 000. D = dentin; P = primer; T = tubule.

In summary, in addition to the chemical bonding provided by GIC-based materials, there is now enough evidence that chemical bonding plays a role in the adhesion of other materials, such as mild self-etch adhesives.

3.6 *In vitro* versus *in vivo* studies

The market is in constant change, with new materials being released every year, or with adhesive formulations being improved frequently, with the aim of achieving improved adhesion combined with a simplified application protocol.

Although clinical trials are the most reliable method to evaluate bonding systems and overall dental materials, clinical tests are expensive and time consuming, making them difficult to implement and complete. This is the principal reason why laboratory tests are more prevalent than clinical trials (De Munck *et al.*, 2005b). For an adhesive to get ADA acceptance (ADA 2001), it must have a retention rate in non-carious cervical lesions (NCCL) of 90% at 18 months. Provisional acceptance can be obtained if at six months their retention in the referred substrate is at least 95% without mechanical retention features.

Laboratory tests are an important tool for measuring and screening experimental adhesives during the development phase and for evaluating the performance of newly developed commercial adhesive systems. These *in vitro* tests should be reliable, reproducible and standardized to allow the results to be compared between different testing centers.

Most dental adhesive materials are launched after *in vitro* testing, but without clinical effectiveness data. Prior to introduction into the dental market, these materials only require FDA approval of the *Section 510(k) – Premarket Notification of Intent to Market the Device*, after the manufacturer submits evidence that the applicant device is substantially equivalent to other legally marketed devices. This usually translates into submission of chemical composition and laboratory tests demonstrating that the new material is equivalent to materials from the same, or other manufacturers, that have been already approved by the FDA (information available online at www.fda.gov).

Despite the improvements in adhesives systems, the bonded interface remains their weakest link. To characterize the bonding interface, imaging methods such as scanning electron microscopy (SEM), transmission electron microscopy (TEM), confocal laser scanning microscopy (CLSM) and atomic force microscopy (AFM) are widely used. Spectroscopic methods such as nuclear magnetic resonance spectroscopy, (NMR) X-ray photoelectron spectroscopy (XPS), electron spectroscopy for chemical analysis (ESCA), Fourier transform infrared spectroscopy (FTIR), Raman spectroscopy or Auger spectroscopy help to identify and to analyze interfacial chemical reactions.

Bond strength tests are still the most widely accepted *in vitro* techniques for analyzing enamel or dentin bond strengths of adhesive resins quantitatively (De Munck *et al.*, 2005b). *In vitro* durability studies are useful but they suffer the limitations of all *in vitro* studies – they are not carried out under clinical conditions, as the teeth are nonvital and not subjected to masticatory stresses. Therefore, *in vivo* long-term studies are required to predict the durability of bonded restorations under function.

In vitro studies examining the durability of bonding after storage require careful control of several factors. They must include antimicrobial agents to inhibit the growth of mold or other non-oral flora. The pH of the storage solution should be kept stable if results at different time periods are to be compared. There is now evidence that a correlation exists between clinical studies and *in vitro* durability tests that include water storage for six months (Heintze *et al.*, 2011). The frequent introduction of new bonding agents makes it difficult to compare time-consuming bond durability studies, as adhesive materials become obsolete very rapidly.

3.7 Incompatibility between adhesives systems and restorative materials

The compatibility between dental adhesives and restorative materials is of prime importance to the success of rehabilitation. Some reports have addressed the adhesive/restorative material compatibility that clinicians must be aware of (Hagge and Lindemuth, 2001; Franco *et al.*, 2002; Cheong *et al.*, 2003; Finger *et al.*, 2005; Bolhuis *et al.*, 2006; Shafiei *et al.*, 2009; Walter *et al.*, 2009) as well as how to prevent the potential incompatibility problems (Reis *et al.*, 2009; Garcia *et al.*, 2010).

Light-cured resins are the material of choice for esthetic direct or indirect restorations, owing to their mechanical, physical and esthetic properties (Willems *et al.*, 1992; Lien and Vandewalle, 2010; Ferracane, 2011). A photoinitiator, usually an α-diketone, is activated to an excited triplet state in light-activated resin-based materials, using a light source, and free radicals are generated. Then, an amine accelerator causes the reduction of the activated photoinitiator, forming an intermediate excited complex, which releases free radicals when dissociation takes place (Ruyter, 1985).

For chemically polymerized resins, a peroxide and a aromatic tertiary amine form a binary, redox curing system that initiates a free radical polymerization mechanism. Chemically activated composites are still important in clinical dentistry, not only in areas of the globe deprived of electrical power, but also as chemically activated resins for luting indirect restorations, endodontic posts, fixed prostheses and construct crown build-ups.

There is evidence that incompatibility may occur between the polymerization mode of adhesive systems and resin composites (Hagge and Lindemuth, 2001). Clinicians have reported some unexpected debondings of chemically polymerized composite build-ups. Recent reports revealed that some light-cured simplified adhesives, either etch-and-rinse or self-etch adhesive systems, have a chemical incompatibility with chemically and dual-cured composite resins (Hagge and Lindemuth, 2001; Cheong *et al.*, 2003). This incompatibility seems to be adhesive-formulation dependent (Hagge and Lindemuth, 2001) and may be attributed to the adverse chemical interaction with acidic monomers, as acidic groups neutralize the self-cured resin amine groups (Finger *et al.*, 2005). Adverse interactions between acidic adhesive resin monomers and tertiary amines in light-cured composites normally do not occur because of the fast rate of free radical generation in photochemical redox reactions (Tay *et al.*, 2001; Suh *et al.*, 2003).

For etch-and-rinse two-step adhesives, the uncured ionic resin monomers in the oxygen-inhibition layer are in direct contact with the composite, as opposed to what occurs with three-step etch-and-rinse adhesives. The latter contain a hydrophobic resin that is applied over the primer to couple the composite resin to the primed dentin/enamel surface (Van Meerbeek *et al.*, 2003a). This hydrophobic bonding layer prevents the ionic monomers in the primed tooth surface coming into contact with the composite resin.

Sanares *et al.* studied the effect of one-bottle adhesives with different acidity – Prime&Bond NT (Dentsply), OptiBond Solo (Kerr), Single Bond (3M ESPE) and One-Step (Bisco) – on bonding to the chemically cured composite resin BisFil 2B (Bisco) and to the light-cured composite resin Z100 (3M) (Sanares *et al.*, 2001). These authors found a significant difference between the factor 'dentin adhesive' and the factor 'curing mode'. The effect of the different type of adhesives on bond strength was dependent on the composite curing mode. The results also showed a negative correlation between the acidity of the adhesives and the bond strengths of the chemically polymerized composites. These results are in agreement with the findings obtained in other studies in which etch-and-rinse one-bottle adhesives resulted in unacceptable dentin bonding ability when combined with chemically polymerized composites (Swift *et al.*, 2001; Hagge and Lindemuth, 2001). There is an adverse chemical interaction between uncured acidic adhesive monomers (carboxylic and phosphate esters) and the tertiary amine in the benzoyl peroxide/amine redox catalyst system (Sanares *et al.*, 2001), as tertiary amines can be neutralized by acidic monomers, losing their reducing agents capacity in redox reactions.

Some manufacturers include an activator (for example, sulfinic acid) in their light-cured adhesive systems to make them dual-cured and provide effective bonding to dual- or chemically polymerized composites (Nyunt and Imai, 1996; Sanares *et al.*, 2001). But even with the presence of these initiators, optimal coupling between dual-cured adhesives and chemically or dual-polymerized composite resins may be difficult to achieve (O'Keefe and Powers, 2001). The use of an activator improves the coupling between OptiBond Solo Plus (Kerr) and the chemically polymerized composite resin Biscore (Bisco) slightly (Tay *et al.*, 2003a). The resin-free sulfinic acid sodium activator completely eliminates the adverse chemical interaction between OptiBond SOLO Plus (Kerr) and Biscore (Bisco), as the activator has good oxygen scavenger proprieties. However, the inherent permeability of the polymerized adhesive precludes the coupling of chemically or dual-polymerized composites in bonding to hydrated dentin (Tay *et al.*, 2003a).

A decrease in bond strengths was also detected with the two-step etch-and-rinse adhesives Prime&Bond NT (Dentsply) and One-Step Plus (Bisco), when coupled to light-cured composites, in case there was a delay in polymerization (Shafiei *et al.*, 2009). The conventional polymerization mode (600 mW cm^{-2}, 40 s) seems to be less affected by the acidity of these adhesives. In a similar fashion, one-step self-etch adhesives contain different types of chemical initiators, but the adhesion of these adhesives to chemically or dual-polymerized composite resins over hydrated dentin is compromised (Tay *et al.*, 2002a), owing to the increased permeability of one-step self-etch adhesives (Tay *et al.*, 2003b). One-step self-etch adhesives absorb and retain water through hydrogen bonds, when applied to hydrated dentin, behaving like semi-permeable membranes (Tay *et al.*, 2002a). These adhesives allow the passage of water and fluids even after polymerization, in a combined adverse effect of evaporative, osmotic and convective water fluxes, from the intertubular dentin and the dentinal tubules (Tay *et al.*, 2005). This water flux is responsible for an intricate pattern of water-filled channels within the adhesive layer referred as water trees (Tay and Pashley, 2003).

When water migrates to the interface adhesive/composite resin it will be trapped by the overlying hydrophobic composite which forms water blisters (Tay *et al.*, 2002a). The water blisters have a detrimental role as they result in mechanical disruption of the coupling between the adhesive and the composite resin (Tay *et al.*, 2003b). Water permeability and blister formation may also occur in light-cured composites when coupled to one-step self-etch adhesives applied to hydrated dentin, in case there is a delay in the composite light polymerization (Tay *et al.*, 2001).

A possible solution to reduce the problem related to dentin permeability when using simplified adhesives is to apply an extra layer of a hydrophobic adhesive (Brackett *et al.*, 2005; Reis *et al.*, 2009). The application of an extra layer of a hydrophobic resin over the cured one-step self-etch adhesive (transforming it in a two-step self-etch adhesive) increases its bonding efficacy *in vitro* and clinically (Reis *et al.*, 2008, 2009).

3.8 Conclusions

While enamel bonding is reliable and easy to achieve as long as enamel is etched with phosphoric acid, dentin bonding is still a challenge. Because of the high hydrophilic nature of the monomers and the high water concentration required for ionization of the acidic monomers in self-etch solutions, it is likely that these materials will have their bonding ability compromised over time.

New techniques have been suggested to prolong the durability of the resin–dentin interface. However, it is still premature to recommend their use without restrictions, as more clinical tests are needed.

Clinicians must be aware of limitations of the materials they use, as well as any existing incompatibility between categories of dental materials that are typically used together.

Numerous simplified adhesives have been introduced to the dental market within the last few years, without comprehensive clinical testing to validate the performance supported by *in vitro* tests. While *in vitro* tests are useful as a triage step, clinical studies are the ultimate test for any biomaterial.

3.9 References

ADA Council on Scientific Affairs (2001) *Revised American Dental Association acceptance program guidelines: dentin and enamel adhesives*. American Dental Association, Chicago, 1–9.

Armstrong SR, Vargas MA, Fang Q and Laffoon JE (2003) 'Microtensile bond strength of a total-etch 3-step, total-etch 2-step, self-etch 2-step, and a self-etch 1-step dentin bonding system through 15-month water storage.' *J Adhes Dent*, **5**, 47–56.

Arola D and Reprogel RK (2005) 'Effects of aging on the mechanical behavior of human dentin'. *Biomaterials*, **26**, 4051–61.

Asmussen E (1985) 'Clinical relevance of physical, chemical, and bonding properties of composite resins'. *Oper Dent*, **10**, 61–73.

Asmussen E and Uno S (1992) 'Adhesion of restorative resin to dentin: chemical and physicochemical aspects'. *Oper Dent*, Suppl. **5**, 68–74.

Baier RE (1992) 'Principles of adhesion'. *Oper Dent*, Suppl. **5**, 1–9.

Barkmeier WW, Shaffer SE and Gwinnett AJ (1986) 'Effects of 15 vs 60 seconds enamel acid conditioning on adhesion and morphology'. *Oper Dent*, **11**, 111–16.

Black GV (1917) *A Work on Operative Dentistry in Two Volumes*, 3rd edition, Medico-Dental Publishing Company, Chicago.

Bolhuis PB, de Gee AJ, Kleverlaan CJ, El Zohairy AA and Feilzer AJ (2006) 'Contraction stress and bond strength to dentin for compatible and incompatible combinations of bonding systems and chemical and light-cured core build-up resin composites'. *Dent Mater*, **22**, 223–33.

Bowen RL, Eick JD, Henderson DA and Anderson DW (1984) 'Smear layer: removal and bonding considerations'. *Oper Dent*, Suppl. **3**, 30–4.

Brackett WW, Ito S, Tay FR, Haisch LD and Pashley DH (2005) 'Microtensile dentin bond strength of self-etching resins: effect of a hydrophobic layer'. *Oper Dent*, **30**, 733–8.

Brackett WW, Tay FR, Looney SW, Ito S, Haisch LD and Pashley DH (2008) 'The effect of subject age on the microtensile bond strengths of a resin and a resin-modified glass ionomer adhesive to tooth structure'. *Oper Dent*, **33**, 282–6.

Brackett MG, Li N, Brackett WW, Sword RJ, Qi YP, Niu LN, Pucci CR, Dib A, Pashley DH and Tay FR (2011) 'The critical barrier to progress in dentine bonding with the etch-and-rinse technique'. *J Dent*, **39**, 238–48.

Brännström M and Nordenvall KJ (1977) 'The effect of acid etching on enamel, dentin, and the inner surface of the resin restoration: a scanning electron microscopic investigation'. *J Dent Res*, **56**, 917–23.

Buonocore MG (1955) 'A simple method of increasing the adhesion of acrylic filling materials to enamel surfaces'. *J Dent Res*, **34**, 849–53.

Buonocore MG, Matsui A and Gwinnett AJ (1968) 'Penetration of resin dental materials into enamel surfaces with reference to bonding'. *Arch Oral Biol*, **13**, 61–70.

Burrow MF, Takakura H, Nakajima M, Inai N, Tagami J and Takatsu T (1994) 'The influence of age and depth of dentin on bonding'. *Dent Mater*, **10**, 241–6.

Carrilho MRO, Carvalho RM, de Goes MF, di Hipólito V, Geraldeli S, Tay FR, Pashley DH, Tjäderhane L (2007) 'Chlorhexidine preserves dentin bond *in vitro*'. *J Dent Res*, **86**, 90–4.

Carvalho RM, Yoshiyama M, Pashley EL and Pashley DH (1996) '*In vitro* study on the dimensional changes of human dentine after demineralization'. *Arch Oral Biol*, **41**, 369–77.

Carvalho RM, Chersoni S, Frankenberger R, Pashley DH, Prati C and Tay FR (2005) 'A challenge to the conventional wisdom that simultaneous etching and resin infiltration always occurs in self-etch adhesives'. *Biomaterials*, **26**, 1035–42.

Causton BE (1984) 'Improved bonding of composite restorative to dentine. A study *in vitro* of the use of a commercial halogenated phosphate ester'. *Br Dent J*, **156**, 93–5.

Ceballos L, Camejo DG, Victoria Fuentes M, Osorio R, Toledano M, Carvalho RM and Pashley DH (2003) 'Microtensile bond strength of total-etch and self-etching adhesives to caries-affected dentine'. *J Dent*, **31**, 469–77.

Cheong C, King NM, Pashley DH, Ferrari M, Toledano M and Tay FR (2003) 'Incompatibility of self-etch adhesives with chemical/dual-cured composites: two-step *vs* one-step systems'. *Oper Dent*, **28**, 747–55.

Costa CAS, Giro EMA, Nascimento ABL, Teixeira HM and Hebling J (2003) 'Short-term evaluation of the pulpo-dentin complex response to a resin-modified glass-ionomer cement and a bonding agent applied in deep cavities'. *Dent Mater*, **19**, 739–46.

Coutinho E, Yoshida Y, Inoue S, Fukuda R, Snauwaert J, Nakayama Y, De Munck J, Lambrechts P, Suzuki K and Van Meerbeek B (2007) 'Gel phase formation at resin-modified glass-ionomer/tooth interfaces'. *J Dent Res*, **86**, 656–61.

Coutinho E, Cardoso MV, De Munck J, Neves AA, Van Landuyt KL, Poitevin A, Peumans M, Lambrechts P and Van Meerbeek B (2009) 'Bonding effectiveness and interfacial characterization of a nano-filled resin-modified glass-ionomer'. *Dent Mater*, **25**, 1347–57.

Cueto EI and Buonocore MG (1967) 'Sealing of pits and fissures with an adhesive resin: its use in caries prevention'. *J Am Dent Assoc*, **75**, 121–8.

Dalton Bittencourt D, Ezecelevski IG, Reis A, Van Dijken JW and Loguercio AD (2005) 'An 18-months' evaluation of self-etch and etch & rinse adhesive in non-carious cervical lesions'. *Acta Odontol Scand*, **63**, 173–8.

Davidson CL, de Gee AJ and Feilzer A (1984) 'The competition between the composite-dentin bond strength and the polymerization contraction stress'. *J Dent Res*, **63**, 1396–9.

De Goes MF, Pachane GC and Garcia-Godoy F (1997) 'Resin bond strength with different methods to remove excess water from the dentin'. *Am J Dent*, **10**, 298–301.

De Munck J, Van Meerbeek B, Yoshida Y, Inoue S, Vargas M, Suzuki K, Lambrechts P and Vanherle G (2003) 'Four-year water degradation of total-etch adhesives bonded to dentin'. *J Dent Res*, **82**, 136–40.
De Munck J, Van Landuyt K, Coutinho E, Poitevin A, Peumans M, Lambrechts P and Van Meerbeek B (2005a) 'Micro-tensile bond strength of adhesives bonded to class-I cavity-bottom dentin after thermo-cycling'. *Dent Mater*, **21**, 999–1007.
De Munck J, Van Landuyt K, Peumans M, Poitevin A, Lambrechts P, Braem M and Van Meerbeek B (2005b) 'A critical review of the durability of adhesion to tooth tissue: Methods and results'. *J Dent Res*, **84**, 118–32.
Eick JD, Wilko RA, Anderson CH and Sorensen SE (1970) 'Scanning electron microscopy of cut tooth surfaces and identification of debris by use of the electron microprobe'. *J Dent Res*, **49**, 1359–68.
Eick JD, Johnson LN, Fromer JR, Good RJ and Neumann AW (1972) 'Surface topography: its influence on wetting and adhesion in a dental adhesive system'. *J Dent Res*, **51**, 780–8.
Eick JD, Cobb CM, Chapell RP, Spencer P and Robinson SJ (1991) 'The dentinal surface: its influence on dentinal adhesion. Part I'. *Quintessence Int*, **22**, 967–77.
Ericson D (2004) 'What is minimally invasive dentistry?'. *Oral Health Prev Dent*, **2**(Supplement 1), 287–92.
Feigal RJ and Quelhas I (2003) 'Clinical trial of a self-etching adhesive for sealant application: success at 24 months with Prompt L-Pop'. *Am J Dent*, **16**, 249–51.
Fejerskov O (2004) 'Changing paradigms in concepts on dental caries: Consequences for oral health care'. *Caries Res*, **38**, 182–91.
Ferracane JL (2011) 'Resin composite – state of the art'. *Dent Mater*, **27**, 29–38.
Finger WJ, Osada T, Tani C and Endo T (2005) 'Compatibility between self-etching adhesive and self-curing resin by addition of anion exchange resin'. *Dent Mater*, **21**, 1044–50.
Franco EB, Lopes LG, D'alpino PH, Pereira JC, Mondelli RF and Navarro MF (2002) 'Evaluation of compatibility between different types of adhesives and dual-cured resin cement'. *J Adhes Dent*, **4**, 271–5.
Franco EB, Benetti AR, Ishikiriama SK, Santiago SL, Lauris JR, Jorge MF and Navarro MF (2006) '5-year clinical performance of resin composite versus resin modified glass ionomer restorative system in non-carious cervical lesions'. *Oper Dent*, **31**, 403–8.
Fukegawa D, Hayakawa S, Yoshida Y, Suzuki K, Osaka A and Van Meerbeek B (2006) 'Chemical interaction of phosphoric acid ester with hydroxyapatite'. *J Dent Res*, **85**, 941–4.
Furuse AY, Peutzfeldt A and Asmussen E (2008) 'Effect of evaporation of solvents from one-step self-etching adhesives'. *J Adhes Dent*, **10**, 35–9.
Fusayama T and Terachima S (1972) 'Differentiation of two layers of carious dentin by staining'. *J Dent Res*, **51**, 866.
Garberoglio R, Brännström M (1976) 'Scanning electron microscopic investigation of human dentinal tubules'. *Arch Oral Biol*, **23**, 355–62.
Garcia EJ, Reis A, Arana-Correa BE, Sepúlved-Navarro WF, Higashi C, Gomes JC and Loguercio AD (2010) 'Reducing the incompatibility between two-step adhesives and resin composite luting cements'. *J Adhes Dent*, **12**, 373–9.
Gendron R, Grenier D, Sorsa T and Mayrand D (1999) 'Inhibition of the activities of matrix metalloproteinases 2, 8, and 9 by chlorhexidine'. *Clin Diagn Lab Immunol*, **6**, 437–43.

Grégoire G and Ahmed Y (2007) 'Evaluation of the enamel etching capacity of six contemporary self-etch adhesives'. *J Dent*, **35**, 388–97.

Gwinnett AJ (1984) 'Smear layer: Morphological considerations'. *Oper Dent*, Suppl. **3**, 3–12.

Gwinnett AJ (1993) 'Quantitative contribution of resin infiltration/hybridization to dentin bonding'. *Am J Dent*, **6**, 7–9.

Gwinnett AJ (1994) 'Dentin bond strengths after air-drying and re-wetting'. *Am J Dent*, **7**, 144–8.

Gwinnett AJ and Jendresen MD (1978) 'Micromorphologic features of cervical erosion after acid conditioning and its relation with composite resin'. *J Dent Res*, **57**, 543–9.

Gwinnett AJ and Kanca J (1992) 'Micromorphology of the bonded dentin interface and its relationship to bond strength'. *Am J Dent*, **5**, 73–7.

Gwinnett AJ and Matsui A (1967) 'A study of enamel adhesives: the physical relationship between enamel and adhesive'. *Arch Oral Biol*, **12**, 1615–20.

Hagge MS and Lindemuth JS (2001) 'Shear bond strength of an autopolymerizing core buildup composite bonded to dentin with 9 dentin adhesive systems'. *J Prosthet Dent*, **86**, 620–3.

Hashimoto M, Ohno H, Kaga M, Sano H, Tay FR, Oguchi H, Arakia Y and Kubota M (2002) 'Over-etching effects on micro-tensile bond strength and failure patterns for two dentin bonding systems'. *J Dent*, **30**, 99–105.

Hebling J, Pashley DH, Tjäderhane L and Tay FR (2005) 'Chlorhexidine arrests subclinical breakdown of dentin hybrid layers *in vivo*'. *J Dent Res*, **84**, 741–6.

Heintze SD, Thunpithayakul C, Armstrong SR and Rousson V (2011) 'Correlation between microtensile bond strength data and clinical outcome of Class V restorations'. *Dent Mater*, **27**, 114–25.

Hosaka K, Nishitani Y, Tagami J, Yoshiyama M, Brackett WW, Agee KA, Tay FR and Pashley DH (2009) 'Durability of resin-dentin bonds to water- *vs.* ethanol-saturated dentin'. *J Dent Res*, **88**, 146–51.

Hudson P (2004) 'Conservative treatment of the Class I lesion – A new paradigm for dentistry'. *J Am Dent Assoc*, **135**, 760–4.

Inoue SE, Vargas MA, Abe Y, Yoshida A, Lambrechts P, Vanherle G, Sano H and Van Meerbeek B (2003) 'Microtensile bond strength of eleven contemporary adhesives to enamel'. *Am J Dent*, **16**, 329–34.

Ito S, Tay FR, Hashimoto M, Yoshiyama M, Saito T, Brackett WW, Waller JL and Pashley DH (2005) 'Effects of multiple coatings of two all-in-one adhesives on dentin bonding'. *J Adhes Dent*, **7**, 133–41.

Kanca J (1992a) 'Resin bonding to wet substrate: I. bonding to dentin'. *Quintessence Int*, **23**, 39–41.

Kanca J (1992b) 'Effect of resin primer solvents and surface wetness on resin composite bond strength to dentin'. *Am J Dent*, **5**, 213–21.

Kanemura N, Sano H and Tagami J (1999) 'Tensile bond strength to and SEM evaluation of ground and intact enamel surfaces'. *J Dent*, **27**, 523–30.

Kenshima S, Francci C, Reis A, Loguercio AD and Filho LE (2006) 'Conditioning effect on dentin, resin tags and hybrid layer of different acidity self-etch adhesives applied to thick and thin smear layer'. *J Dent*, **34**, 775–83.

Kidd EAM (2004) 'How 'clean' must a cavity be before restoration?'. *Caries Res*, **38**, 305–13.

Kinney JH, Nalla RK, Pople JA, Breunig TM and Ritchie RO (2005) 'Age-related transparent root dentin: mineral concentration, crystallite size, and mechanical properties'. *Biomaterials*, **26**, 3363–76.

Koshiro K, Sidhu SK, Inoue S, Ikeda T and Sano H (2006) 'New concept of resin-dentin interfacial adhesion: the nanointeraction zone'. *J Biomed Mater Res, Part B: Appl Biomater*, **77**, 401–8.

Kramer IRH (1952) 'Alterations in the staining reactions of dentin resulting from a constituent of a new self-polymerising resin'. *Br Dent J*, **93**, 150–2.

Kubo S, Kawasaki K, Yokota H and Hayashi Y (2006) 'Five-year clinical evaluation of two adhesive systems in non-carious cervical lesions'. *J Dent*, **34**, 97–105.

Kuboki Y, Ohgushi K and Fusayama T (1977) 'Collagen biochemistry of the two layers of carious dentin'. *J Dent Res*, **56**, 1233–37.

Kwong SM, Cheung GS, Kei LH, Itthagarun A, Smales RJ, Tay FR and Pashley DH (2002) 'Micro-tensile bond strengths to sclerotic dentin using a self-etching and a total-etching technique'. *Dent Mater*, **18**, 359–69.

Lien W and Vandewalle KS (2010) 'Physical properties of a new silorane-based restorative system'. *Dent Mater*, **26**, 337–44.

Lin A, McIntyre NS and Davidson RD (1992) 'Studies on the adhesion of glass–ionomer cements to dentin'. *J Dent Res*, **71**, 1836–41.

Loesche WJ, Svanberg ML and Pape HR (1979) 'Intraoral transmission of *Streptococcus mutans* by a dental explorer'. *J Dent Res*, **58**, 1765–70.

Loguercio AD, Bittencourt DD, Baratieri LN and Reis A (2007) 'A 36-month evaluation of self-etch and etch-and-rinse adhesives in noncarious cervical lesions'. *J Am Dent Assoc*, **138**, 507–14.

Lopes GC, Vieira LC, Araujo E, Bruggmann T, Zucco J and Oliveira G (2011) 'Effect of dentin age and acid etching time on dentin bonding'. *J Adhes Dent*, **13**, 139–45.

Lussi A (1991) 'Validity of diagnostic and treatment decisions of fissure caries'. *Caries Res*, **25**, 296–303.

Lussi A and Francescut P (2003) 'Performance of conventional and new methods for the detection of occlusal caries in deciduous teeth'. *Caries Res*, **37**, 2–7.

Maciel KT, Carvalho RM, Ringle RD, Preston CD, Russell CM and Pashley DH (1996) 'The effect of acetone, ethanol, HEMA, and air on the stiffness of human decalcified dentin matrix'. *J Dent Res*, **75**, 1851–8.

Marshall Jr GW, Chang YJ, Saeki K, Gansky SA and Marshall SJ (2000) 'Citric acid etching of cervical sclerotic dentin lesions: an AFM study'. *J Biomed Mater Res*, **49**, 338–44.

Martin-De Las Heras S, Valenzuela A and Overall CM (2000) 'The matrix metalloproteinase gelatinase A in human dentine'. *Arch Oral Biol*, **45**, 757–65.

Mazzoni A, Pashley DH, Nishitani Y, Breschi L, Tjaderhane L, Toledano M, Pashley EL and Tay FR (2006) 'Reactivation of quenched endogenous proteolytic activities in phosphoric acid-etched dentine by etch-and-rinse adhesives'. *Biomaterials*, **27**, 4470–6.

McCullock AJ and Smith BGN (1986) '*In vitro* studies of cuspal movement produced by adhesive restorative materials'. *Br Dent J*, **161**, 405–9.

McLean JW and Kramer IRH (1952) 'A clinical and pathological evaluation of a sulphinic acid activated resin for use in restorative dentistry'. *Br Dent J*, **93**, 255–69.

Mine A, De Munck J, Cardoso MV, Van Landuyt KL, Poitevin A, Kuboki T, Yoshida Y, Suzuki K, Lambrechts P, Van Meerbeek B (2009) 'Bonding effectiveness of two contemporary self-etch adhesives to enamel and dentin'. *J Dent*, **37**, 872–83.

Mitchem JC and Gronas DG (1986) 'Effects of time after extraction and depth of dentin on resin dentin adhesives'. *J Am Dent Assoc*, **113**, 285–7.

Mitra SB, Lee CY, Bui HT, Tantbirojn D and Rusin RP (2009) 'Long-term adhesion and mechanism of bonding of a paste-liquid resin-modified glass–ionomer'. *Dent Mater*, **25**, 459–66.

Mixson JM, Richards ND and Mitchell RJ (1993) 'Effects of dentin age and bonding on microgap formation'. *Am J Dent*, **6**, 72–6.

Miyazaki M, Sato M and Onose H (2000) 'Durability of enamel bond strength of simplified bonding systems'. *Oper Dent*, **25**, 75–80.

Morin D, Delong R and Douglas WH (1984) 'Cusp reinforcement by the acid-etch technique'. *J Dent Res*, **63**, 1075–8.

Mount GJ (2007) 'A new paradigm for operative dentistry'. *Aust Dent J*, **52**, 264–70.

Murray PE, Stanley HR, Matthews JB, Sloan AJ and Smith AJ (2002) 'Age-related odontometric changes of human teeth'. *Oral Surg Oral Med Oral Pathol Oral Radiol Endod*, **93**, 474–82.

Nakabayashi N, Kojima K and Masuhara E (1982) 'The promotion of adhesion by the infiltration of monomers into tooth substrates'. *J Biomed Mater Res*, **16**, 265–73.

Nakamichi I, Iwaku M and Fusayama T (1983) 'Bovine teeth as possible substitutes in the adhesion test'. *J Dent Res*, **62**, 1076–81.

Nishitani Y, Yoshiyama M, Wadgaonkar B, Breschi L, Manello F, Mazzoni A, Carvalho RM, Tjäderhane L, Tay FR and Pashley DH (2006) 'Activation of gelatinolytic activity in dentin by self-etching adhesives'. *Eur J Oral Sci*, **114**, 160–6.

Nyunt MM and Imai Y (1996) 'Adhesion to dentin with resin using sulfinic acid initiator system'. *Dent Mater J*, **15**, 75–182.

O'Keefe KL and Powers JM (2001) 'Adhesion of resin composite core materials to dentin'. *Int J Prosthodont*, **14**, 451–6.

Ohgushi K and Fusayama T (1975) 'Electron microscopic structure of the two layers of carious dentin'. *J Dent Res*, **54**, 1019–26.

Opdam NJ, Roeters FJ, Feilzer AJ and Verdonschot EH (1998) 'Marginal integrity and postoperative sensitivity in Class 2 resin composite restorations *in vivo*'. *J Dent*, **26**, 555–62.

Packham DE (1992) 'Adhesion'. In *Handbook of Adhesion*, DE Packham (ed.), Longman Scientific & Technical, Essex, 18–20.

Pashley DH (1992) 'The effects of acid etching on the pulpodentin complex'. *Oper Dent*, **17**, 229–42.

Pashley DH (1996) 'Dynamics of the pulpo-dentin complex'. *Crit Rev Oral Biol Med*, **7**, 104–33.

Pashley DH and Tay FR (2001) 'Aggressiveness of contemporary self-etching adhesives. Part II: etching effects on unground enamel'. *Dent Mater*, **17**, 430–44.

Pashley DH, Ciucchi B, Sano H, Carvalho RM and Russell CM (1995) 'Bond strength versus dentine structure: a modelling approach'. *Arch Oral Biol*, **40**, 1109–18.

Pashley DH, Tay FR, Yiu C, Hashimoto M, Breschi L, Carvalho RM and Ito S (2004) 'Collagen degradation by host-derived enzymes during aging'. *J Dent Res*, **83**, 216–21.

Pashley DH, Tay FR, Carvalho RM, Rueggeberg FA, Agee KA, Carrilho M, Donelly A and García-Godoy F (2007) 'From dry bonding to water wet bonding to ethanol-wet bonding. A review of the interactions between dentin matrix and solvated resins using a macromodel of the hybrid layer'. *Am J Dent*, **20**, 7–20.

Perdigão J (2002) 'Dentin bonding as function of dentin structure'. *Dent Clin North Am*, **46**, 1–25.

Perdigão J and Geraldeli S (2003) 'Bonding characteristics of self-etching adhesives to intact versus prepared enamel'. *J Esthet Restor Dent*, **15**, 32–42.

Perdigão J, Denehy GE, Swift EJ Jr. (1994) 'Effects of chlorhexidine on dentin surfaces and shear bond strengths'. *Am J Dent*, **7**, 81–4.

Perdigão J, Lambrechts P, Van Meerbeek B, Braem M, Yildiz E, Yücel T and Vanherle G (1996) 'The interaction of adhesive systems with human dentin'. *Am J Dent*, **9**, 167–73.

Perdigão J, Van Meerbeek B, Lopes MM and Ambrose WW (1999) 'The effect of a re-wetting agent on dentin bonding'. *Dent Mater*, **15**, 282–95.

Perdigão J, Fundingsland JW, Duarte S and Lopes MM (2005a) 'Microtensile adhesion of sealants to intact enamel'. *Int J Paediatr Dent*, **15**, 342–8.

Perdigão J, Carmo APR and Geraldeli S (2005b) 'Eighteen-month clinical evaluation of two dentin adhesives applied on dry vs. moist dentin'. *J Adhes Dent*, **7**, 253–8.

Perdigão J, Carmo APR, Anauate-Netto C, Amore R, Lewgoy HR, Cordeiro HJD, Dutra-Correa M and Castilhos N (2005c) 'Clinical performance of a self-etching adhesive at 18 months'. *Am J Dent*, **18**, 135–40.

Perdigão J, Gomes G and Lopes MM (2006) 'The influence of conditioning time on enamel adhesion'. *Quintessence Int*, **37**, 41–7.

Perdigão J, Lopes MM and Gomes G (2008) 'In vitro bonding performance of self-etch adhesives: II – ultramorphological evaluation'. *Oper Dent*, **33**, 534–49.

Perdigão J, Dutra-Correa M, Anauate-Netto C, Castilhos N, Carmo APR, Lewgoy HR, Amore R and Cordeiro HJD (2009) 'Two-year clinical evaluation of self-etch adhesives in posterior restorations'. *J Adhes Dent*, **11**, 149–59.

Perdigão J, Sezinando A and Monteiro P (2012) 'Effect of substrate age and adhesive composition on dentin bonding'. *submitted.*

Peumans M, Kanumilli P, De Munck J, Van Landuyt K, Lambrechts P and Van Meerbeek B (2005) 'Clinical effectiveness of contemporary adhesives: a systematic review of current clinical trials'. *Dent Mater*, **21**, 864–81.

Peumans M, De Munck J, Van Landuyt KL, Poitevin A, Lambrechts P, Van Meerbeek B (2010) 'Eight-year clinical evaluation of a 2-step self-etch adhesive with and without selective enamel etching'. *Dent Mater*, **26**, 1176–84.

Platt JA, Almeida J, Gonzalez-Cabezas C, Rhodes B and Moore BK (2001) 'The effect of double adhesive application on the shear bond strength to dentin of compomers using three one-bottle adhesive systems'. *Oper Dent*, **26**, 313–17.

Prati C and Pashley DH (1992) 'Dentin wetness, permeability, thickness and bond strength of adhesive systems'. *Am J Dent*, **5**, 33–8.

Reis A, Albuquerque M, Pegoraro M, Mattei G, Bauer JR, Grande RH, Klein-Junior CA, Baumhardt-Neto R and Loguercio AD (2008) 'Can the durability of one-step self-etch adhesives be improved by double application or by an extra layer of hydrophobic resin?'. *J Dent*, **36**, 309–15.

Reis A, Leite TM, Matte K, Michels R, Amaral RC, Geraldeli S and Loguercio AD (2009) 'Improving clinical retention of one-step self-etching adhesive systems with an additional hydrophobic adhesive layer'. *J Am Dent Assoc*, **140**, 877–85.

Ricci HA, Sanabe ME, De Souza Costa CA, Pashley DH and Hebling J (2010) 'Chlorhexidine increases the longevity of *in vivo* resin-dentin bonds'. *Eur J Oral Sci*, **118**, 411–16.

Roberts HW, Charlton DG and Murchison DF (2001) 'Repair of non-carious amalgam margin defects'. *Oper Dent*, **26**, 273–6.

Rock W and Kidd E (1988) 'The electronic detection of demineralization in occlusal fissures'. *Br Dent J*, **164**, 243–7.

Ruyter IE (1985) 'Monomer systems and polymerization'. In: *Posterior Composite Resin Dental Restorative Materials*, Vanherle G and Smith DC (eds), Peter Szulc Publishing, Ultecht, 109–35.

Sadek FT, Castellan CS, Braga RR, Mai S, Tjäderhane L, Pashley DH and Tay FR (2010) 'One-year stability of resin-dentin bonds created with a hydrophobic ethanol-wet bonding technique'. *Dent Mater*, **26**, 380–6.

Sanares AME, Itthagarun A, King NM, Tay FR and Pashley DH (2001) 'Adverse surface interactions between one-bottle light-cured adhesives and chemical-cured composites'. *Dent Mater*, **17**, 542–56.

Say EC, Nakajima M, Senawongse P, Soyman M, Ozer F and Tagami J (2005) 'Bonding to sound vs. caries-affected dentin using photo- and dual-cure adhesives'. *Oper Dent*, **30**, 90–8.

Shafiei F, Saffarpour A, Moradmand M and Alavi AA (2009) 'Effect of light activation mode on the incompatibility between one-bottle adhesives and light-cured composites: an *in vitro* shear bond strength study'. *Oper Dent*, **34**, 558–64.

Shinchi MJ, Soma K and Nakabayashi N (2000) 'The effect of phosphoric acid concentration on resin tag length and bond strength of a photo-cured resin to acid-etched enamel'. *Dent Mater*, **16**, 324–29.

Silverstone L (1974) 'Fissure sealants'. *Caries Res*, **8**, 2–26.

Spreafico D, Semeraro S, Mezzanzanica D, Re D, Gagliani M, Tanaka T, Sano H and Sidhu SK (2006) The effect of the air-blowing step on the technique sensitivity of four different adhesive systems'. *J Dent*, **34**, 237–44.

Stanford JW, Sabri Z and Jose S (1985) 'A comparison of the effectiveness of dentin bonding agents'. *Int Dent J*, **35**, 139–44.

Stanislawczuk R, Amaral RC, Zander-Grande C, Gagler D, Reis A and Loguercio AD (2009) 'Chlorhexidine-containing acid conditioner preserves the longevity of resin–dentin bonds'. *Oper Dent*, **34**, 481–90.

Stanislawczuk R, Reis A and Loguercio AD (2011) 'A 2-year *in vitro* evaluation of a chlorhexidine-containing acid on the durability of resin–dentin interfaces'. *J Dent*, **39**, 40–7.

Stanley HR, Pereira JC, Spiegel E, Broom C and Schultz M (1983) 'The detection and prevalence of reactive and physiologic sclerotic dentin, reparative dentin and dead tracts beneath various types of dental lesions according to tooth surface and age'. *J Oral Pathol*, **12**, 257–89.

Suh BI, Feng L, Pashley DH and Tay FR (2003) 'Factors contributing to the incompatibility between simplified-step adhesives and chemically-cured or dual-cured composites. Part III. Effect of acidic resin monomers'. *J Adhes Dent*, **5**, 267–82.

Sulkala M, Larmas M, Sorsa T, Salo T and Tjäderhane L (2002) 'The localization of matrix metalloproteinase-20 (MMP-20, enamelysin) in mature human teeth'. *J Dent Res*, **81**, 603–38.

Suzuki T and Finger WJ (1988) 'Dentin adhesives: site of dentin *vs.* bonding of composite resins'. *Dent Mater*, **4**, 379–83.
Swift EJ, Perdigão J and Heymann HO (1995) 'Bonding to enamel and dentin: a brief history and state of the art. *Quintessence Int*, **26**, 95–110.
Swift EJ Jr, Perdigão J, Combe EC, Simpson CH and Nunes MF (2001) 'Effects of restorative and adhesive curing methods on dentin bond strengths'. *Am J Dent*, **14**, 137–40.
Tao L and Pashley DH (1988) 'Shear bond strengths to dentin: effects of surface treatments, depth and position'. *Dent Mater*, **4**, 371–8.
Tay FR and Pashley DH (2001) 'Aggressiveness of contemporary self-etching systems. I: Depth of penetration beyond smear layers'. *Dent Mater*, **17**, 296–308.
Tay FR and Pashley DH (2003) 'Water treeing – a potential mechanism for degradation of dentin adhesives'. *Am J Dent*, **16**, 6–12.
Tay FR and Pashley DH (2004) 'Resin bonding to cervical sclerotic dentin: a review'. *J Dent*, **32**, 173–96.
Tay FR, Gwinnett AJ, Pang KM and Wei SHY (1995) 'Micromorphologic relationship of the resin-dentin interface following a total-etch technique *in vivo* using a dentinal bonding system'. *Quintessence Int*, **26**, 63–70.
Tay FR, Gwinnett AJ and Wei SHY (1996) 'Micromorphological spectrum from over-drying to overwetting acid-conditioned dentin in water-free, acetone-based, single-bottle primer/adhesives'. *Dent Mater*, **12**, 236–44.
Tay FR, Gwinnett AJ and Wei SHY (1997) 'Ultrastructure of the resin–dentin interface following reversible and irreversible rewetting'. *Am J Dent*, **10**, 77–82.
Tay FR, King NM, Suh BI and Pashley DH (2001) 'Effect of delayed activation light-cured resin composites on bonding of all-in-one adhesives'. *J Adhes Dent*, **3**, 207–25.
Tay FR, Pashley DH, Suh BI, Carvalho RM and Itthagarun A (2002a) 'Single-step adhesives are permeable membranes'. *J Dent*, **30**, 371–82.
Tay FR, Pashley DH and Yoshiyama M (2002b) 'Two modes of nanoleakage expression in single-step adhesives'. *J Dent Res*, **81**, 472–6.
Tay FR, Suh BI, Pashley DH, Prati C, Chuang S-F and Li F (2003a) 'Factors contributing to the incompatibility between simplified-step adhesives and self-cured or dual-cured composites. Part II. Single-bottle, total-etch adhesive'. *J Adhes Dent*, **5**, 91–105.
Tay FR, Pashley DH, Yiu CKY, Sanares AME and Wei SHY (2003b) 'Factors contributing to the incompatibility between simplified-step adhesives and chemically-cured or dual-cured composites. Part I. Single-step self-etching adhesive'. *J Adhes Dent*, **5**, 27–40.
Tay FR, Lai CNS, Chersoni S, Pashley DH, Mak YF, Suppa P, Prati C and King NM (2004a) 'Osmotic blistering in enamel bonded with one-step self-etch adhesives'. *J Dent Res*, **83**, 290–5.
Tay FR, Frankenberger R, Krejci I, Bouillaguet S, Pashley DH, Carvalho RM and Lai CNS (2004b) 'Single-bottle adhesives behave as permeable membranes after polymerization. I. *In vivo* evidence'. *J Dent*, **32**, 611–21.
Tay FR, Sidhu SK, Watson TF and Pashley DH (2004c) 'Water-dependent interfacial transition zone in resin-modified glass-ionomer cement/dentin interfaces'. *J Dent Res*, **83**, 644–9.

Tay FR, Pashley DH, Suh BI, Hiraishi N and Tiu CKY (2005) 'Buonocore memorial lecture: Water treeing in simplified dentin adhesives – *déjà vu?*'. *Oper Dent*, **30**, 561–79.

Tay FR, Pashley DH, Kapur RR, Carrilho MRO, Hur YB, Garrett LV and Tay KCY (2007) 'Bonding BisGMA to dentin – a proof of concept for hydrophobic dentin bonding'. *J Dent Res*, **86**, 1034–9.

Tyas MJ, Anusavice KJ, Frencken JE and Mount GJ (2000) 'Minimal intervention dentistry – A review'. *Int Dent J*, **50**, 1–12.

Van der Graaf ER and ten Bosch JJ (1993) 'Changes in dimension and weight of human dentine after different drying procedures and during subsequent rehydration'. *Arch Oral Biol*, **38**, 97–9.

van Dijken JW (2004) 'Durability of three simplified adhesive systems in Class V non-carious cervical dentin lesions'. *Am J Dent*, **17**, 27–32.

van Dijken JW (2005) 'Retention of a resin-modified glass ionomer adhesive in non-carious cervical lesions. A 6-year follow-up'. *J Dent*, **33**, 541–7.

van Dijken JW (2010) 'A prospective 8-year evaluation of a mild two-step self-etching adhesive and a heavily filled two-step etch-and-rinse system in non-carious cervical lesions'. *Dent Mater*, **26**, 940–6.

van Dorp CSE, Exterkate AM and ten Cate JM (1988) 'The effect of dental probing on subsequent enamel demineralization'. *J Dent Child*, **55**, 343–7.

Van Landuyt KL, De Munck J, Snauwaert J, Coutinho E, Poitevin A, Yoshida Y, Inoue S, Peumans M, Suzuki K, Lambrechts P and Van Meerbeek B (2005) 'Monomer-solvent phase separation in one-step self-etch adhesives'. *J Dent Res*, **84**, 183–8.

Van Landuyt KL, Yoshida Y, Hirata I, Snauwaert J, De Munck J, Okazaki M, Suzuki K, Lambrechts P and Van Meerbeek B (2008) 'Influence of the chemical structure of functional monomers on their adhesive performance'. *J Dent Res*, **87**, 757–61.

Van Meerbeek B, Inokoshi S, Braem M, Lambrechts P and Vanherle G (1992) 'Morphologycal aspects of the resin-dentin interdiffusion zone with different dentin adhesive systems'. *J Dent Res*, **71**, 1530–40.

Van Meerbeek B, Perdigão J, Lambrechts P and Vanherle G (1998) 'The clinical performance of dentin adhesives'. *J Dent*, **26**, 1–20.

Van Meerbeek B, De Munck J, Yoshida Y, Inoue S, Vargas M, Vijay P, Van Landuyt K, Lambrechts P and Vanherle G (2003a) 'Buonocore memorial lecture. Adhesion to enamel and dentin: current status and future challenges'. *Oper Dent*, **28**, 215–35.

Van Meerbeek B, De Munck J, Mattar D, Van Landuyt K and Lambrechts P (2003b) 'Microtensile bond strength of an etch&rinse and self-etch adhesive to enamel and dentin as a function of surface treatment'. *Oper Dent*, **28**, 647–60.

Van Meerbeek B, Yoshihara K, Yoshida Y, Mine A, De Munck J and Van Landuyt KL (2011) 'State of the art of self-etch adhesives'. *Dent Mater*, **27**, 17–28.

Vasiliadis L, Darling AI and Levers BG (1983) 'The amount and distribution of sclerotic human root dentine'. *Arch Oral Biol*, **28**, 645–9.

Walshaw PR and McComb D (1994) 'SEM evaluation of the resin–dentin interface with proprietary bonding agents in human subjects'. *J Dent Res*, **73**, 1079–87.

Walter R, Macedo GV, Oliveira GM and Swift EJ Jr. (2009) 'Adhesive bond strengths using self- and light-cured composites'. *J Contemp Dent Pract*, **10**, E025–032.

Wei S, Sadr A, Shimada Y and Tagami J (2008) 'Effect of caries-affected dentin hardness on the shear bond strength of current adhesives'. *J Adhes Dent*, **10**, 431–40.

Wendt LK, Koch G and Birkhed D (1998) 'Replacements of restorations in the primary and young permanent dentition'. *Swed Dent J*, **22**, 149–55.
Willems G, Lambrechts P, Braem M, Celis JP and Vanherle G (1992)'A classification of dental composites according to their morphological and mechanical characteristics'. *Dent Mater*, **8**, 310–19.
Wolf MS, Allen K and Kaim J (2007) 'A 100-year journey from GV Black to minimal surgical intervention'. *Comp Contin Educ Dent*, **28**, 130–5.
Yassin OM (1995) '*In vitro* studies of the effect of a dental explorer on the formation of an artificial carious lesion'. *J Dent Child*, **62**, 111–17.
Yoshida Y, Van Meerbeek B, Nakayama Y, Snauwaert J, Hellemans L, Lambrechts P, Vanherle G and Wakasa K (2000) 'Evidence of chemical bonding at biomaterial-hard tissues interface'. *J Dent Res*, **79**, 709–14.
Yoshida Y, Van Meerbeek B, Nakayama Y, Yoshioka M, Snauwaert J, Abe Y, Lambrechts P, Vanherle G and Okazaki M (2001) 'Adhesion to and decalcification of hydroxyapatite by carboxylic acids'. *J Dent Res*, **80**, 1565–9.
Yoshihara K, Yoshida Y, Nagaoka N, Fukegawa D, Hayakawa S, Mine A, Nakamura M, Minagi S, Osaka A, Suzuki K and Van Meerbeek B (2010) Nano-controlled molecular interaction at adhesive interfaces for hard tissue reconstruction'. *Acta Biomater*, **6**, 3573–82.
Yoshioka M, Yoshida Y, Inoue S, Lambrechts P, Vanherle G, Nomura Y, Okazaki M, Shintani H and Van Meerbeek B (2002) 'Adhesion/decalcification mechanisms of acid interactions with human hard tissues'. *J Biomed Mater Res*, **59**, 56–62.
Yoshiyama M, Sano H, Ebisu S, Tagami J, Ciucchi B, Carvalho RM, Johnson MH and Pashley DH (1996) 'Regional strengths of bonding agents to cervical sclerotic root dentin'. *J Dent Res*, **75**, 1404–13.
Yoshiyama M, Tay FR, Doi J, Nishitani Y, Yamada T, Itou K, Carvalho RM, Nakajima M and Pashley DH (2002) 'Bonding of self-etch and total-etch adhesives to carious dentin'. *J Dent Res*, **81**, 556–60.
Zander-Grande C, Ferreira SQ, da Costa TRF, Loguercio AD and Reis A (2011) 'Application of etch-and-rinse adhesives on dry and rewet dentin under rubbing action – A 24-month clinical evaluation'. *J Am Dent Assoc*, **142**, 828–35.

4
Enamel matrix proteins (EMP) for periodontal regeneration

N. DONOS, UCL-Eastman Dental Institute, UK,
X. DEREKA, National and Kapodistrian University of Athens, Greece and
H. D. AMIN, Imperial College London, UK

DOI: 10.1533/9780857096432.1.90

Abstract: Periodontal therapy aims to restore a healthy and functional periodontium. Several non-surgical and surgical techniques have been applied so far mainly leading to periodontal repair. Recently, a new therapeutic approach has been proposed in order to achieve regeneration of the lost periodontal tissues which is the ultimate goal of the periodontal treatment. Human histological studies provided evidence that the application of enamel matrix derivatives (EMD) to the diseased root surface promotes the formation of new cementum and new perpendicularly inserting collagen fibres. Although the underlying biological mechanism is not well clarified, it seems that a variety of patient-related as well as defect-related factors determine the clinical outcomes. The present review will present knowledge of EMD use on the various types of periodontal defects based on *in vitro* findings and on preclinical and clinical studies.

Key words: cementum regeneration, enamel matrix derivative, enamel matrix proteins, new attachment, periodontal regeneration, periodontal stem cells.

4.1 Introduction to principles of periodontal regeneration

The main goal of periodontal therapy is to restore healthy and normal periodontal function. The initial phase of periodontal treatment aims to eliminate infection and inflammation by removing root surface deposits and to control the bacterial infection by an effective oral hygiene programme (Garrett, 1996). However, if the periodontal defect still persists, surgical procedures need to be undertaken. The ultimate goal of periodontal treatment in all types of periodontal defects would be the complete regeneration of the periodontal tissues which have been lost owing to inflammatory periodontal disease (Caton and Greenstein, 1993).

A series of experiments whose aim was to clarify the role of the four distinct tissue compartments (oral epithelium, gingival connective tissue, alveolar bone, periodontal ligament) comprising the periodontium showed that only the periodontal ligament cells are capable of forming a layer of new cementum on the root surface (Karring *et al.*, 1993). This observation resulted in the development of the biological principle of 'guided tissue regeneration' (GTR) which is nowadays routinely applied successfully in the treatment of various types of periodontal defects (Jepsen *et al.*, 2002; Murphy and Gunsolley, 2003; Needleman *et al.*, 2005).

Recently, the use of enamel matrix derivatives (EMD) was introduced as a new treatment alternative for periodontal regeneration (Trombelli and Farina, 2008). It was suggested that the application of enamel matrix derived proteins on a previously diseased root surface promotes periodontal regeneration because they mimic events that take place during the development of the periodontal tissues.

4.2 Periodontal ligament (PDL) stem/progenitor cells

Tissue regeneration is considered to be dependent on three fundamental elements: (i) appropriate signalling molecules; (ii) progenitor cells; and (iii) sufficient blood supply. Each of these factors is of crucial importance in the healing process and is internally dependent on each of the others for successful regeneration of damaged/diseased tissues. Stem/progenitor cells provide the basis for tissue growth and differentiation. Signalling molecules, such as growth factors and biological mediators, modulate cell proliferation activity and stimulate cell differentiation and the production of extracellular matrix (ECM). At the same time, newly created vascular networks promoted by angiogenic signals provide blood supply for the new tissue growth (Taba *et al.*, 2005).

Stem cells are defined functionally as cells that are able to give rise to at least one differentiated cell type throughout the lifetime of the organism as well as having the unique capacity to self-renew. In contrast to the large majority of the cell population of adult tissues that are committed to a specific function, stem cells are uncommitted and remain as such, until they receive signals from the environment to generate specialised cells (Lemoli *et al.*, 2005). Thus, stem cells are considered to play a key role in tissue homeostasis and the replenishment of cells that have died (Weissman, 2000).

Adult stem cells have been isolated from various types of human and animal tissues including bone marrow (Haynesworth *et al.*, 1992; Jiang *et al.*, 2002), the central nervous system (Johe *et al.*, 1996), olfactory epithelium (Barnett and Chang, 2004), dental pulp (Gronthos *et al.*, 2002), epidermis of the skin (Cotsarelis *et al.*, 1990; Niemann and Watt, 2002), the gastrointestinal tract (Potten, 1998), blood vessels (BV) (Asahara *et al.*, 1997), skeletal muscle (Collins *et al.*, 2005), cornea (Chen *et al.*, 2004), adipose tissue (Zuk *et al.*, 2001), lung (Wu and Wei, 2004) and PDL (Singhatanadgit *et al.*, 2009; Amin *et al.*, 2011).

During embryogenesis, PDL is suggested to be formed by cells residing within the dental follicle (for review see Amin, 2011). These cells are considered to be derived from the ectomesenchyme. The most compelling evidence that such cells are present in the PDL was provided by McCulloch *et al.* (1987), who identified a small population of progenitor cells adjacent to BV within the PDL. These cells demonstrated some typical cytological features of a stem cell-like population, including small size, responsiveness to stimulatory growth factors, slow cell cycle time, a higher number of population doublings and colony forming capacity (McCulloch *et al.*, 1987). More recently, it has been confirmed that the adult PDL contains an adult stem cell-like population that exhibits certain characteristic features of mesenchymal stem cells, and expresses embryonic stem cell-associated antigenic markers such as Oct3/4, nanog and Sox-2 (Singhatanadgit *et al.*, 2009; Kawanabe *et al.*, 2010). Whether the stem cells isolated from adult human PDL are comparable to bone marrow derived mesenchymal stem cells (BMSC) is still unclear, but it is notable that the putative stem cell marker, STRO-1, used to isolate and purify BMSC, has been shown to be expressed by human PDL cells (Fujii *et al.*, 2008; Xu *et al.*, 2009). In contrast, other reports have suggested that this stem cell-like population residing in adult PDL does not express STRO-1 and may be a more primitive cell population that differs from BMSC (Chen *et al.*, 2006; Singhatanadgit *et al.*, 2009). Nevertheless, adult PDL stem cells share with BMSC the common expression of the perivascular cell marker CD146, alpha-smooth muscle actin and the pericyte-associated antigen 3G5 (Singhatanadgit *et al.*, 2009), suggesting a possible perivascular origin for these cells, as reported previously (McCulloch *et al.*, 1987).

PDL stem cell-like populations have been shown to differentiate into some of the mesoderm-associated lineages (i.e. osteogenic, adipogenic, chondrogenic). Seo *et al.* (2004) isolated PDL 'stem-like' cells using ring-cloning technique (Seo *et al.*, 2004). These were capable of undergoing osteogenesis and to form bone-like mineralised nodules *in vitro* and, moreover, when cultured under adipogenic differentiation conditions, they were also capable of forming lipid-like droplets, a key feature of mature adipocytes *in vitro*. In addition, under chondrogenic differentiation conditions, these cells underwent chondrogenic differentiation, staining positive for proteoglycans (Singhatanadgit *et al.*, 2009; Xu *et al.*, 2009; Amin *et al.*, 2011).

While PDL stem cells have been reported to be able to differentiate to various extents into these three mesenchymal lineages a number of times, 'non-mesenchymal' vasculogenic, angiogenic, neurogenic and gliogenic lineage-associated differentiation capability has recently been studied by Amin (2011). In this study, it was shown that PDL contains cells capable of differentiating into endothelial cells and appears to form aligned angiogenic structures, neuronal cells with apparent bipolar proprioceptive nerve-like morphology and all three types of glial cells (astrocytes, oligodendrocytes and Schwann cells). These non-mesenchymal lineages are of physiological, structural and fundamental importance in the PDL tissue and therefore such wide range of cell plasticity *in vitro* might be useful for further identifying growth factors/biological mediators for 'true' periodontal regeneration (for review see Amin, 2011) (Amin *et al.*, 2011). However, further studies are clearly needed in this area of research.

4.3 Secretion and composition of enamel matrix proteins (EMP)

4.3.1 Secretion of EMP

Enamel, a unique and highly mineralised ectodermal tissue covering vertebrate teeth, is synthesised and secreted by specialised cells called ameloblasts (for review see Amin, 2011). During the process of enamel development ameloblasts secrete EMP that bind to hydroxyapatite to structure the enamel and to modulate crystal growth (Heritier, 1982; Deutsch *et al.*, 1995; Ten Cate, 1996). The secretion of EMP can be observed during three distinct stages of enamel formation: (i) the presecretory stage (Ten Cate, 1996); (ii) the secretory stage (also called the forming stage) (Heritier, 1982); and (iii) the maturing stage (also called the secondary mineralisation stage). Although the major biosynthesis and secretion of EMP has been reported to take place in the secretory stage, full-length amelogenin and its splicing forms (e.g. leucine-rich amelogenin peptide, LRAP), major protein components of EMP, are also secreted in the early presecretory and late maturation stages (Deutsch *et al.*, 1995). In addition to EMP, growth factors such as bone morphogenetic protein (BMP) and transforming growth factor beta (TGF-β) have also been shown to be secreted during enamel development (Heritier, 1982; Deutsch *et al.*, 1995; Ten Cate, 1996). Within hours of secretion, progressive proteolytic clipping of amelogenin peptides has been shown to give rise to breakdown products of amelogenin, and secreted EMP components have also been shown to be gradually degraded by enzymatic digestion (Deutsch *et al.*, 1991, 1995), suggesting that the secretion of EMP components varies between different stages of enamel development.

EMP secreted by ameloblasts has been shown to play a crucial role in enamel formation and biomineralisation (Deutsch *et al.*, 1995). Other findings indicate that EMP also has a function other than enamel development, such as in dentine root formation (Hammarstrom, 1997; Heijl, 1997). The involvement of EMP in root cementum formation was first proposed by Slavkin (1974), who suggested that Hertwig epithelial root sheath (HERS) cells produce a basement membrane containing EMP that directs the induction of cementoblast differentiation from dental follicle cells (Slavkin, 1974). Several hypotheses explaining the role of EMP in root cementum formation have been proposed: (i) it is involved in the attachment of root dentine; (ii) it initiates cementogenesis; and (iii) it serves as an inducer of dental follicle cell differentiation into cementoblasts (Slavkin, 1974). EMP may also have a significant role in periodontal development and regeneration since it has been demonstrated that porcine EMP placed in experimentally created defects on teeth of monkeys led to formation of new cementum and alveolar bone (Hammarstrom *et al.*, 1997).

The major EMP components secreted by ameloblasts, have been partly identified and characterised and comprise the hydrophobic amelogenins, sheathlins, acidic tuftelin, a high molecular weight enamelin and various isoforms of these proteins. However, as described above, the content of EMP varies between different stages of enamel development and it is therefore a possibility that there are also variations between different EMP preparations (for review see Amin, 2011). A commercial product derived from EMP, called enamel matrix derivative (EMD) which has been designated as a FDA approved 'material' for periodontal regeneration since 1997, has been obtained via a rigidly controlled industrial process of purification and heat-treatment of an acidic extract of developing enamel from six-month-old piglets. In this chapter, EMP designation refers to the relatively crude and non-heat-treated mixture of proteins that are obtained from developing porcine enamel, whereas EMD designation refers to the commercially prepared heat-treated lyophilised proteins isolated from porcine enamel during a specific stage of development.

4.3.2 Composition of EMP

The major components of EMP are amelogenins, a family of hydrophobic proteins that accounts for more than 90% of the organic matter in the enamel matrix (Brookes *et al.*, 1995). The amelogenins have been remarkably conserved through evolution, suggesting that they may be of critical biological importance (Brookes *et al.*, 1995). Other abundant 'non-amelogenin' components in EMP include enamelins (Brookes *et al.*, 1995), tuftelin (Deutsch *et al.*, 1991) and sheathlin proteins (Hu *et al.*, 1997b). As shown in Fig. 4.1, these four matrix proteins, amelogenins (Hu *et al.*, 1996), enamelins (Hu *et al.*, 1997a), tuftelin (Deutsch *et al.*, 1991) and sheathlins (also called ameloblastin or amelin) (Hu *et al.*, 1997b) together with two enzymes, matrix metalloproteinase (MMP)-20 and enamel matrix serine proteinase (EMSP)-1 (Fukae and Tanabe, 1987), are present in EMP.

Investigation of possible growth factors in EMP concluded that they were not present in such preparations (Gestrelius *et al.*, 1997), but other studies

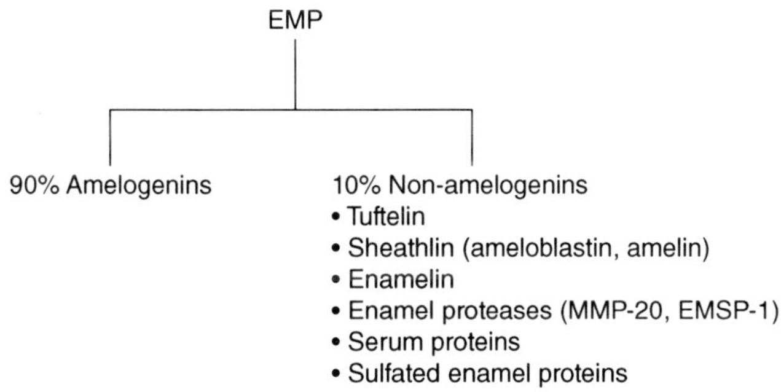

4.1 Composition of enamel matrix proteins (EMPs) (adapted by Amin, 2011).

indicated the presence of low levels of TGF-β1 and BMP-2 (Kawase *et al.*, 2001; Iwata *et al.*, 2002). These growth factors have been shown to be secreted along with EMP during the enamel developmental process (Heritier, 1982; Deutsch *et al.*, 1995; Ten Cate, 1996) and, as noted above, they can also vary between different stages of enamel development.

Amelogenins

Amelogenin is a major protein component of EMD, accounting for approximately 90% of the protein secreted by ameloblasts (Gestrelius *et al.*, 2000). It is a hydrophobic protein, rich in proline, glutamine, leucine and histidine and exhibiting a very high degree of sequence homology (>80%) among the higher vertebrates examined (Fincham *et al.*, 1999). The multiple amelogenin peptides present in EMD are the products of alternative splicing of the amelogenin gene and also of proteolytic processing of the parent proteins. Although the primary transcript of the amelogenin gene is highly conserved between species, the alternative splicing forms vary in number and structure between species. For example, five different splicing variants of amelogenin have been identified in the human, whereas in the mouse there are at least 14 different splicing isoforms. In the pig, four different splicing forms of amelogenins have been identified, each translated into the four corresponding amelogenin peptide isoforms (27, 25, 18 and 6.5 kDa), as shown in Fig. 4.2 (for review see Amin, 2011). The smallest splicing variant is a 6.5 kDa (56-amino acid) leucine-rich amelogenin peptide (LRAP) containing the N-terminal (33 amino acids) and C-terminal (23 amino acids) sequences of the full-length amelogenin (Fincham *et al.*, 1994; Ten Cate, 1996).

The 25 kDa splicing variant of amelogenin is the main source of the majority of the proteolytic products of amelogenin. It is converted either to the 20 kDa amelogenin, which is the most abundant amelogenin in secretory porcine enamel, and in EMD, and to the 23 kDa amelogenin. It has been shown that the 20 kDa amelogenin is further processed proteolytically to 5.3 and 5.1 kDa tyrosine-rich amelogenin peptides (TRAP) (Fincham *et al.*, 1994). The N-terminal of TRAP has been shown to be identical to the N-terminal of the 20 kDa amelogenin. Other pathways of proteolytic degradation of the 18 kDa splicing variant also produce a 5 kDa TRAP as well as additional uncharacterised proteins. All these different forms of amelogenins shown in Fig. 4.2 have been reported to be present in EMD (Fincham *et al.*, 1994), although their precise functions are not yet known.

Non-amelogenins

Enamelin is the largest enamel protein and is concentrated along the secretory face of the ameloblasts. Following secretion by ameloblasts, it is processed to other low-molecular weight proteins associated with progressive enamel mineralisation and is also suggested to have a role in enamel biomineralisation (Brookes *et al.*, 1995).

Tuftelin is an anionic non-amelogenin enamel protein first fully characterised by Deutsch *et al.* (1991). It is expressed as early as the bud stage of tooth development and may be involved in crystal formation of the tooth and also in ameloblast differentiation and/or extracellular matrix secretion (Paine *et al.*, 2000).

Sheathlin (also known as ameloblastin and amelin) represents 5% of the non-amelogenin mRNA and has a domain homologous to the $\alpha2\beta1$ integrin recognition site present in collagen type I (Cerny *et al.*, 1996). It is localised in ameloblasts and in the sheath space in enamel and may have a role in enamel biomineralisation. The sheathlin gene is localised in the region where the autosomal dominant *amelogenesis imperfecta* gene has been identified (Forsman *et al.*, 1994), again suggesting that this protein is important for enamel formation (for review see Amin, 2011).

4.4 Modulation of cell differentiation by EMP and enamel matrix derivatives (EMD) *in vitro*

4.4.1 Mesenchymal lineages

A number of investigations have been carried out to clarify the effects of EMD on bone regeneration (Schwartz *et al.*, 2000; Tokiyasu *et al.*, 2000; Jiang *et al.*, 2001; Ohyama *et al.*, 2002; Yoneda *et al.*, 2003), using several different types of cell *in vitro*. For example, Schwartz *et al.* (2000) showed that EMD induced proliferation and stimulated the osteogenic markers

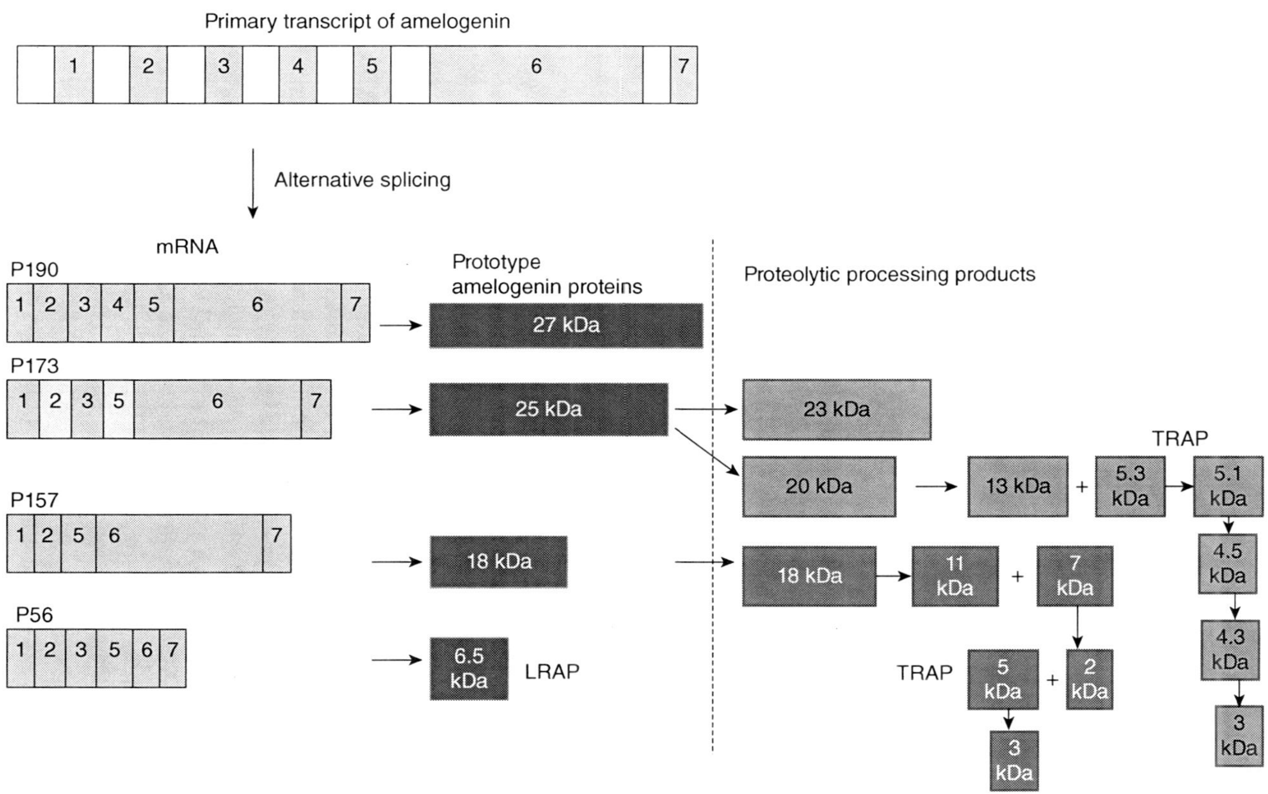

4.2 Schematic diagram of extracellular porcine amelogenin mRNA splicing and proteolytic processing. Numbers in grey boxes represent exons, (adapted by Amin, 2011).

osteocalcin (OC) and alkaline phosphatase (ALP) in a normal human osteoblast cell line although in the same study it was also observed that EMD induced proliferation but suppressed OC and ALP expression of a pre-osteoblast cell line 2T9 (Schwartz *et al.*, 2000). Moreover, it was also shown that EMD suppressed proliferation but induced OC and ALP expression by the osteosarcoma cell line MG63 (Schwartz *et al.*, 2000), whereas it suppressed OC gene expression and mineralisation by the osteoblast and cementoblast cell lines OCT-1 and MC3T3 (Tokiyasu *et al.*, 2000). In addition, EMD enhanced the proliferation of primary osteoblasts but stimulated the bone resorption markers IL-6 and prostaglandin G/H synthase 2, while failing to stimulate OC gene expression (Jiang *et al.*, 2001). The studies noted above clearly indicate discrepancies in the effects of EMD on osteogenic differentiation *in vitro*, possibly because of the use of different cell types, varying culture conditions and varying length of incubation time.

Similarly, in studies of other lineages, it has been shown that the osteogenic and chondrogenic markers (ALP, OC, Col X (type X collagen)) of a pluripotent mesenchymal cell line C2C12 were stimulated by EMD, whereas EMD suppressed the myogenic markers (myoD1 and desmin), indicating that at least some components in EMD were capable of differentially regulating these pathways in C2C12 cells (Ohyama *et al.*, 2002). In contrast, it has also been shown that although EMD increased proliferation of premature chondrocytes, it inhibited chondrogenic differentiation, as measured by ALP activity, and had no measurable effects of collagen synthesis, proteoglycan secretion and TGF-β production (Dean *et al.*, 2002). Another study using pre-chondrocytes also concluded that EMD up-regulated proliferation but failed to increase ALP activity and prostaglandin E_2 (PGE_2) production (Yoneda *et al.*, 2003), again indicating discrepancies in the effects of EMD on chondrogenesis.

Several studies using PDL cells to investigate the effects of EMD on osteogenesis found that it stimulated ALP activity and bone-like nodule formation under growth as well as differentiation conditions (Gestrelius *et al.*, 1997; Van der Pauw *et al.*, 2000). Similarly, in a study by Nagano *et al.* (2004), expression of ALP mRNA and ALP activity were dose-dependently increased when PDL cells were treated with EMD under growth conditions (Nagano *et al.*, 2004). In contrast, Cattaneo *et al.* (2003) observed a lack of ALP activity stimulation in human PDL cells cultured on EMD-coated tissue culture dishes (Cattaneo *et al.*, 2003). Hakki *et al.* (2001) showed that EMD suppressed OC gene expression and blocked mineralisation of murine dental follicle cells under differentiation conditions *in vitro* (Hakki *et al.*, 2001). Thus, in some cases EMD appeared to stimulate osteogenic marker genes and terminal osteogenic differentiation, indicating the possible presence of osteoinductive component(s) in EMD. However, other contradictory results have demonstrated the lack of consistency between studies of the effects of EMD on osteogenic differentiation, possibly due to differences in cell type and varying experimental conditions.

Because of the discrepancies observed in the responses of PDL and other bone-forming cells *in vitro*, several attempts have been made to fractionate freshly isolated porcine EMP in order to evaluate the specific component which could have osteoinductive activity. Iwata *et al.* (2002) fractionated EMP from developing porcine teeth and reported that the osteoinductive fraction contained mainly 20 kDa proteins. This fraction enhanced ALP activity and mineralised nodule formation, and up-regulated OC, BSP and ALP gene expression in the mouse bone marrow stromal cell line ST2. However, the methodology used in this study could not exclude the possibility that the osteoinductive fraction might contain additional low-molecular weight amelogenins and other proteins. In addition, crude extracts of EMP derived from developing pigs are known to contain growth factors such as BMPs and TGF-β, which may have also contributed to the osteoinductive effects observed in this report (Iwata *et al.*, 2002). Nagano *et al.* (2006) used crude EMP fractions to look at osteogenic differentiation by ST2 cells and concluded that the crude EMP contained TGF-β1, again demonstrating the importance of using more purified EMP components to examine biological activity (Nagano *et al.*, 2006). There is therefore a need for less heterogeneous and more consistent preparations of EMP, such as EMD, in order to understand the mechanism(s) by which specific components influence PDL cell differentiation *in vitro* and may lead to successful regeneration of damaged periodontal tissues *in vivo*.

4.4.2 Non-mesenchymal lineages

Periodontal ligament comprises primarily fibroblasts, osteoblasts and osteoclasts and has recently also been reported to contain a progenitor/stem cell-like population that can undergo multilineage differentiation, as described above (Nagano *et al.*, 2006; Tomokiyo *et al.*, 2007; Huang *et al.*, 2008; Cheng *et al.*, 2009; Singhatanadgit *et al.*, 2009; Xu *et al.*, 2009; Amin, 2011). The homeostasis, repair and regeneration of PDL tissue are considered to be dependent on such progenitor cells and also the appropriate biological mediators and a sufficient blood supply (Cochran and Wozney, 1999; Molloy *et al.*, 2003; Taba *et al.*, 2005; Huang *et al.*, 2008; Cheng *et al.*, 2009). Thus, growth factors, cytokines and morphogens have been shown to modulate the proliferation and differentiation of PDL cells and the production of extracellular matrix (ECM) *in vitro* (Karring *et al.*, 1993; Cochran and Wozney, 1999; Molloy *et al.*, 2003; Messenger *et al.*, 2007; Huang *et al.*, 2008; Cheng *et al.*, 2009), while new vascular networks formed by progenitor cells ensure the supply of sufficient blood for repair/wound healing of damaged PDL and the regeneration of healthy new tissue *in vivo* (Brey *et al.*, 2005; Taba *et al.*, 2005).

It is now recognised that blood vessel (BV) formation, the complex process of neo-vasculogenesis, comprises both vasculogenic and angiogenic differentiation during adult wound healing as well as in developing micro-environments (Flamme *et al.*, 1997; Brey *et al.*, 2005). The former process, vasculogenesis, the differentiation of progenitor/stem cells into endothelial cells (Flamme *et al.*, 1997; Brey *et al.*, 2005; Demir *et al.*, 2007) and the latter, angiogenesis, the development of an organised network of tubular structures originating from endothelial precursors (D'Amore and Thompson, 1987; Flamme *et al.*, 1997; Brey *et al.*, 2005), are regulated *in vitro* and *in vivo* by a number of biological mediators, including vascular endothelial growth factor (VEGF), platelet-derived growth factor (PDGF), insulin-like growth factor (IGF), transforming growth factor-beta (TGF-β), basic fibroblast growth factor (bFGF) and epidermal growth factor (EGF) (Lynch *et al.*, 1991; Cochran and Wozney, 1999; Nomi *et al.*, 2002; Molloy *et al.*, 2003; Brey *et al.*, 2005; Pandya *et al.*, 2006) and also by enamel matrix proteins (EMP) (Messenger *et al.*, 2007; Schlueter *et al.*, 2007; Bertl *et al.*, 2009; Johnson *et al.*, 2009; Kauvar *et al.*, 2010).

Several clinical studies carried out to evaluate the effects of EMP and EMD on periodontal soft tissue wound healing have led to a number of discrepancies (Wennstrom and Lindhe, 2002; Hagenaars *et al.*, 2004). For example, periodontal wounds treated topically with EMP exhibited rapid and complete healing, compared with the control sites that were not treated with EMP which exhibited only partial healing (Wennstrom and Lindhe, 2002). In contrast, it was shown that the test patient group treated with EMD exhibited only partial healing, similar to the control group that did not receive EMD (Hagenaars *et al.*, 2004). The reason(s) for this discrepancy are not known, but it may be at least partly due to lack of sufficient blood supply, that is differences in BV formation activity/neovasculogenic activity.

A number of attempts have therefore been made *in vitro* to understand these apparent clinical discrepancies by examining the effects of EMD on angiogenic differentiation *in vitro*. However, such studies have been limited because some have used freshly isolated and non-heat treated EMP while others have used commercially prepared and heat-treated EMD (Yuan *et al.*, 2003; Schlueter *et al.*, 2007; Bertl *et al.*, 2009; Johnson *et al.*, 2009; Thoma *et al.*, 2011). For example, while freshly extracted EMP has been found to strongly stimulate migration/chemotaxis and formation of a tubular network of human microvascular endothelial cells (HMVEC) *in vitro* (Yuan *et al.*, 2003; Johnson *et al.*, 2009), both Schlueter *et al.* (2007) and Bertl *et al.* (2009) showed that commercially prepared EMD did not induce HMVEC migration/chemotaxis in an *in vitro* monolayer cell wound healing assay (Schlueter *et al.*, 2007; Bertl *et al.*, 2009). Since the components of EMP preparations are likely to vary qualitatively and quantitatively, a number of attempts have also been made to delineate the specific protein fractions in freshly isolated (and non-heat-treated) EMP and commercially prepared EMD that have angiogenic activity (Johnson *et al.*, 2009; Thoma *et al.*, 2011). For example, Johnson *et al.* (2009) examined the effects of EMP fractions on HMVEC angiogenesis *in vitro* and observed that both low and high molecular weight fractions stimulate chemotaxis and tube formation of HMVEC, but the EMP fractions used contained proteins of differing sizes, with all the fractions containing some low molecular weight peptides. In addition, Thoma *et al.* (2011) examined the effects of EMD in a murine angiogenesis model *in vivo* and reported that both the low (<6 KDa) and high (<15 kDa) molecular weight fractions of heat-treated EMD exhibited angiogenic activity, but could not identify specific component(s). Again, low molecular weight proteins were found to be present in all the fractions isolated from EMD (Thoma *et al.*, 2011) indicating that discrepancies in the effects of EMP and EMD on angiogenesis *in vitro* and *in vivo* could be associated with the use of heterogeneous fractions whose components could have differential effects on angiogenesis.

There is therefore a need for less heterogeneous and more consistent preparations of EMP/EMD, in order to understand the mechanism(s) by which specific components influence PDL cell differentiation *in vitro* and may lead to successful regeneration of damaged periodontal soft and hard tissue and BV *in vivo*.

4.5 *In vivo* studies (for bone regeneration)

The osteoinductive activity of EMD has been examined using immune-deficient (nude) mice in a heterotopic (outside the skeletal tissue) bone formation model (Boyan *et al.*, 2000; Kawana *et al.*, 2001). Although no bone formation was observed when EMD alone (used at a significantly higher concentration (4 mg) than the recommended concentration for clinical use (300 μg) was implanted into muscle, when the same amount of EMD was implanted together with osteoinductive demineralised freeze-dried bone allograft (DFDBA), enhanced bone stimulation was observed compared with the osteoinductive DFDBA alone. These results thus indicated that high concentrations of EMD might increase the osteoinductive properties of the bone graft material. In contrast, a study evaluating the osteoinductive properties of EMD and deproteinised bovine bone mineral (DBBM) in the muscle of rats reported that EMD alone, DBBM alone or both combined did not stimulate bone (Donos *et al.*, 2006). The lack of osteogenic potential of EMD has also been demonstrated in two established preclinical models of bone regeneration (Donos *et al.*, 2004b, 2005), again indicating the inconsistent effects of EMD on bone regeneration, possibly due to varying experimental conditions including different preclinical models/defects, varying age and healing conditions.

4.6 Treatment of periodontal osseous defects with enamel matrix derivatives

4.6.1 Intrabony defects: Preclinical and clinical studies

Intrabony defects are defined as vertical periodontal breakdown characterised by the apical location of the base of the pocket with respect to the residual alveolar crest. These defects whose intrabony component affects one tooth are classified according to their morphology in terms of the residual bony walls and the width of the defect (or radiographic angle). Based on the number of residual bony walls, the defects are defined as three-wall, two-wall and one-wall defects. Frequently enough, after flap elevation, the defects are shown to have a more complex anatomy presenting a three-wall component at the apical portion and a two- or one-wall component at the cervical portion of the defect (Lang, 2000; Karring and Lindhe, 2008).

The effectiveness of EMD in periodontal regeneration has been evaluated in preclinical studies (Hammarstrom *et al.*, 1997; Sculean *et al.*, 2002) and clinical trials (Sculean *et al.*, 2003; Aspriello *et al.*, 2011) using different experimental designs. EMD has been proved to create an environment favourable for periodontal regeneration when applied to the treatment of intrabony defects.

In vivo studies

In a number of preclinical studies, the use of EMD had resulted predictably in significant amounts of regenerated cementum with inserting collagen fibres (Sculean *et al.*, 2000b; Cochran *et al.*, 2003). More specifically, in the defects treated with EMD the formation of new acellular cementum was observed at the apical (lower) part of the defect and a mixed acellular and cellular cementum at the more coronal part of the defect (Sculean *et al.*, 2000b). The collagen fibres were perpendicularly oriented to the root surface inserting into the newly formed cementum. The results demonstrated that periodontal regeneration occurred to a varying extent in the defects treated with EMD and/or GTR, while the control defects healed by long junctional epithelium and limited periodontal regeneration in the bottom of the defect. Although research data provide evidence that EMD promotes periodontal regeneration, the underlying biological process is not yet fully understood or evident from these studies. In another preclinical study it has been shown that the application of EMD to reimplanted roots that have been extracted and deprived of vital cementoblasts was characterised by processes that included root resorption and ankylosis (Araujo *et al.*, 2003). Thus, the authors noted that in these experimental conditions, EMD was unable to 'protect' the root from resorption and had no effect on cell migration and cell repopulation of the instrumented root surface.

In conclusion, it could be suggested that preclinical studies provide evidence that periodontal regeneration of intrabony defects might be successfully attempted by the EMD treatment approach (for review see Bosshardt, 2008; Bosshardt and Sculean, 2009).

Clinical safety of EMD use

The clinical adverse reactions, immune compatibility and allergic reactions that could be attributed to EMD application have been evaluated (Zetterstrom *et al.*, 1997; Heard *et al.*, 2000; Nikolopoulos *et al.*, 2002; Froum *et al.*, 2004). In a study performed in 10 Swedish specialist clinics with a test group of 107 patients treated repeatedly with EMD in conjunction with periodontal surgery (Zetterstrom *et al.*, 1997), none of the blood samples from treated patients, not even from allergy prone patients after two treatments, indicated deviations from the normal ranges established for a control group of blood donors matched for gender, age and frequency of smoking. Furthermore, EMD is well tolerated by the immune system of the host even one year after the application (Nikolopoulos *et al.*, 2002). In a multicentre study, where the potential for sensitisation to EMD was evaluated in 376 periodontally affected patients treated at least twice with a period of two months between treatments, no clinical adverse reactions were noted (Froum *et al.*, 2004).

Clinical studies

The clinical efficacy of EMD in the treatment of intrabony defects is well documented. Reduction of pocket depth (PD), clinical attachment (CAL) gain and bone filling of the intrabony component of the defect have been confirmed by a series of controlled clinical studies and case reports.

EMD in combination with different types of periodontal flaps

The earliest study conducted to evaluate clinically the treatment of one- and two-wall intrabony defects with EMD compared the long-term effect of EMD treatment as an adjunct to modified Widman flap (MWF) to the effect of MWF and placebo (Heijl *et al.*, 1997). The sites treated with EMD demonstrated significantly better effectiveness of the MWF with the adjunctive use of EMD compared to MWF alone. CAL gain (2.2 mm) and bone level gain (66% defect fill) at the EMD-treated sites after 36 months were characterised as predictable and clinically relevant.

The additional application of EMD in the surgical treatment of intrabony defects was compared to placebo or open flap debridement (OFD) (Pontoriero *et al.*, 1999; Okuda *et al.*, 2000; Froum *et al.*, 2001; Rosing *et al.*, 2005; Chambrone *et al.*, 2010a), to the MWF (Heijl *et al.*, 1997; Silvestri *et al.*, 2000) and to a simplified papilla preservation flap (SPPF) technique (Tonetti *et al.*, 2002; Wachtel *et al.*, 2003; Francetti *et al.*, 2004; Francetti *et al.*, 2005; Fickl *et al.*, 2009). These studies have shown that the use of EMD resulted in significantly more favourable clinical improvement in intrabony periodontal defects (Okuda *et al.*, 2000) and the average percentage of defect fill was more than three times greater for EMD versus control-treated sites (Froum *et al.*, 2001). On the other hand, in one study the use of EMD did not result in more improvement in clinical and radiographic parameters compared to placebo (Rosing *et al.*, 2005).

In a multicentre randomised controlled clinical trial, the treatment of intrabony defects with SPPF surgery with or without application of EMD was studied (Tonetti *et al.*, 2002). One hundred and seventy-two patients with at least one intrabony defect of ≥3 mm were recruited in 12 centres in seven countries. The average CAL gain observed in the test group was 3.1 ± 1.5 mm. The authors noted that the probability of obtaining CAL gains of ≥3 mm following application of EMD was improved in non-smokers and in defects with a predominantly three-wall anatomy. Moreover, EMD combined with SPPF led to a significant improvement in PD and radiographic bone fill compared to OFD and SPPF alone (Wachtel *et al.*, 2003; Fickl *et al.*, 2009) and an enhanced periodontal regeneration rate (Francetti *et al.*, 2004). Furthermore, periodontal pockets with an initial depth of ≥6 mm showed major improvement when treated with EMD (Francetti *et al.*, 2005).

EMD versus guided tissue regeneration (GTR)

The treatment of intrabony defects with EMD was also compared to guided tissue regeneration (GTR) (Pontoriero *et al.*, 1999; Sculean *et al.*, 1999a; Sculean *et al.*, 2001b; Minabe *et al.*, 2002; Windisch *et al.*, 2002; Zucchelli *et al.*, 2002; Silvestri *et al.*, 2003; Sanz *et al.*, 2004; Cortellini and Tonetti, 2005; Crea *et al.*, 2008). In a prospective, randomised, controlled clinical trial, 40 patients were included who presented an intrabony component of the defect (as assessed in radiographs) ≥3 mm (Pontoriero *et al.*, 1999). The patients were divided into four groups and were treated with either EMD or GTR with a non-resorbable membrane or GTR with two different resorbable membranes. After 12 months, the findings demonstrated that all regenerative modalities enhanced probing pocket depth and probing attachment gain. The combined treatment of intrabony defects performed by EMD+GTR did not seem to improve the outcome of the regenerative procedure (Sculean *et al.*, 1999a, 2001b; Minabe *et al.*, 2002). A statistically greater amount of CAL gain was demonstrated in the GTR-treated sites compared to EMD-treated sites and the two surgical procedures were found to be almost equally satisfactory in terms of efficacy; however EMD treatment was recommended especially for the resolution of deep defects in aesthetically sensitive sites as a more simple, less risky and less invasive technique (Zucchelli *et al.*, 2002).

In a multicentre study including 98 patients with interproximal intrabony defects of PD ≥6 mm and an intrabony component ≥4 mm, the application of EMD was compared to GTR (Silvestri *et al.*, 2003). No statistically significant difference between GTR and EMD treatments in terms of CAL gain, PD reduction and recession variation was found, whereas the statistical analysis revealed a strong correlation between CAL gain and a full mouth bleeding score, and between CAL gain and defect morphology and depth in both groups. Similarly, the results of a prospective multicentre, randomised, controlled clinical trial that compared the clinical outcomes of EMD to GTR failed to demonstrate superiority of one treatment modality over the other, after 12 months (Sanz *et al.*, 2004). The CAL gain for the EMD group was 3.1 ± 1.8 mm compared with 2.5 ± 1.9 mm for the GTR group and PD reduction was 3.8 ± 1.5 mm and 3.3 ± 1.5 mm, respectively. According to the authors, the results were influenced by the high frequency of post-operative complications; in the GTR group 100% of cases had at least one complication, while in the EMD group the incidence was 6%. The absence of complications was related to a 0.85 mm greater CAL gain.

Combination of EMD and bone grafts

EMD formulation has a fluid consistency which is related to limitations in the use of the material. Thus, combining EMD with bone grafts was suggested in order to overcome the fact that in deep and not self-contained defects viscous EMD does not support the flap. The effectiveness of EMD combined with bovine porous bone mineral (BPBM) compared to OFD in the treatment of intrabony defects was evaluated in a split-mouth design study. Statistically and clinically significant results were obtained by the EMD+BPBM treatment compared to OFD alone. Surgical re-entry of the defects at six months revealed a significantly greater amount of defect fill in favour of the experimental sites (Camargo *et al.*, 2001). In a controlled clinical trial, the sites treated with EMD+BPBM showed improved clinical and radiographic outcomes compared to sites treated with EMD alone

(Zucchelli *et al.*, 2003). The findings were attributed to the ability of space maintenance of the graft to optimise the space available for regeneration.

The adjunctive use of DFDBA to EMD led to greater bone fill and percentage of bone fill (50% and 90%) and less crestal resorption (Gurinsky *et al.*, 2004), although, the combination of EMD with a bioactive glass did not seem additionally to improve the clinical results (Sculean *et al.*, 2005). Furthermore, according to the results from a multicentre randomised controlled study, the treatment of wide (≥2 mm) and deep (≥4 mm) intrabony defects with EMD cannot be improved by the additional use of a synthetic bone graft (Meyle *et al.*, 2011).

Minimally invasive surgical technique (MIST)

A minimally invasive surgical technique (MIST) was proposed to reduce surgical trauma, to increase wound stability, to reduce surgical time and to minimise intra- and post-operative patient discomfort (Harrel, 1999; Cortellini *et al.*, 2009). The healing response to EMD combined with MIST was evaluated in isolated deep two- or three-wall intrabony defects (Cortellini *et al.*, 2009) and led to significant reduction in probing depths and improvements in attachment levels and to little or no increase of gingival recession (Harrel *et al.*, 2005). These results remained stable for more than six years (Harrel *et al.*, 2010). In contrast, others reported that the use of EMD did not provide superior benefits for the outcome of the MIST approach for the treatment of intrabony defects (Ribeiro *et al.*, 2011).

Human histological data from the treatment of intrabony defects with EMD

The ultimate proof for a biomaterial that fulfils the requirements for a true periodontal regeneration is human histological studies. Histological data from studies in humans imply the potential of EMD to promote periodontal regeneration by the formation of new cementum which can be acellular (Heijl, 1997; Mellonig, 1999), cellular (Sculean *et al.*, 1999b) or both (Yukna and Mellonig, 2000; Bosshardt *et al.*, 2006). The earliest histological evidence derived from a study that assessed the application of EMD in one human experimental defect (Heijl, 1997). In this acute surgically created defect, periodontal healing was characterised by the formation of acellular cementum firmly attached to the underlying dentin surface with an associated periodontal ligament and alveolar bone. It was assumed that the use of EMD adjunctive to periodontal surgery may provide the matrix proteins necessary to induce a cementoblast phenotype expression on the cells that chemotactically colonise the intrabony defect area and root surface (Heijl,

1997; Mellonig, 1999). In a study where human biopsies of teeth presenting hopeless prognosis were treated with EMD, GTR or OFD and following treatment they were histologically evaluated, it was demonstrated that the quality of periodontal regeneration in terms of new cementum with inserting fibres was qualitatively similar for GTR and EMD and occupied a large surface of the denuded root surface (Sculean *et al.*, 2000a). However, the cementum in the EMD treated defects was not acellular but rather of a mixed cellular/acellular nature.

In order to clarify whether the newly formed mineralised tissue is more cementum-like or more bone-like, a study was designed on human periodontally affected teeth scheduled for extraction (Bosshardt *et al.*, 2006). In this study, the ultrastructural evaluation of the samples revealed a combination of bone-like and cellular intrinsic fibre cementum characteristics (CIFC) in the newly formed tissues, while the immunohistochemical results suggested that the mineralisation pattern resembled bone more than CIFC.

In conclusion, the histological findings of the studies provide evidence that the EMD treatment approach to intrabony defects might lead to regenerative response by the formation of new cementum, new alveolar bone and perpendicularly oriented/inserting collagen fibres.

Conclusion

The application of EMD to the treatment of intrabony defects is documented by a variety of clinical studies; although the underlying biological mechanism of its action is not yet well clarified. From the published research evidence it might be assumed that the treatment of intrabony defects with EMD might be proposed over GTR when the surgical site is not easily accessible, the surgical manipulation is rather difficult and a small band of keratinised tissue exists; furthermore, challenges due to anatomical reasons or defect characteristics such as inability to fix the membrane or to cover it completely with soft tissue could be overcome with the use of EMD. In a recent meta-analysis of randomised controlled trials, additional benefits for EMD in conjunction with bone grafts or barrier membranes in the treatment of intrabony defects were not found, whereas EMD achieved better treatment outcomes compared to OFD (Tu *et al.*, 2010).

4.6.2 Furcation defects: Preclinical and clinical studies

The lesions within the interradicular area of multi-rooted teeth are defined as furcation involvements and are classified as degree I, II and III according to the extent of horizontal loss of periodontal support in relation to the width of the tooth. The presence of furcation involvement in a multi-rooted tooth constitutes a risk for tooth loss, even when patients are well-maintained (Hirschfeld and Wasserman, 1978; McFall, 1982; Goldman *et al.*, 1986; Wood *et al.*, 1989; Wang *et al.*, 1994; McGuire and Nunn, 1996a, 1996b). Therefore, a number of treatment modalities have been used in the past for the resolution of the furcation defects. However, none of these techniques result in predictable periodontal regeneration.

Mandibular molars

There are not many preclinical or clinical studies in the literature where EMD has been used for the treatment of mandibular degree II furcation involvement. In an investigation in experimental animals (Regazzini *et al.*, 2004), the use of EMD alone or in combination with GTR was evaluated in surgically created degree II furcation involvements. EMD has been proved suitable for regeneration of buccal degree II furcation involvement resulting in 67% new bone formation and 94% new cementum while the combined approach with GTR resulted in compromised healing owing to the exposure of the membranes.

Clinical studies

In terms of clinical trials there is still not a large number of studies where EMD has been used for the treatment of degree II mandibular furcation involvements. In a case series study with 36 months follow-up, the use of EMD in both buccal and lingual furcation involvements was evaluated (Donos *et al.*, 2003a). At the buccal furcation defects, a mean change in the probing attachment level in the horizontal direction (PAL-H) of 1.4 ± 1.2 mm was demonstrated at six months while the change was reduced to 0.8 ± 1.2 and 0.6 ± 1.4 mm at 12 and 36 months, respectively, and as such the PAL-H changes were not adequate to transform the degree II furcation involvement to degree I. At the lingual sites, the PAL-H changes were minimal.

A multicentre randomised controlled clinical trial was performed comparing EMD and GTR in the treatment of degree II buccal furcation defects in mandibular molars. EMD demonstrated a median reduction of PAL-H of 2.8 mm whereas the GTR treated sites showed a reduction of 1.8 mm. Complete furcation closure was achieved in 8/45 furcation defects treated with EMD and at 3/45 defects treated with GTR. Partial closure (change from degree II to degree I) was the same in both groups (27/45). The results indicated that both regenerative procedures led predictably to clinical improvement. Furthermore, following the use of EMD there was less post-operative pain and swelling reported which could be explained by the antibacterial (Sculean *et al.*, 2001a) or anti-inflammatory potential that EMD might possess (Myhre *et al.*, 2006).

Maxillary molars

In a double-blind randomised controlled clinical trial with a split-mouth design, the use of EMD for the treatment of proximal degree II furcation involvements of maxillary molars was compared to OFD in conjunction with conditioning of the root surfaces with EDTA gel (Casarin *et al.*, 2008). At six months, a statistically significant difference in the number of remaining degree II furcation involvements in favour of EMD was observed. Of 15 proximal degree II furcations, following EMD application, two were completely closed and nine converted into degree I. In contrast, in the OFD group, five furcations were converted into degree I, while all the remaining 10 defects remained degree II.

Conclusion

Clinical improvement in buccal degree II furcation defects of mandibular molars could be achieved with the use of EMD. However, the EMD application might lead to complete resolution in the minority of the cases. The selection of the case is of paramount importance; defect associated factors such as the defect size (Klinge *et al.*, 1981; Pontoriero *et al.*, 1988, 1992), the presence of proximal bone to the level of fornix and the thickness/biotype and amount of keratinised tissues should be considered. Furthermore, patient-related factors such as oral hygiene and smoking should also be evaluated. Currently, the available results do not encourage the use of EMD for the treatment of lingual degree II mandibular molar furcation defects. There is some evidence indicating that the use of EMD in maxillary molars might result in conversion of degree II furcation involvements to degree I which could be important in terms of the future prognosis of the tooth.

4.6.3 Treatment of degree III furcation involvement in mandibular molars

Periodontal regeneration of degree III furcation involvements is doubtful owing to the anatomical characteristics and the amount of tissue destruction that is usually present in this type of defect. The complete closure of degree III furcation involvements with GTR is unpredictable (for review see Karring and Cortellini, 1999) and the clinical outcome is often related to the size of the entrance of the defect (Pontoriero *et al.*, 1989, 1992), the height of the defect and the complete flap coverage of the membrane during the healing period (Lindhe *et al.*, 1995).

Preclinical studies

Araujo and Lindhe (1998) performed the first study in a preclinical model evaluating the effect of EMD in combination with GTR in degree III furcation defects (Araujo and Lindhe, 1998). After four months of healing, it was histologically observed that the central portion of both test and control furcation defects was closed and the relative amounts of mineralised bone, bone marrow and periodontal ligament were similar in both control (GTR) and test (GTR+EMD) sites. However, the new cementum was of a cellular nature at the control sites whereas at the test sites a thin acellular cementum at the apical portion of the defect and a thick cellular cementum at the coronal portion of the defect were present. The authors suggested that EMD, when combined with GTR, might have the potential to promote formation of acellular cementum.

Similar outcomes were reported in another preclinical study with a similar design (Donos *et al.*, 2003b) at the sites that were treated with GTR alone or combination of GTR and EMD. However, the application of EMD alone resulted in unpredictable amounts of regenerated periodontal tissues and newly formed bone. At the sites that were treated only with EMD or a combination of GTR and EMD, the cementum was characterised apically as acellular extrinsic fibre and coronally as mixed stratified (Gkranias *et al.*, 2012).

Clinical studies

There is only one case series study in a limited number of patients where the treatment of degree III mandibular furcation defects was evaluated following the use of EMD alone or in combination with a bioresorbable membrane (Donos *et al.*, 2004a). No obvious difference between the various treatment modalities was observed. Within the limits of this case series study it can be suggested that the use of EMD alone or in combination with GTR does not result in a predictable regeneration of degree III mandibular defects.

Conclusion

EMD can be used for the treatment of degree II buccal furcation involvements. However, the available evidence does not support the use of EMD either in lingual degree II or degree III furcation defects in mandibular or maxillary molars.

4.6.4 Recession defects: preclinical and clinical studies

Gingival recession is defined as the periodontal defect in which 'location of marginal periodontal tissues apical to the cemento-enamel junction' is clinically observed (AAP, 2001). In many cases, localised gingival recessions and root exposure represent not only an aesthetic problem for the patient but also a functional one because of the accompanied root sensitivity and reduction of the keratinised tissue band. It has been suggested that anatomic factors, mechanical trauma, iatrogenic factors and periodontal disease are associated with the development of the gingival recessions (Wennstrom, 1996).

According to the classification proposed by Miller (1985), gingival recessions are divided in four categories considering the root coverage that could be possibly obtained: (i) class I: marginal tissue recession not extending to the mucogingival junction; no loss of interdental bone or soft tissue, (ii) class II: marginal tissue recession extends to or beyond the mucogingival junction; no loss of interdental bone or soft tissue, (iii) class III: marginal tissue recession extends to or beyond the mucogingival junction; loss of interdental bone or soft tissue is apical to the cemento-enamel junction, but coronal to the apical extent of the marginal tissue recession and (iv) class IV: marginal tissue recession extends beyond the mucogingival junction; loss of interdental bone extends to a level apical to the extent of the marginal tissue recession (Miller, 1985). Complete root coverage can be achieved in class I and II defects, partial coverage in class III, while class IV defects are not amenable to root coverage (Wennstrom, 1996; Wennstrom *et al.*, 2008).

A variety of surgical techniques for the treatment of recession defects have been proposed which include rotational flaps (laterally sliding flap, double papilla flap and oblique rotated flap), advanced flap procedures (coronally advanced and semilunar coronally advanced flap) and free soft tissue graft procedures (epithelialised graft or subepithelial connective tissue graft). The grafts are harvested from the palate resulting in an additional wound area and increased morbidity of the patient. Regenerative procedures aiming at root coverage and new connective tissue attachment are also applied involving the placement of a barrier membrane or the application of EMD (Wennstrom *et al.*, 2008).

The ultimate goal of recession treatment is the complete coverage of the root and the new connective tissue attachment. In this context, several clinical studies assessing the application of EMD in the treatment of recessions with conflicting results have been published while a limited number of histological data proving the nature of attachment are available.

Preclinical and human biopsies

The nature of the attachment following treatment of gingival recessions was investigated in human biopsies (Rasperini *et al.*, 2000; Carnio *et al.*, 2002; McGuire and Cochran, 2003) and animal studies (de Oliveira *et al.*, 2005; Fujita *et al.*, 2011). Evidence of formation of new cementum, islands of new woven bone and new collagen fibres inserting into the new cementum was found in the histological evaluation of denuded root surfaces treated with either coronally advanced flap (CAF)+EMD (McGuire and Cochran, 2003) or subepithelial connective tissue graft (SCTG)+EMD (Rasperini *et al.*, 2000; Carnio *et al.*, 2002). It was of interest that long junctional epithelium was minimal, implying that EMD may act on epithelial cells by inhibiting their proliferation and migration.

Clinical studies

An overall estimation of the treatment findings of the studies comparing the combination of CAF with EMD to CAF alone leads to conflicting outcomes. Clinical trials demonstrated that CAF+EMD increases the percentage of root coverage and significantly improves the width of keratinised tissue when applied to the treatment of class I and II recession defects (Cueva *et al.*, 2004; Spahr *et al.*, 2005; Castellanos *et al.*, 2006; Pilloni *et al.*, 2006). A systematic review (Cheng *et al.*, 2007) and a meta-analysis (Cairo *et al.*, 2008) also confirmed that EMD in conjunction with CAF enhances the probability of obtaining complete root coverage and more keratinised tissue in apico-coronal dimensions (Chambrone *et al.*, 2010b) compared to CAF alone.

Furthermore, the potential of EMD in the treatment of recessions has also been compared to SCTG. The application of EMD was superior to SCTG in terms of early healing and patient morbidity, whereas with regard to percentage of root coverage the results showed that both procedures had a similar clinical outcome (McGuire and Nunn, 2003) or showed superiority of SCTG over EMD (Nemcovsky *et al.*, 2004; Moses *et al.*, 2006). The additional application of EMD to SCTG did not lead to statistically significant differences between the control and test group (Berlucchi *et al.*, 2002), while a decreased root coverage was also observed (Gunay *et al.*, 2008). In a recent multicentre study, the combination of EMD+SCTG was compared to SCTG alone providing evidence that the additional use of EMD does not produce a beneficial clinical outcome in terms of root coverage (Rasperini *et al.*, 2011).

Conclusion

There is conflicting evidence concerning the clinical benefit of EMD in the treatment of Miller class I and II recession defects. Two recent systematic reviews revealed that EMD in conjunction with CAF procedure enhances the probability of obtaining complete root coverage and improving recession reduction (Cairo *et al.*, 2008; Chambrone *et al.*, 2010b). It has also been demonstrated that EMD may prevent long junctional epithelium healing and promote periodontal regeneration.

4.7 Acknowledgement

Sections of this chapter describing EMP/EMD compositions and the effects of these proteins on precursor cell differentiation pathways have been extracted and modified from the PhD thesis of one of the co-authors (Amin, 2011) with his approval.

4.8 References

AAP (2001), *Glossary of Periodontal Terms*, The American Academy of Periodontology, USA.

Amin HD (2011). *Effects of Enamel Matrix Derivative Components on PDL Cell Differentiation.* Doctoral thesis, University College London.

Amin HD, Olsen I, Knowles J and Donos N (2011), 'A procedure for identifying stem cell compartments with multi-lineage differentiation potential', *Analyst*, **136**, 1440–9.

Araujo MG and Lindhe J (1998), 'GTR treatment of degree III furcation defects following application of enamel matrix proteins. An experimental study in dogs', *J Clin Periodontol*, **25**, 524–30.

Araujo M, Hayacibara R, Sonohara M, Cardaropoli G and Lindhe J (2003), 'Effect of enamel matrix proteins (Emdogain') on healing after re-implantation of "periodontally compromised" roots. An experimental study in the dog', *J Clin Periodontol*, **30**, 855–61.

Asahara T, Murohara T, Sullivan A, Silver M, van der Zee R, Li T, Witzenbichler B, Schatteman G and Isner JM (1997), 'Isolation of putative progenitor endothelial cells for angiogenesis', *Science*, **275**, 964–7.

Aspriello SD, Zizzi A, Spazzafumo L, Rubini C, Lorenzi T, Marzioni D, Bullon P and Piemontese M (2011), 'Effects of enamel matrix derivative on vascular endothelial growth factor expression and microvessel density in gingival tissues of periodontal pocket: a comparative study', *J Periodontol*, **82**, 606–12.

Barnett SC and Chang L (2004), 'Olfactory ensheathing cells and CNS repair: going solo or in need of a friend?', *Trends Neurosci*, **27**, 54–60.

Berlucchi I, Francetti L, Del Fabbro M, Testori T and Weinstein RL (2002), 'Enamel matrix proteins (Emdogain) in combination with coronally advanced flap or subepithelial connective tissue graft in the treatment of shallow gingival recessions', *Int J Periodontics Restorative Dent*, **22**, 583–93.

Bertl K, An N, Bruckmann C, Dard M, Andrukhov O, Matejka M and Rausch-Fan X (2009), 'Effects of enamel matrix derivative on proliferation/viability, migration, and expression of angiogenic factor and adhesion molecules in endothelial cells *in vitro*', *J Periodontol*, **80**, 1622–30.

Bosshardt DD (2008), 'Biological mediators and periodontal regeneration: a review of enamel matrix proteins at the cellular and molecular levels', *J Clin Periodontol*, **35**, 87–105.

Bosshardt DD and Sculean A (2009), 'Does periodontal tissue regeneration really work?', *Periodontology 2000*, **51**, 208–19.

Bosshardt DD, Sculean A, Donos N and Lang NP (2006), 'Pattern of mineralization after regenerative periodontal therapy with enamel matrix proteins', *Eur J Oral Sci*, **114** (Suppl 1), 225–31; discussion 254–26, 381–222.

Boyan BD, Weesner TC, Lohmann CH, Andreacchio D, Carnes DL, Dean DD, Cochran DL and Schwartz Z (2000), 'Porcine fetal enamel matrix derivative enhances bone formation induced by demineralized freeze dried bone allograft *in vivo*', *J Periodontol*, **71**, 1278–86.

Brey EM, Uriel S, Greisler HP and McIntire LV (2005), 'Therapeutic neovascularization: contributions from bioengineering', *Tissue Eng*, **11**, 567–84.

Brookes SJ, Robinson C, Kirkham J and Bonass WA (1995), 'Biochemistry and molecular biology of amelogenin proteins of developing dental enamel', *Arch Oral Biol*, **40**, 1–14.

Cairo F, Pagliaro U and Nieri M (2008), 'Treatment of gingival recession with coronally advanced flap procedures: a systematic review', *J Clin Periodontol*, **35**, 136–62.

Camargo PM, Lekovic V, Weinlaender M, Vasilic N, Kenney EB and Madzarevic M (2001), 'The effectiveness of enamel matrix proteins used in combination with bovine porous bone mineral in the treatment of intrabony defects in humans', *J Clin Periodontol*, **28**, 1016–22.

Carnio J, Camargo PM, Kenney EB and Schenk RK (2002), 'Histological evaluation of 4 cases of root coverage following a connective tissue graft combined with an enamel matrix derivative preparation', *J Periodontol*, **73**, 1534–43.

Casarin RC, Del Peloso Ribeiro E, Nociti FH, Jr., Sallum AW, Sallum EA, Ambrosano GM and Casati MZ (2008), 'A double-blind randomized clinical evaluation of enamel matrix derivative proteins for the treatment of proximal class-II furcation involvements', *J Clin Periodontol*, **35**, 429–37.

Castellanos A, de la Rosa M, de la Garza M and Caffesse RG (2006), 'Enamel matrix derivative and coronal flaps to cover marginal tissue recessions', *J Periodontol*, **77**, 7–14.

Caton JG and Greenstein G (1993), 'Factors related to periodontal regeneration', *Periodontology 2000*, **1**, 9–15.

Cattaneo V, Rota C, Silvestri M, Piacentini C, Forlino A, Gallanti A, Rasperini G and Cetta G (2003), 'Effect of enamel matrix derivative on human periodontal fibroblasts: proliferation, morphology and root surface colonization. An *in vitro* study', *J Periodontal Res*, **38**, 568–74.

Cerny R, Slaby I, Hammarstrom L and Wurtz T (1996), 'A novel gene expressed in rat ameloblasts codes for proteins with cell binding domains', *J Bone Miner Res*, **11**, 883–91.

Chambrone D, Pasin IM, Chambrone L, Pannuti CM, Conde MC and Lima LA (2010a), 'Treatment of infrabony defects with or without enamel matrix proteins: a 24-month follow-up randomized pilot study', *Quintessence Int*, **41**, 125–34.

Chambrone L, Sukekava F, Araujo MG, Pustiglioni FE, Chambrone LA and Lima LA (2010b), 'Root-coverage procedures for the treatment of localized recession-type defects: a Cochrane systematic review', *J Periodontol*, **81**, 452–78.

Chen SC, Marino V, Gronthos S and Bartold PM (2006), 'Location of putative stem cells in human periodontal ligament', *J Periodontal Res*, **41**, 547–53.

Chen Z, de Paiva CS, Luo L, Kretzer FL, Pflugfelder SC and Li DQ (2004), 'Characterization of putative stem cell phenotype in human limbal epithelia', *Stem Cells*, **22**, 355–66.

Cheng MT, Yang HW, Chen TH and Lee OKS (2009), 'Isolation and characterization of multipotent stem cells from human cruciate ligaments', *Cell Proliferation*, **42**, 448–60.

Cheng YF, Chen JW, Lin SJ and Lu HK (2007), 'Is coronally positioned flap procedure adjunct with enamel matrix derivative or root conditioning a relevant predictor for achieving root coverage? A systemic review', *J Periodontal Res*, **42**, 474–85.

Cochran DL and Wozney JM (1999), 'Biological mediators for periodontal regeneration', *Periodontology 2000*, **19**, 40–58.

Cochran DL, King GN, Schoolfield J, Velasquez-Plata D, Mellonig JT and Jones A (2003), 'The effect of enamel matrix proteins on periodontal regeneration as determined by histological analyses', *J Periodontol*, **74**, 1043–55.

Collins CA, Olsen I, Zammit PS, Heslop L, Petrie A, Partridge TA and Morgan JE (2005), 'Stem cell function, self-renewal, and behavioral heterogeneity of cells from the adult muscle satellite cell niche', *Cell*, **122**, 289–301.

Cortellini P and Tonetti MS (2005), 'Clinical performance of a regenerative strategy for intrabony defects: scientific evidence and clinical experience', *J Periodontol*, **76**, 341–50.

Cortellini P, Pini-Prato G, Nieri M and Tonetti MS (2009), 'Minimally invasive surgical technique and enamel matrix derivative in intrabony defects: 2. Factors associated with healing outcomes', *Int J Periodontics Restorative Dent*, **29**, 257–65.

Cotsarelis G, Sun TT and Lavker RM (1990), 'Label-retaining cells reside in the bulge area of pilosebaceous unit: implications for follicular stem cells, hair cycle, and skin carcinogenesis', *Cell*, **61**, 1329–37.

Crea A, Dassatti L, Hoffmann O, Zafiropoulos GG and Deli G (2008), 'Treatment of intrabony defects using guided tissue regeneration or enamel matrix derivative: a 3-year prospective randomized clinical study', *J Periodontol*, **79**, 2281–9.

Cueva MA, Boltchi FE, Hallmon WW, Nunn ME, Rivera-Hidalgo F and Rees T (2004), 'A comparative study of coronally advanced flaps with and without the addition of enamel matrix derivative in the treatment of marginal tissue recession', *J Periodontol*, **75**, 949–56.

D'Amore PA and Thompson RW (1987), 'Mechanisms of angiogenesis', *Ann Rev Physiol*, **49**, 453–64.

de Oliveira CA, Spolidorio LC, Cirelli JA and Marcantonio RA (2005), 'Acellular dermal matrix allograft used alone and in combination with enamel matrix protein in gingival recession: histologic study in dogs', *Int J Periodontics Restorative Dent*, **25**, 595–603.

Dean DD, Lohmann CH, Sylvia VL, Cochran DL, Liu Y, Boyan BD and Schwartz Z (2002), 'Effect of porcine fetal enamel matrix derivative on chondrocyte proliferation, differentiation, and local factor production is dependent on cell maturation state', *Cells Tissues Organs*, **171**, 117–27.

Demir R, Seval Y and Huppertz B (2007), 'Vasculogenesis and angiogenesis in the early human placenta', *Acta Histochem*, **109**, 257–65.

Deutsch D, Palmon A, Fisher LW, Kolodny N, Termine JD and Young MF (1991), 'Sequencing of bovine enamelin ("tuftelin") a novel acidic enamel protein', *J Biol Chem*, **266**, 16021–28.

Deutsch D, Catalano-Sherman J, Dafni L, David S and Palmon A (1995), 'Enamel matrix proteins and ameloblast biology', *Connect Tissue Res*, **32**, 97–107.

Donos N, Glavind L, Karring T and Sculean A (2003a), 'Clinical evaluation of an enamel matrix derivative in the treatment of mandibular degree II furcation involvement: a 36-month case series', *Int J Periodontics Restorative Dent*, **23**, 507–12.

Donos N, Sculean A, Glavind L, Reich E and Karring T (2003b), 'Wound healing of degree III furcation involvements following guided tissue regeneration and/or Emdogain. A histologic study', *J Clin Periodontol*, **30**, 1061–8.

Donos N, Glavind L, Karring T and Sculean A (2004a), 'Clinical evaluation of an enamel matrix derivative and a bioresorbable membrane in the treatment of degree III mandibular furcation involvement: a series of nine patients', *Int J Periodontics Restorative Dent*, **24**, 362–9.

Donos N, Lang NP, Karoussis IK, Bosshardt D, Tonetti M and Kostopoulos L (2004b), 'Effect of GBR in combination with deproteinized bovine bone mineral and/or enamel matrix proteins on the healing of critical-size defects', *Clin Oral Implants Res*, **15**, 101–11.

Donos N, Bosshardt D, Lang N, Graziani F, Tonetti M, Karring T and Kostopoulos L (2005), 'Bone formation by enamel matrix proteins and xenografts: an experimental study in the rat ramus', *Clin Oral Implants Res*, **16**, 140–6.

Donos N, Kostopoulos L, Tonetti M, Karring T and Lang NP (2006), 'The effect of enamel matrix proteins and deproteinized bovine bone mineral on heterotopic bone formation', *Clin Oral Implants Res*, **17**, 434–8.

Fickl S, Thalmair T, Kebschull M, Bohm S and Wachtel H (2009), 'Microsurgical access flap in conjunction with enamel matrix derivative for the treatment of intra-bony defects: a controlled clinical trial', *J Clin Periodontol*, **36**, 784–90.

Fincham AG, Moradian-Oldak J and Sarte PE (1994), 'Mass-spectrographic analysis of a porcine amelogenin identifies a single phosphorylated locus', *Calcif Tissue Int*, **55**, 398–400.

Fincham AG, Moradian-Oldak J, Simmer JP (1999), 'The structural biology of the developing dental enamel matrix', *J Struct Biol*, **126**, 270–99.

Flamme I, Frolich T and Risau W (1997), 'Molecular mechanisms of vasculogenesis and embryonic angiogenesis', *J Cell Physiol*, **173**, 206–10.

Forsman K, Lind L, Backman B, Westermark E and Holmgren G (1994), 'Localization of a gene for autosomal dominant amelogenesis imperfecta (ADAI) to chromosome 4q', *Hum Mol Genet*, **3**, 1621–5.

Francetti L, Del Fabbro M, Basso M, Testori T and Weinstein R (2004), 'Enamel matrix proteins in the treatment of intra-bony defects. A prospective 24-month clinical trial', *J Clin Periodontol*, **31**, 52–9.

Francetti L, Trombelli L, Lombardo G, Guida L, Cafiero C, Roccuzzo M, Carusi G and Del Fabbro M (2005), 'Evaluation of efficacy of enamel matrix derivative in the treatment of intrabony defects: a 24-month multicenter study', *Int J Periodontics Restorative Dent*, **25**, 461–73.

Froum S, Lemler J, Horowitz R and Davidson B (2001), 'The use of enamel matrix derivative in the treatment of periodontal osseous defects: a clinical decision tree based on biologic principles of regeneration', *Int J Periodontics Restorative Dent*, **21**, 437–49.

Froum S, Weinberg M, Novak J, Mailhot J, Mellonig J, Van Dyke T, McClain P, Papapanou PN, Childers G, Ciancio S, Blieden T, Polson A, Greenstein G, Yukna R, Wallace ML, Patters M and Wagener C (2004), 'A multicenter study evaluating the sensitization potential of enamel matrix derivative after treatment of two infrabony defects', *J Periodontol*, **75**, 1001–8.

Fujii S, Maeda H, Wada N, Tomokiyo A, Saito M and Akamine A (2008), 'Investigating a clonal human periodontal ligament progenitor/stem cell line *in vitro* and *in vivo*', *J Cell Physiol*, **215**, 743–9.

Fujita T, Yamamoto S, Ota M, Shibukawa Y and Yamada S (2011), 'Coverage of gingival recession defects using guided tissue regeneration with and without adjunctive enamel matrix derivative in a dog model', *Int J Periodontics Restorative Dent*, **31**, 247–53.

Fukae M and Tanabe T (1987), 'Nonamelogenin components of porcine enamel in the protein fraction free from the enamel crystals', *Calcif Tissue Int*, **40**, 286–93.

Garrett S (1996), 'Periodontal regeneration around natural teeth', *Ann Periodontol*, **1**, 621–66.

Gestrelius S, Andersson C, Lidstrom D, Hammarstrom L and Somerman M (1997), '*In vitro* studies on periodontal ligament cells and enamel matrix derivative', *J Clin Periodontol*, **24**, 685–92.

Gestrelius S, Lyngstadaas SP and Hammarstrom L (2000), 'Emdogain–periodontal regeneration based on biomimicry', *Clin Oral Investig*, **4**, 120–5.

Gkranias ND, Graziani F, Sculean A and Donos N (2012), 'Wound healing following regenerative procedures in furcation degree III defects: histomorphometric outcomes', *Clin Oral Investig*, **16**, 239–49.

Goldman MJ, Ross IF and Goteiner D (1986), 'Effect of periodontal therapy on patients maintained for 15 years or longer. A retrospective study', *J Periodontol*, **57**, 347–53.

Gronthos S, Brahim J, Li W, Fisher LW, Cherman N, Boyde A, DenBesten P, Robey PG and Shi S (2002), 'Stem cell properties of human dental pulp stem cells', *J Dent Res*, **81**, 531–5.

Gunay H, Dogan S and Geurtsen W (2008), 'Harvesting technique using a mucotome and modified surgical procedure for root coverage with enamel matrix derivatives with and without a connective tissue graft', *Int J Periodontics Restorative Dent*, **28**, 497–507.

Gurinsky BS, Mills MP and Mellonig JT (2004), 'Clinical evaluation of demineralized freeze-dried bone allograft and enamel matrix derivative versus enamel matrix derivative alone for the treatment of periodontal osseous defects in humans', *J Periodontol*, **75**, 1309–18.

Hagenaars S, Louwerse PHG, Timmerman MF, Van der Velden U and Van der Weijden GA (2004), 'Soft tissue wound healing following periodontal surgery and Emdogain application', *J Clin Periodontol*, **31**, 850–6.

Hakki SS, Berry JE and Somerman MJ (2001), 'The effect of enamel matrix protein derivative on follicle cells *in vitro*', *J Periodontol*, **72**, 679–87.

Hammarstrom L (1997), 'Enamel matrix, cementum development and regeneration', *J Clin Periodontol*, **24**, 658–68.

Hammarstrom L, Heijl L and Gestrelius S (1997), 'Periodontal regeneration in a buccal dehiscence model in monkeys after application of enamel matrix proteins', *J Clin Periodontol*, **24**, 669–77.

Harrel SK (1999), 'A minimally invasive surgical approach for periodontal regeneration: surgical technique and observations', *J Periodontol*, **70**, 1547–57.

Harrel SK, Wilson TG and Nunn ME (2005), 'Prospective assessment of the use of enamel matrix proteins with minimally invasive surgery', *J Periodontol*, **76**, 380–4.

Harrel SK, Wilson TG, Jr. and Nunn ME (2010), 'Prospective assessment of the use of enamel matrix derivative with minimally invasive surgery: 6-year results', *J Periodontol*, **81**, 435–41.

Haynesworth SE, Goshima J, Goldberg VM and Caplan AI (1992), 'Characterization of cells with osteogenic potential from human marrow', *Bone*, **13**, 81–8.

Heard RH, Mellonig JT, Brunsvold MA, Lasho DJ, Meffert RM and Cochran DL (2000), 'Clinical evaluation of wound healing following multiple exposures to enamel matrix protein derivative in the treatment of intrabony periodontal defects', *J Periodontol*, **71**, 1715–21.

Heijl L (1997), 'Periodontal regeneration with enamel matrix derivative in one human experimental defect. A case report', *J Clin Periodontol*, **24**, 693–6.

Heijl L, Heden G, Svardstrom G and Ostgren A (1997), 'Enamel matrix derivative (EMDOGAIN) in the treatment of intrabony periodontal defects', *J Clin Periodontol*, **24**, 705–14.

Heritier M (1982), 'Experimental induction of cementogenesis on the enamel of transplanted mouse tooth germs', *Arch Oral Biol*, **27**, 87–97.

Hirschfeld L and Wasserman B (1978), 'A long-term survey of tooth loss in 600 treated periodontal patients', *J Periodontol*, **49**, 225–37.

Hu CC, Bartlett JD, Zhang CH, Qian Q, Ryu OH and Simmer JP (1996), 'Cloning, cDNA sequence, and alternative splicing of porcine amelogenin mRNAs', *J Dent Res*, **75**, 1735–41.

Hu CC, Fukae M, Uchida T, Qian Q, Zhang CH, Ryu OH, Tanabe T, Yamakoshi Y, Murakami C, Dohi N, Shimizu M and Simmer JP (1997a), 'Cloning and characterization of porcine enamelin mRNAs', *J Dent Res*, **76**, 1720–9.

Hu CC, Fukae M, Uchida T, Qian Q, Zhang CH, Ryu OH, Tanabe T, Yamakoshi Y, Murakami C, Dohi N, Shimizu M and Simmer JP (1997b), 'Sheathlin: cloning, cDNA/polypeptide sequences, and immunolocalization of porcine enamel sheath proteins', *J Dent Res*, **76**, 648–57.

Huang TF, Chen YT, Yang TH, Chen LL, Chiou SH, Tsai TH, Tsai CC, Chen MH, Ma HL and Hung SC (2008), 'Isolation and characterization of mesenchymal stromal cells from human anterior cruciate ligament', *Cytotherapy*, **10**, 806–14.

Iwata T, Morotome Y, Tanabe T, Fukae M, Ishikawa I and Oida S (2002), 'Noggin blocks osteoinductive activity of porcine enamel extracts', *J Dent Res*, **81**, 387–91.

Jepsen S, Eberhard J, Herrera D and Needleman I (2002), 'A systematic review of guided tissue regeneration for periodontal furcation defects. What is the effect of guided tissue regeneration compared with surgical debridement in the treatment of furcation defects?', *J Clin Periodontol*, **29** (Suppl 3), 103 16; discussion 160-102.

Jiang J, Safavi KE, Spangberg LS and Zhu Q (2001), 'Enamel matrix derivative prolongs primary osteoblast growth', *J Endod*, **27**, 110–12.

Jiang Y, Jahagirdar BN, Reinhardt RL, Schwartz RE, Keene CD, Ortiz-Gonzalez XR, Reyes M, Lenvik T, Lund T, Blackstad M, Du J, Aldrich S, Lisberg A, Low WC, Largaespada DA and Verfaillie CM (2002), 'Pluripotency of mesenchymal stem cells derived from adult marrow', *Nature*, **418**, 41–9.

Johe KK, Hazel TG, Muller T, Dugich-Djordjevic MM and McKay RD (1996), 'Single factors direct the differentiation of stem cells from the fetal and adult central nervous system', *Genes Dev*, **10**, 3129–40.

Johnson DL, Carnes D, Steffensen B and Cochran DL (2009), 'Cellular effects of enamel matrix derivative are associated with different molecular weight fractions following separation by size-exclusion chromatography', *J Periodontol*, **80**, 648–56.

Karring T and Cortellini P (1999), 'Regenerative therapy: furcation defects', *Periodontology 2000*, **19**, 115–37.

Karring T and Lindhe J (2008), 'Concepts in periodontal tissue regeneration', in *Clinical Periodontology and Implant Dentistry*, Lindhe J, Lang N P and Karring T (eds), Blackwell Munskgaard, 541–69.

Karring T, Nyman S, Gottlow J and Laurell L (1993), 'Development of the biological concept of guided tissue regeneration–animal and human studies', *Periodontology 2000*, **1**, 26–35.

Kauvar AS, Thoma DS, Carnes DL and Cochran DL (2010), '*In vivo* angiogenic activity of enamel matrix derivative', *J Periodontol*, **81**, 1196–201.

Kawana F, Sawae Y, Sahara T, Tanaka S, Debari K, Shimizu M and Sasaki T (2001), 'Porcine enamel matrix derivative enhances trabecular bone regeneration during wound healing of injured rat femur', *Anat Rec*, **264**, 438–46.

Kawanabe N, Murata S, Murakami K, Ishihara Y, Hayano S, Kurosaka H, Kamioka H, Takano-Yamamoto T and Yamashiro T (2010), 'Isolation of multipotent stem cells in human periodontal ligament using stage-specific embryonic antigen-4', *Differentiation*, **79**, 74–83.

Kawase T, Okuda K, Momose M, Kato Y, Yoshie H and Burns DM (2001), 'Enamel matrix derivative (EMDOGAIN) rapidly stimulates phosphorylation of the MAP kinase family and nuclear accumulation of smad2 in both oral epithelial and fibroblastic human cells', *J Periodontal Res*, **36**, 367–76.

Klinge B, Nilveus R, Kiger RD and Egelberg J (1981), 'Effect of flap placement and defect size on healing of experimental furcation defects', *J Periodontal Res*, **16**, 236–48.

Lang NP (2000), 'Focus on intrabony defects–conservative therapy', *Periodontology 2000*, **22**, 51–8.

Lemoli RM, Bertolini F, Cancedda R, De Luca M, Del Santo A, Ferrari G, Ferrari S, Martino G, Mavilio F and Tura S (2005), 'Stem cell plasticity: time for a reappraisal?', *Haematologica*, **90**, 360–81.

Lindhe J, Pontoriero R, Berglundh T and Araujo M (1995), 'The effect of flap management and bioresorbable occlusive devices in GTR treatment of degree III furcation defects. An experimental study in dogs', *J Clin Periodontol*, **22**, 276–83.

Lynch SE, De Castilla GR, Williams RC, Kiritsy CP, Howell TH, Reddy MS and Antoniades HN (1991), 'The effects of short-term application of a combination of platelet-derived and insulin-like growth factors on periodontal wound healing', *J Periodontol*, **62**, 458–67.

McCulloch CA, Nemeth E, Lowenberg B and Melcher AH (1987), 'Paravascular cells in endosteal spaces of alveolar bone contribute to periodontal ligament cell populations', *Anat Rec*, **219**, 233–42.

McFall WT, Jr. (1982), 'Tooth loss in 100 treated patients with periodontal disease. A long-term study', *J Periodontol*, **53**, 539–49.

McGuire MK and Cochran DL (2003), 'Evaluation of human recession defects treated with coronally advanced flaps and either enamel matrix derivative or connective tissue. Part 2: Histological evaluation', *J Periodontol*, **74**, 1126–35.

McGuire MK and Nunn ME (1996a), 'Prognosis versus actual outcome. II. The effectiveness of clinical parameters in developing an accurate prognosis', *J Periodontol*, **67**, 658–65.

McGuire MK and Nunn ME (1996b), 'Prognosis versus actual outcome. III. The effectiveness of clinical parameters in accurately predicting tooth survival', *J Periodontol*, **67**, 666–74.

McGuire MK and Nunn M (2003), 'Evaluation of human recession defects treated with coronally advanced flaps and either enamel matrix derivative or connective tissue. Part 1: Comparison of clinical parameters', *J Periodontol*, **74**, 1110–25.

Mellonig JT (1999), 'Enamel matrix derivative for periodontal reconstructive surgery: technique and clinical and histologic case report', *Int J Periodontics Restorative Dent*, **19**, 8–19.

Messenger MP, Raif EM, Seedhom BB and Brookes SJ (2007), 'The potential use of enamel matrix derivative for *in situ* anterior cruciate ligament tissue engineering: a translational *in vitro* investigation', *Tissue Eng*, **13**, 2041–51.

Meyle J, Hoffmann T, Topoll H, Heinz B, Al-Machot E, Jervoe-Storm PM, Meiss C, Eickholz P and Jepsen S (2011), 'A multi-centre randomized controlled clinical trial on the treatment of intra-bony defects with enamel matrix derivatives/synthetic bone graft or enamel matrix derivatives alone: results after 12 months', *J Clin Periodontol*, **38**, 652–60.

Miller PD, Jr. (1985), 'A classification of marginal tissue recession', *Int J Periodontics Restorative Dent*, **5**, 8–13.

Minabe M, Kodama T, Kogou T, Takeuchi K, Fushimi H, Sugiyama T and Mitarai E (2002), 'A comparative study of combined treatment with a collagen membrane and enamel matrix proteins for the regeneration of intraosseous defects', *Int J Periodontics Restorative Dent*, **22**, 595–605.

Molloy T, Wang Y and Murrell GAC (2003), 'The roles of growth factors in tendon and ligament healing', *Sports Med*, **33**, 381–94.

Moses O, Artzi Z, Sculean A, Tal H, Kozlovsky A, Romanos GE and Nemcovsky CE (2006), 'Comparative study of two root coverage procedures: a 24-month follow-up multicenter study', *J Periodontol*, **77**, 195–202.

Murphy KG and Gunsolley JC (2003), 'Guided tissue regeneration for the treatment of periodontal intrabony and furcation defects. A systematic review', *Ann Periodontol*, **8**, 266–302.

Myhre AE, Lyngstadaas SP, Dahle MK, Stuestol JF, Foster SJ, Thiemermann C, Lillcaascn P, Wang JE and Aasen AO (2006), 'Anti inflammatory properties of enamel matrix derivative in human blood', *J Periodontal Res*, **41**, 208–13.

Nagano T, Iwata T, Ogata Y, Tanabe T, Gomi K, Fukae M, Arai T and Oida S (2004), 'Effect of heat treatment on bioactivities of enamel matrix derivatives in human periodontal ligament (HPDL) cells', *J Periodontal Res*, **39**, 249–56.

Nagano T, Oida S, Suzuki S, Iwata T, Yamakoshi Y, Ogata Y, Gomi K, Arai T and Fukae M (2006), 'Porcine enamel protein fractions contain transforming growth factor-beta1', *J Periodontol*, **77**, 1688–94.

Needleman I, Tucker R, Giedrys-Leeper E and Worthington H (2005), 'Guided tissue regeneration for periodontal intrabony defects – a Cochrane Systematic Review', *Periodontology 2000*, **37**, 106–23.

Nemcovsky CE, Artzi Z, Tal H, Kozlovsky A and Moses O (2004), 'A multicenter comparative study of two root coverage procedures: coronally advanced flap with addition of enamel matrix proteins and subpedicle connective tissue graft', *J Periodontol*, **75**, 600–7.

Niemann C and Watt FM (2002), 'Designer skin: lineage commitment in postnatal epidermis', *Trends Cell Biol*, **12**, 185–92.

Nikolopoulos S, Peteinaki E and Castanas E (2002), 'Immunologic effects of emdogain in humans: one-year results', *Int J Periodontics Restorative Dent*, **22**, 269–77.

Nomi M, Atala A, Coppi PD and Soker S (2002), 'Principals of neovascularization for tissue engineering', *Mol Aspects Med*, **23**, 463–83.

Ohyama M, Suzuki N, Yamaguchi Y, Maeno M, Otsuka K and Ito K (2002), 'Effect of enamel matrix derivative on the differentiation of C2C12 cells', *J Periodontol*, **73**, 543–50.

Okuda K, Momose M, Miyazaki A, Murata M, Yokoyama S, Yonezawa Y, Wolff LF and Yoshie H (2000), 'Enamel matrix derivative in the treatment of human intrabony osseous defects', *J Periodontol*, **71**, 1821–8.

Paine CT, Paine ML, Luo W, Okamoto CT, Lyngstadaas SP and Snead ML (2000), 'A tuftelin-interacting protein (TIP39) localizes to the apical secretory pole of mouse ameloblasts', *J Biol Chem*, **275**, 22284–92.

Pandya NM, Dhalla NS and Santani DD (2006), 'Angiogenesis – a new target for future therapy', *Vascular Pharmacology*, **44**, 265–74.

Pilloni A, Paolantonio M and Camargo PM (2006), 'Root coverage with a coronally positioned flap used in combination with enamel matrix derivative: 18-month clinical evaluation', *J Periodontol*, **77**, 2031–9.

Pontoriero R, Lindhe J, Nyman S, Karring T, Rosenberg E and Sanavi F (1988), 'Guided tissue regeneration in degree II furcation-involved mandibular molars. A clinical study', *J Clin Periodontol*, **15**, 247–54.

Pontoriero R, Lindhe J, Nyman S, Karring T, Rosenberg E and Sanavi F (1989), 'Guided tissue regeneration in the treatment of furcation defects in mandibular molars. A clinical study of degree III involvements', *J Clin Periodontol*, **16**, 170–4.

Pontoriero R, Nyman S, Ericsson I and Lindhe J (1992), 'Guided tissue regeneration in surgically-produced furcation defects. An experimental study in the beagle dog', *J Clin Periodontol*, **19**, 159–63.

Pontoriero R, Wennstrom J and Lindhe J (1999), 'The use of barrier membranes and enamel matrix proteins in the treatment of angular bone defects. A prospective controlled clinical study', *J Clin Periodontol*, **26**, 833–40.

Potten CS (1998), 'Stem cells in gastrointestinal epithelium: numbers, characteristics and death', *Philos Trans R Soc, B*, **353**, 821–30.

Rasperini G, Silvestri M, Schenk RK and Nevins ML (2000), 'Clinical and histologic evaluation of human gingival recession treated with a subepithelial connective tissue graft and enamel matrix derivative (Emdogain): a case report', *Int J Periodontics Restorative Dent*, **20**, 269–75.

Rasperini G, Roccuzzo M, Francetti L, Acunzo R, Consonni D and Silvestri M (2011), 'Subepithelial connective tissue graft for treatment of gingival recessions with and without enamel matrix derivative: a multicenter, randomized controlled clinical trial', *Int J Periodontics Restorative Dent*, **31**, 133–9.

Regazzini PF, Novaes AB, Jr., de Oliveira PT, Palioto DB, Taba M, Jr., de Souza SL and Grisi MF (2004), 'Comparative study of enamel matrix derivative with or without GTR in the treatment of class II furcation lesions in dogs', *Int J Periodontics Restorative Dent*, **24**, 476–87.

Ribeiro FV, Casarin RC, Junior FH, Sallum EA and Casati MZ (2011), 'The role of enamel matrix derivative protein in minimally invasive surgery in treating intrabony defects in single-rooted teeth: a randomized clinical trial', *J Periodontol*, **82**, 522–32.

Rosing CK, Aass AM, Mavropoulos A and Gjermo P (2005), 'Clinical and radiographic effects of enamel matrix derivative in the treatment of intrabony periodontal defects: a 12-month longitudinal placebo-controlled clinical trial in adult periodontitis patients', *J Periodontol*, **76**, 129–33.

Sanz M, Tonetti MS, Zabalegui I, Sicilia A, Blanco J, Rebelo H, Rasperini G, Merli M, Cortellini P and Suvan JE (2004), 'Treatment of intrabony defects with enamel matrix proteins or barrier membranes: results from a multicenter practice-based clinical trial', *J Periodontol*, **75**, 726–33.

Schlueter SR, Carnes Jr DL and Cochran DL (2007), 'In vitro effects of enamel matrix derivative on microvascular cells', *J Periodontol*, **78**, 141–51.

Schwartz Z, Carnes DL, Jr., Pulliam R, Lohmann CH, Sylvia VL, Liu Y, Dean DD, Cochran DL and Boyan BD (2000), 'Porcine fetal enamel matrix derivative stimulates proliferation but not differentiation of pre-osteoblastic 2T9 cells, inhibits proliferation and stimulates differentiation of osteoblast-like MG63 cells, and increases proliferation and differentiation of normal human osteoblast NHOst cells', *J Periodontol*, **71**, 1287–96.

Sculean A, Donos N, Blaes A, Lauermann M, Reich E and Brecx M (1999a), 'Comparison of enamel matrix proteins and bioabsorbable membranes in the treatment of intrabony periodontal defects. A split-mouth study', *J Periodontol*, **70**, 255–62.

Sculean A, Donos N, Windisch P, Brecx M, Gera I, Reich E and Karring T (1999b), 'Healing of human intrabony defects following treatment with enamel matrix proteins or guided tissue regeneration', *J Periodontal Res*, **34**, 310–22.

Sculean A, Chiantella GC, Windisch P and Donos N (2000a), 'Clinical and histologic evaluation of human intrabony defects treated with an enamel matrix protein derivative (Emdogain)', *Int J Periodontics Restorative Dent*, **20**, 374–81.

Sculean A, Donos N, Brecx M, Reich E and Karring T (2000b), 'Treatment of intrabony defects with guided tissue regeneration and enamel-matrix-proteins. An experimental study in monkeys', *J Clin Periodontol*, **27**, 466–72.
Sculean A, Blaes A, Arweiler N, Reich E, Donos N and Brecx M (2001a), 'The effect of postsurgical antibiotics on the healing of intrabony defects following treatment with enamel matrix proteins', *J Periodontol*, **72**, 190–5.
Sculean A, Windisch P, Chiantella GC, Donos N, Brecx M and Reich E (2001b), 'Treatment of intrabony defects with enamel matrix proteins and guided tissue regeneration. A prospective controlled clinical study', *J Clin Periodontol*, **28**, 397–403.
Sculean A, Junker R, Donos N, Berakdar M, Brecx M and Dunker N (2002), 'Immunohistochemical evaluation of matrix molecules associated with wound healing following regenerative periodontal treatment in monkeys', *Clin Oral Investig*, **6**, 175–82.
Sculean A, Junker R, Donos N, Windisch P, Brecx M and Dunker N (2003), 'Immunohistochemical evaluation of matrix molecules associated with wound healing following treatment with an enamel matrix protein derivative in humans', *Clin Oral Investig*, **7**, 167–74.
Sculean A, Pietruska M, Schwarz F, Willershausen B, Arweiler NB and Auschill TM (2005), 'Healing of human intrabony defects following regenerative periodontal therapy with an enamel matrix protein derivative alone or combined with a bioactive glass. A controlled clinical study', *J Clin Periodontol*, **32**, 111–17.
Seo BM, Miura M, Gronthos S, Bartold PM, Batouli S, Brahim J, Young M, Robey PG, Wang CY and Shi S (2004), 'Investigation of multipotent postnatal stem cells from human periodontal ligament', *Lancet*, **364**, 149–55.
Silvestri M, Ricci G, Rasperini G, Sartori S and Cattaneo V (2000), 'Comparison of treatments of infrabony defects with enamel matrix derivative, guided tissue regeneration with a nonresorbable membrane and Widman modified flap. A pilot study', *J Clin Periodontol*, **27**, 603–10.
Silvestri M, Sartori S, Rasperini G, Ricci G, Rota C and Cattaneo V (2003), 'Comparison of infrabony defects treated with enamel matrix derivative versus guided tissue regeneration with a nonresorbable membrane', *J Clin Periodontol*, **30**, 386–93.
Singhatanadgit W, Donos N and Olsen I (2009), 'Isolation and characterization of stem cell clones from adult human ligament', *Tissue Eng, Part A*, **15**, 2625–36.
Slavkin HC (1974), 'Cementum: an epithelial secretory product?', *J Dent Res*, **53**, 157.
Spahr A, Haegewald S, Tsoulfidou F, Rompola E, Heijl L, Bernimoulin JP, Ring C, Sander S and Haller B (2005), 'Coverage of Miller class I and II recession defects using enamel matrix proteins versus coronally advanced flap technique: a 2-year report', *J Periodontol*, **76**, 1871–80.
Taba M, Jr., Jin Q, Sugai JV and Giannobile WV (2005), 'Current concepts in periodontal bioengineering', *Orthod Craniofacial Res*, **8**, 292–302.
Ten Cate AR (1996), 'The role of epithelium in the development, structure and function of the tissues of tooth support', *Oral Dis*, **2**, 55–62.
Thoma DS, Villar CC, Carnes DL, Dard M, Chun YH and Cochran DL (2011), 'Angiogenic activity of an enamel matrix derivative (EMD) and EMD-derived proteins: an experimental study in mice', *J Clin Periodontol*, **38**, 253–60.

Tokiyasu Y, Takata T, Saygin E and Somerman M (2000), 'Enamel factors regulate expression of genes associated with cementoblasts', *J Periodontol*, **71**, 1829–39.

Tomokiyo A, Maeda H, Fujii S, Wada N, Shima K and Akamine A (2007), 'Development of a multipotent clonal human periodontal ligament cell line', *Differentiation*, **76**, 337–47.

Tonetti MS, Lang NP, Cortellini P, Suvan JE, Adriaens P, Dubravec D, Fonzar A, Fourmousis I, Mayfield L, Rossi R, Silvestri M, Tiedemann C, Topoll H, Vangsted T and Wallkamm B (2002), 'Enamel matrix proteins in the regenerative therapy of deep intrabony defects', *J Clin Periodontol*, **29**, 317–25.

Trombelli L and Farina R (2008), 'Clinical outcomes with bioactive agents alone or in combination with grafting or guided tissue regeneration', *J Clin Periodontol*, **35**, 117–35.

Tu YK, Woolston A and Faggion CM, Jr. (2010), 'Do bone grafts or barrier membranes provide additional treatment effects for infrabony lesions treated with enamel matrix derivatives? A network meta-analysis of randomized-controlled trials', *J Clin Periodontol*, **37**, 59–79.

Van der Pauw MT, Van den Bos T, Everts V and Beertsen W (2000), 'Enamel matrix-derived protein stimulates attachment of periodontal ligament fibroblasts and enhances alkaline phosphatase activity and transforming growth factor beta1 release of periodontal ligament and gingival fibroblasts', *J Periodontol*, **71**, 31–43.

Wachtel H, Schenk G, Bohm S, Weng D, Zuhr O and Hurzeler MB (2003), 'Microsurgical access flap and enamel matrix derivative for the treatment of periodontal intrabony defects: a controlled clinical study', *J Clin Periodontol*, **30**, 496–504.

Wang HL, Burgett FG, Shyr Y and Ramfjord S (1994), 'The influence of molar furcation involvement and mobility on future clinical periodontal attachment loss', *J Periodontol*, **65**, 25–9.

Weissman IL (2000), 'Stem cells: units of development, units of regeneration, and units in evolution', *Cell*, **100**, 157–68.

Wennstrom JL (1996), 'Mucogingival therapy', *Ann Periodontol*, **1**, 671–701.

Wennstrom JL and Lindhe J (2002), 'Some effects of enamel matrix proteins on wound healing in the dento gingival region', *J Clin Periodontol*, **29**, 9–14.

Wennstrom J, Zucchelli G and Pini-Prato G (2008), 'Mucogingival therapy-Periodontal plastic surgery', in *Clinical Periodontology and Implant Dentistry*, Lindhe J, Lang N and Karring T (eds), Blackwell Munskgaard, 971–91.

Windisch P, Sculean A, Klein F, Toth V, Gera I, Reich E and Eickholz P (2002), 'Comparison of clinical, radiographic, and histometric measurements following treatment with guided tissue regeneration or enamel matrix proteins in human periodontal defects', *J Periodontol*, **73**, 409–17.

Wood WR, Greco GW and McFall WT, Jr. (1989), 'Tooth loss in patients with moderate periodontitis after treatment and long-term maintenance care', *J Periodontol*, **60**, 516–20.

Wu M and Wei YQ (2004), 'Development of respiratory stem cells and progenitor cells', *Stem Cells Dev*, **13**, 607–13.

Xu J, Wang W, Kapila Y, Lotz J and Kapila S (2009), 'Multiple differentiation capacity of STRO-1+/CD146+ PDL mesenchymal progenitor cells', *Stem Cells Dev*, **18**, 487–96.

Yoneda S, Itoh D, Kuroda S, Kondo H, Umezawa A, Ohya K, Ohyama T and Kasugai S (2003), 'The effects of enamel matrix derivative (EMD) on osteoblastic cells in culture and bone regeneration in a rat skull defect', *J Periodontal Res*, **38**, 333–42.

Yuan K, Chen CL and Lin MT (2003), 'Enamel matrix derivative exhibits angiogenic effect in vitro and in a murine model', *J Clin Periodontol*, **30**, 732–8.

Yukna RA and Mellonig JT (2000), 'Histologic evaluation of periodontal healing in humans following regenerative therapy with enamel matrix derivative. A 10-case series', *J Periodontol*, **71**, 752–9.

Zetterstrom O, Andersson C, Eriksson L, Fredriksson A, Friskopp J, Heden G, Jansson B, Lundgren T, Nilveus R, Olsson A, Renvert S, Salonen L, Sjostrom L, Winell A, Ostgren A and Gestrelius S (1997), 'Clinical safety of enamel matrix derivative (EMDOGAIN) in the treatment of periodontal defects', *J Clin Periodontol*, **24**, 697–704.

Zucchelli G, Bernardi F, Montebugnoli L and De SM (2002), 'Enamel matrix proteins and guided tissue regeneration with titanium-reinforced expanded polytetrafluoroethylene membranes in the treatment of infrabony defects: a comparative controlled clinical trial', *J Periodontol*, **73**, 3–12.

Zucchelli G, Amore C, Montebugnoli L and De Sanctis M (2003), 'Enamel matrix proteins and bovine porous bone mineral in the treatment of intrabony defects: a comparative controlled clinical trial', *J Periodontol*, **74**, 1725–35.

Zuk PA, Zhu M, Mizuno H, Huang J, Futrell JW, Katz AJ, Benhaim P, Lorenz HP and Hedrick MH (2001), 'Multilineage cells from human adipose tissue: implications for cell-based therapies', *Tissue Eng*, **7**, 211–28.

Part II

Dental ceramics and glasses for tooth repair and replacement

5
Processing and bonding of dental ceramics

J. P. MATINLINNA, The University of Hong Kong, PR China

DOI: 10.1533/9780857096432.2.129

Abstract: This chapter gives readers a concise introduction to ceramic dental biomaterials, draws attention to their surface pretreatment and to silane primers used before cementation, and discusses several findings based on experimental laboratory studies. Chemical aspects related to ceramic materials, their pretreatment (conditioning) and their cementation with resin cements are discussed. Ceramics (porcelains) form a very popular and safe group of restorative materials in contemporary dentistry because of their aesthetics and high biocompatibility and they are discussed elsewhere in this book in detail. Ceramics used in dentistry are mostly based on silicon, Si, a metalloid element that is predominantly found in the form of silica and various silicate minerals in the Earth's crust. No contraindications have been reported for ceramics. Ceramic materials have three major indications: (i) ceramic–metal crowns and fixed partial dentures, (ii) all-ceramic restorations consisting of short-span anterior bridges, onlays, inlays, crowns and veneers (laminates), and (iii) ceramic denture teeth. The chemistry of zirconia, a contemporary dental material of choice, is also discussed. For durable cementation, it is mandatory to acid etch enamel and dentin with *ortho*-phosphoric acid, H_3PO_4. On the other hand, the ceramic (porcelain) surface need to be etched with hydrofluoric acid, HF, followed by silanization. Silanes are key primer monomers owing to their special, unique chemistry and are therefore discussed in detail. Some other acidic agents used in dentistry are introduced. Resin zirconia bonding concepts and related laboratory studies finalize this chapter.

Key words: alumina, dental ceramics, dental porcelain, primers, silanes, zirconia.

5.1 Introduction to dental ceramics

Ceramics (porcelains) are widely used as restorative materials in dentistry because of their high biocompatibility and aesthetics. Ceramic materials in prosthetic dentistry have three major indications: (i) ceramic–metal crowns and fixed partial dentures; (ii) all-ceramic restorations consisting of short-span anterior bridges, crowns, onlays, inlays and veneers; and (iii) ceramic denture teeth (Garber and Goldstein, 1994; van Noort, 2007). A ceramic veneer (porcelain laminate) is used to cover an unsightly area by bonding to the facial surface of the tooth. No contraindications have been reported for ceramics.

It is well understood that direct bonding of ceramic to natural teeth is inadequate because ceramics do not have a natural affinity for teeth. Thus, to obtain sufficient adhesion, it is vital to etch the tooth enamel with *ortho*-phosphoric acid, H_3PO_4, before priming and cementation. The porcelain surface to be bonded should be etched with an etchant, which is usually hydrofluoric acid, HF. After this mandatory step, the surface must be rinsed and dried. Next, when the surface is silanized (Lung and Matinlinna, 2012), the luting resin cement is able to penetrate into the surface pores and ensure adequate bonding between the ceramic restoration and flowable resin composite cement (Ho and Matinlinna, 2011a). Resin composite-based dental biomaterials are discussed elsewhere in this book.

5.1.1 Classification of dental ceramics

Ceramics (porcelains) in dentistry may be categorized according to the firing temperature. Firing temperature ranges of between 870°C and 1065°C referred to as low-fusing ceramics, temperature ranges of 1090–1260°C referred to as medium-fusing ceramics and, finally, temperature ranges between 1315°C and 1370°C are attributed to high-fusing ceramics. High-fusing ceramics are used for denture teeth, medium-fusing ceramics for porcelain jacket restorations and low-fusing ceramics for metal–ceramic (i.e. porcelain fused-to-metal, PFM) restorations. High-fusing dental ceramics are superior in translucency, strength, insolubility and accuracy during repeated firing steps in comparison to medium- and low-fusing ceramics (Touati *et al.*, 1999; Powers and Sakaguchi, 2006).

All-ceramic materials used in dentistry are composed of a wide range of crystalline phases and they may even contain up to 99% by volume of crystalline phase. Their aesthetical appearance and biomechanical properties are determined by the particle size distribution and the amount of crystalline phase. All-ceramic restorations can be fabricated by four diverse methods: (i) sintering; (ii) heat-pressing; (iii) slip-casting; and (iv) machining. A clinical disadvantage of all-ceramic restorations may be that more tooth tissue needs to be removed to maximize the wall thickness of the restoration. On the other hand, this reduces the risk of fracture and failure. Also, this has been reported to increase pulpal pathology in some individuals (Schmalz and Arenholt-Bindslev, 2009; Kaminski and Easton, 2009).

The most traditional type of dental ceramic (porcelain) is feldspar-based, that is containing silica, SiO_2, glasses. This type of ceramic is also known as feldspathic-based (feldspar, $KAlSi_3O_8$) or silica-based ceramic. Actually, porcelain is a term often used to describe this type of ceramic owing to its high silica content (Powers and Sakaguchi, 2006). The most notable properties of feldspathic ceramics are their resistance to chemical attack and full biocompatibility (Hämmerle *et al.*, 2008; Ho and Matinlinna, 2011a; Lung and Matinlinna, 2012). Interestingly, some calcium phosphate materials used for coating subgingival dental Ti-implants (to promote biointegration and osseointegration) are also considered to be ceramics (Schmalz and Arenholt-Bindslev, 2009), but will not be discussed in this chapter.

5.1.2 Biomechanical properties

The compressive strength of porcelain is on the scale 350–550 MPa. However, its tensile strength is very low, only 20–60 MPa, owing to the brittle glassy nature of porcelain. Feldspar-based ceramics lack fracture toughness and are sensitive to surface microcracks (Garber and Goldstein, 1994; Touati *et al.*, 1999). The shear strength of porcelain is reported to be about 110 MPa and its diametric tensile strength is about 34 MPa. Its flexural strength is reported to be about 50–75 MPa, its elastic modulus is about 69–70 GPa and its average surface hardness is about 460 KHN (Knoop Hardness Number) compared to 340 KHN for enamel (Powers and Sakaguchi, 2006). Feldspar-based ceramics have a coefficient of thermal expansion of about 13×10^{-6} per °C, which surprisingly matches enamel and dentin (Kaminski and Easton, 2009).

5.1.3 High strength core ceramics

The hostile oral environment with its temperature shocks, pH fluctuations, masticatory forces, parafunctions and so on, creates stressful conditions for dental biomaterials. The inner porcelain surfaces are subjected to tensile stresses, allowing microcracks to propagate. These cracks may reach the outer surface leading to catastrophic failure (Powers and Sakaguchi, 2006; van Noort, 2007). For these reasons, several ways were developed to strengthen dental ceramics, such as (i) to reinforce the core of the ceramic and (ii) to combine feldspar-based ceramics with a metallic substructure (van Noort 2007; Clelland *et al.*, 2007). The so-called core ceramics consist of an aesthetic ceramic supported by another, underlying ceramic matrix that provides the core and strength, but this configuration may lack the desired aesthetics owing to its opacity. These contemporary oxide ceramics are pure alumina and zirconia (Kaminski and Easton, 2009; Matinlinna and Mittal, 2009) (see below).

All-ceramic restorations may in general be described as pleasant looking, even though they are in principle brittle and may fracture in the stressful oral environment. All metal/alloy restorations are strong, yet they lack aesthetics. By combining both materials, metal and porcelain, together a composite structure can be made that possesses the strength and toughness of metal with the aesthetics of porcelain. This composite system is known as porcelain-fused-to-metal, PFM, or ceramic–metal system (Powers and

Wataha, 2008; Ubassy, 1993). PFMs are prepared with cast base metal alloys, such as Co-Cr, Ni-Cr, or Au-Pd, and porcelain which is fused onto the metal surface to shield the unpleasant appearance of metal or alloy. An opaque shade, such as intensely white TiO_2, is usually applied to mask the metal appearance of the metal substructure. However, the opaque shade makes the restoration look unnatural compared to all-ceramic restorations, and some base metal alloys may elicit allergic reactions (Touati *et al.*, 1999; Powers and Sakaguchi, 2006).

The most common clinical failures in all-ceramic and PFM restorations are delamination (also called chipping) of porcelain off the zirconia core and crack initiation in the porcelain matrix. Bearing this in mind, careful attention must be paid to good adhesion between the restoration and tooth tissues. The direction of dental ceramics is shifting away from using base and noble metal alloys because they may contain allergens (such as Be and Ni). It seems that more research needs to be devoted to all-ceramic materials because of their highly promising biocompatibility (Ho and Matinlinna, 2011a). PFM restorations are not discussed further in this chapter.

Zirconia, ZrO_2, and spinel, $MgAl_2O_4$, can be substituted for alumina as the core material. Spinel has better aesthetics than alumina, but a compromise is its lower flexural strength, 300 MPa. Zirconia has a higher flexural strength, about 700 MPa, than alumina but it is less translucent (van Noort, 2007; Matinlinna and Mittal, 2009) (see below).

5.1.4 Chemistry of dental ceramics

The structure of ceramics exists in the form of crystalline solid or amorphous glasses. Ceramics used in dentistry are mostly based on silicon, Si, usually found in the form of silica (silicon dioxide), SiO_2, owing to the high affinity of silicon for oxygen. In general terms, however, ceramics may formally be defined as compounds of metallic and non-metallic elements consisting of oxides, nitrides, carbides and silicates, such as SiO_4^{4-}, $Si_3O_8^{4-}$ and $Si_2O_5^{2-}$. Silicates consist of Si-tetrahedrons, SiO_4 and a vast array of ≡Si-O-type compounds. Silicate minerals exist abundantly in the Earth's crust. When silica occurs as a crystalline material, it can be in the form of quartz, crystobalite and tridymite. Silica in dental ceramics is usually in the form of quartz. Owing to the black appearance of nitrides and carbides, they are not used as biomaterials in dentistry (Shriver and Atkins, 2001).

The traditional type of dental ceramics is feldspar-based and composed of a tectosilicate mineral feldspar ($KAlSi_3O_8$), quartz (SiO_2), or kaolin ($Al_2O_3 \cdot 2SiO_2 \cdot 2H_2O$), and fired at above 870°C. Because feldspar-based ceramics were prone to failure owing to their inherent brittle nature, ceramics with a higher crystalline content such as alumina (Al_2O_3) and zirconia were developed to improve their biomechanical properties (Touati *et al.*,

Table 5.1 Ceramic materials used in dentistry

Type	Quality	Indications
Glass-ceramics	SiO_2 based. High aesthetic qualities, but generally weak	Veneering ceramics, laminate veneers, inlays, and onlays
Hybrid ceramics	Glass-infiltrated porous alumina. Infiltration glass is used to fill the porosity associated with alumina	Core, frameworks
Polycrystalline ceramics	Alumina and zirconia	Frameworks. Nowadays zirconia predominantly used. When combined with porcelain veneer, both are known as core veneered all-ceramic restorations.

1999). High crystalline content ceramics are commonly used as the core (or framework), while feldspar-based ceramics are used as veneers to shield the core in prosthetic dentistry (Hämmerle *et al.*, 2008).

For convenience, based on their chemical compositions, ceramic materials used in dentistry and dental technology are usually divided into three categories, as presented in Table 5.1 (Liu *et al.*, 2012).

5.2 Alumina and zirconia chemistry

5.2.1 Alumina

Aluminium trioxide, Al_2O_3 (alumina), sometimes called 'aluminium oxide', occurs in nature as the minerals bauxite, corundum, gibbsite and diaspore. Native alumina is crystalline, very hard and insoluble in water. When heated above 800°C, it becomes insoluble in acids and its specific gravity increases from 2.8 to 4.0. Alumina can be called the predecessor of zirconium dioxide, ZrO_2, as a biomaterial in dentistry. Alumina was first introduced as a reinforcing inclusion for dental porcelain in the mid-1960s. However, the inherently low tensile strength of porcelain, does not allow it to be used in areas subjected to high stresses. However, alumina has found an application in dentistry as orthodontic brackets. Today, alumina is still used to some extent as a framework for the construction of crowns and small all-ceramic fixed restorations. Another biomaterial application has been found in orthopaedics, where aluminium trioxide is used in ball and socket replacements of the hip joint (McLean, 2001).

Interestingly, when zirconia particles are added to alumina and mixed properly, alumina will be toughened and will become harder. The combination of these two materials is called ZrO_2-toughened alumina, ZTA. The zirconia content varies between 10% and 20% in ZTA (Claussen, 1976).

Alumina and zirconia are single-phase microstructures without a glassy phase as such. Both are true inorganic crystalline ceramic materials. Pure alumina core materials on the market contain about 99.5% alumina and their flexural strength ranges between 487 and 699 MPa. Alumina's fracture toughness is reported to be around 4.48–6 MPa $m^{1/2}$. In comparison, pure zirconia has a flexural strength of 1000 MPa and a fracture toughness of about 10.00 MPa $m^{1/2}$ (Raigrodski, 2004; Hefferman *et al.*, 2002). It is noteworthy that alumina in powder form is widely used as a grit-blasting material in dentistry and dental technology (see below).

5.2.2 Zirconia

Zirconia (zirconium dioxide), ZrO_2, has a remarkably dense and hard surface that is, in a way, ideal for wear resistance and contact damage. In addition, zirconia is highly biocompatible. In nature zirconia occurs as the mineral baddeleyite. Dental zirconia is white, heavy, odourless, tasteless, virtually insoluble in water, slightly soluble in hydrochloric acid, HCl, and nitrous acid, HNO_3, but slowly soluble in hydrofluoric acid, HF. Zirconia forms tetragonal crystals above ~1100°C and cubic crystals above ~1900°C. Biomechanical properties, such as Young's modulus, compressive strength, and hardness are lower for zirconia than for alumina; on the other hand, zirconia has a higher bending strength (Matinlinna and Mittal, 2009; Liu *et al.*, 2012). These properties have made it the contemporary dental biomaterial of choice when high functional demands are required. Previously, one of the main risks associated with zirconia has been its potential radioactivity but this has been proved to be negligible (Piconi and Maccauro, 1999). When zirconia was used as a femural head material, it was observed that about 400 femoral heads failed in a very short period in 2001. This took place in two unsuccessful production batches of Prozyr® zirconia and it was explained by its sensitivity to low temperature degradation, LTD (Chevalier, 2006).

Feldspar-based veneers are applied because zirconia and alumina are opaque and dull in colour as substructures. Zirconia is usually manufactured as presintered blocks that may shrink by up to 20% upon firing. With attractive biomechanical properties, however, there comes a drawback, *viz.* highly crystalline ceramics cannot be acid etched for bonding with resin composite luting cements (Kaminski and Easton, 2009).

Zirconia currently has multiple clinical applications such as root canal posts which have been used to reinforce non-vital teeth since the mid-1990s

(Meyenberg *et al.*, 1995), subgingival dental implant abutments (Canullo, 2007), orthodontic brackets (Keith *et al.*, 1994), dental subgingival implant fixtures with adequate osteo-integration (Tete *et al.*, 2009) and frameworks for all-ceramic fixed dental prostheses (FDPs) where it is expected to resist areas of stress concentration (Rosentritt *et al.*, 2008; Hjerppe *et al.*, 2008). Usually, zirconia structures are veneered with porcelain to give a tooth-like appearance and finish. The bond strength between the veneering porcelain and zirconia was reported to be inferior compared to other all-ceramic systems. There are studies reporting delamination (chipping) of the veneer ceramic from intact zirconia frameworks (Piconi and Maccauro, 1999; Choi *et al.*, 2009).

5.2.3 Pretreatment of dental ceramics

Direct bonding of ceramic to natural teeth is obviously inadequate because ceramics do not have a natural affinity for teeth. To obtain sufficient retention, it is essential to etch the tooth enamel with phosphoric acid. The bonding surface of the ceramic is etched with an acid etchant. Then, the ceramic surface is rinsed with water and necessarily silanized to ensure good bonding between the ceramic veneer and the luting resin cement. Etching also provides a retentive topography on the surface so that the luting resin cement can penetrate into the pores (Matinlinna *et al.*, 2004; Hämmerle *et al.*, 2008; Ho and Matinlinna, 2011b; Lung and Matinlinna, 2012). When the ceramic restoration is cemented with a resin composite cement, fracture resistance is increased (Garber and Goldstein, 1994). It is noteworthy that in many *in vitro* studies, resin composite is used as a custom substitute for enamel or dentin because of their similar biomechanical properties (Ho and Matinlinna, 2011c).

It is widely accepted that etching with acids is the most effective procedure in enhancing retention and bonding between feldspar-based ceramic restoration and resin composite cement, compared with sandblasting the ceramic surface (Yen *et al.*, 1993). Etching with hydrofluoric acid, HF, creates a porous structure that facilitates micromechanical retention between the resin composite and ceramic. It has been shown that uncured flowable resin composite luting cements may penetrate into the porous surface structure (Matinlinna and Mittal, 2009). Another function of etching is to cleanse the ceramic surface by removing unwanted oxides and debris. Etching enhances the wettability of the ceramic surface by a silane coupling agent (Touati *et al.*, 1999; Matinlinna *et al.*, 2004). It has been claimed that etching is the most significant step and factor in improving bond strengths in dentistry. Some examples of acidic etchants (i.e. at pH <7) include hydrofluoric acid, acidulated phosphate fluoride and ammonium hydrogen difluoride (Stangel *et al.*, 1987; Ho and Matinlinna, 2011b; Lung and Matinlinna, 2012).

5.2.4 Acid etching with hydrofluoric acid

There is a general, though not unanimous, agreement that hydrofluoric acid (hydrogen fluoride), HF, etching followed by the so-called silanization (Lung and Matinlinna, 2012) generates higher bond strengths than either treatment alone. Application of a silane coupling agent, a procedure called silanization, is understood to create hydrogen bonds and covalent bonds between the resin cement and the ceramic substrate, while etching *per se* provides micromechanical interlocking (Canay *et al.*, 2001; Matinlinna and Vallittu, 2007a; Ho and Matinlinna, 2011b).

Hydrogen fluoride, HF, is actually a colourless, aggressively reactive gas that fumes in air. HF is very soluble in ethanol and water. Its solution in water is called hydrofluoric acid. This acid is strongly corrosive, is an excellent ionizing solvent and dissolves many inorganic and organic compounds. The ionization (acidity) constant K_a for hydrofluoric acid is surprisingly low, only 7.2×10^{-4} that is, by definition a weak acid, because it is very strongly hydrogen-bonded. It is noteworthy that the weakly acidic nature of HF is largely due to the very strong bond in the HF molecule, which reduces its tendency to dissociate into ions in aqueous solution (Heslop and Robinson, 1967; Shriver and Atkins, 2001).

Strong (i.e. concentrated) solutions of hydrofluoric acid readily attack silica and glass and create a porous structure on the ceramic surface by reacting with the silica matrix of the ceramic to produce SiF_4, which is volatile (Matinlinna and Vallittu, 2007a; Lung and Matinlinna, 2012):

$$\underset{\text{hydrofluoric acid}}{4HF}\ (l) + \underset{\text{silica matrix}}{SiO_2}\ (s) \rightarrow \underset{\text{silicon tetrafluoride}}{SiF_4}\ (l) + 2H_2O\ (l) \qquad [5.1]$$

In the next stage, silicon tetrafluoride reacts further with the hydrofluoric acid again to form a soluble complex ion, hexafluorosilicate:

$$2HF\ (l) + \underset{\text{silicon tetrafluoride}}{SiF_4}\ (l) \rightarrow \underset{\text{hexafluorosilicate}}{[SiF_6]^{2-}}\ (aq) + 2H^+\ (aq) \qquad [5.2]$$

The hydrogen ions in the solution then react further with the hexafluorosilicate complex ion that can be rinsed off with water:

$$\underset{\text{hexafluorosilicate}}{[SiF_6]^{2-}}\ (aq) + 2H^+\ (aq) \rightarrow \underset{\text{fluorosilisic acid}}{H_2SiF_6}\ (l) \qquad [5.3]$$

Given this, hydrofluoric acid may attack ceramics such as leucite-reinforced, glass-infiltrated alumina, lithium disilicate ($Li_2Si_2O_5$) and low alumina ceramic (Fig. 5.1). In this way, a deep porous structure with an average pore size of 3–4 μm may be created on a feldspar-based ceramic

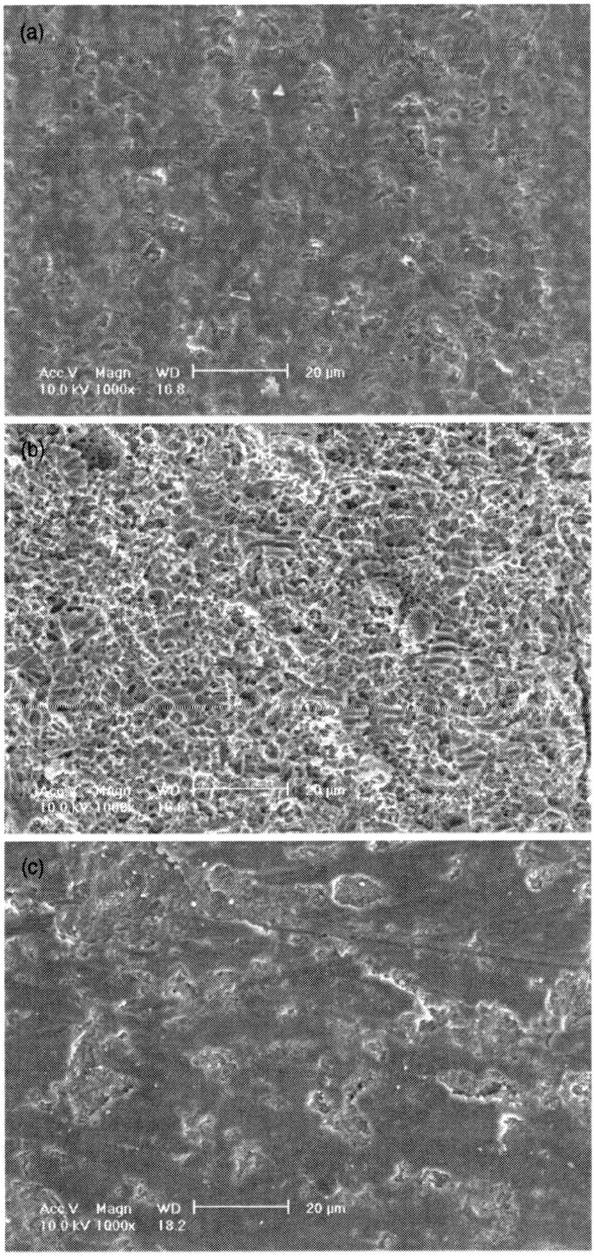

5.1 (a) Unetched leucite-reinforced ceramic at 1000× magnification. (b) Etched leucite-reinforced ceramic at 1000× magnification. (c) Unetched lithium disilicate ceramic at 1000× magnification. (d) Etched lithium disilicate ceramic at 1000× magnification (all by courtesy of Mr Gary Ho, 2011).

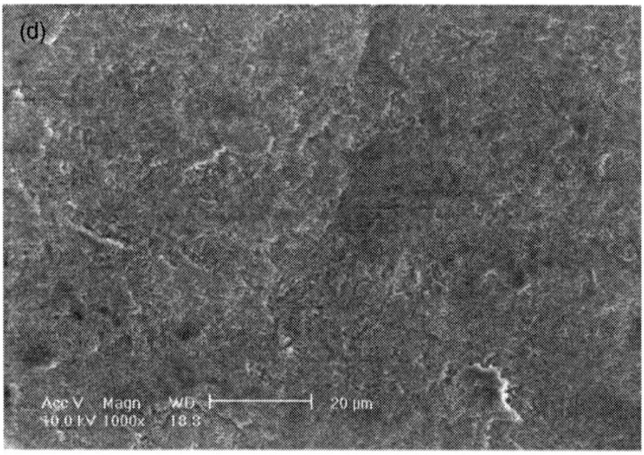

5.1 Continued

by removing and dissolving the glassy phase matrix that contains silicates, silica and leucite, $K_2O \cdot Al_2O_3 \cdot 4SiO_2$, crystals. Feldspar-based ceramics have a larger glassy phase that enables more etching to take place, creating more porous structures and creating more micromechanical interlocking by the penetration of resin composite cement (Della Bona *et al.*, 2003). As a rule of thumb, etching the surface for 5 min with HF may result in a depth of 5–7 μm; in the case of glass ceramics, the etching depth may be 10 μm after 5 min etching (Yen *et al.*, 1993).

Ceramics etched with a higher concentration of hydrofluoric acid, such as 52% for 1.5 min, dissolved more of the glassy phase and produced uniformly crystalline patterns, while a lower concentration (20%) of HF dissolved more of the crystalline phase and displayed a more amorphous structure with large porosity (Stangel *et al.*, 1987). A laboratory study found that the optimum etching time was 2 min using 5% HF etching, as evidenced by the highest mean shear bond strength after 24 h water storage at 37°C, *viz.* 44.5 ± 7.6 MPa, for feldspar-based ceramic bonded to resin composite. A scanning electron microscope (SEM) analysis revealed that ceramic surfaces etched for 2–3 min resulted in deeper, rougher and a larger number of pore sites, enabling more resin to penetrate to provide micromechanical interlocking for retention (Chen and Brauer, 1982). Given this, the best advice is to follow the manufacturer's recommendation or, if no specific instruction is given, a good rule of thumb is to etch for between 1 and 2 min. It is suggested that as low a concentration of HF as possible be used, to neutralize hydrofluoric acid before disposal and to keep hydrofluoric acid containers sealed and closed, and in cold and dark conditions, at all times when not in use.

5.2.5 Alternative acid etchants

There are, indeed, some other etching agents that have been studied in dentistry. Ammonium hydrogen difluoride, NH_4HF_2, may be used as a glass etchant. Interestingly, it can also be used as an intermediate for preparing hydrofluoric acid, HF. Now, NH_4HF_2 readily attacks the SiO_2 component of glass or porcelain (Tylka and Stewart, 1994):

$$SiO_2 + 4NH_4HF_2 \rightarrow SiF_4 + 4NH_4F + 2H_2O \quad [5.4]$$

Another known etchant, acidulated phosphate fluoride, APF, contains 1.23% fluoride ions. These fluoride ions are released from HF and NaF. Before use, this etchant is further acidified by the addition of dilute, 0.1 mol L^{-1} H_3PO_4 (Capelli and Mobley, 2008). Both of these etchants are thixotropic gels, that is a state of material with no stable three-dimensional network. It has been reported, however, that etching feldspar-based ceramics with 23% APF for 10 min is insufficient to generate the amount of micromechanical interlocking in comparison with 9.5% HF etching for 4 min. An SEM study showed a shallow and smooth homogeneous surface with acidulated phosphate fluoride (APF) in contrast to a deep, three-dimensional lattice, and uniformly porous channels using hydrofluoric acid (Canay *et al.*, 2001; Della Bona *et al.*, 2002). Increasing etching time for APF is reported to increase shear bond strength *in vitro* (Kukiattrakoon and Thammasitboon, 2007). Reported laboratory micro-tensile bond strength values for lithium disilicate ceramics etched with 9.6% HF for 2 min had higher bond strength, 41.7 ± 6.7 MPa, than those etched with 4.0% APF for 2 min, 19.1 ± 2.6 MPa (Della Bona *et al.*, 2000).

It was also found that ceramics etched with either 1.23% acidulated phosphate fluoride for 7–10 min or 9.6% HF for 4 min and bonded with a resin composite did not produce a significant difference in shear bond strengths between the two surface treatment approaches. Nevertheless, etching with HF for 4 min still yielded the highest shear bond strength, 17.64 ± 1.48 MPa, compared to etching with acidulated phosphate fluoride, 17.33 ± 1.43 MPa (Kukiattrakoon and Thammasitboon, 2007). A couple of words of warning to readers may be timely. It is important to regard bond strength results only study by study, bearing in mind that mutual comparisons between separately reported studies are cumbersome to interpret and may not be exactly justified. Usually, the standard deviations are high, even up to 50% of the mean bond strength results, owing to several factors.

5.2.6 Resin ceramics bonding without acid etching

The hazards of hydrofluoric acid as an etchant for ceramics in dentistry have been well identified and recognized. Potential symptoms of overexposure to HF are irritation to the eyes, skin, nose and throat. These symptoms may manifest as skin and eye burns, pulmonary oedema and bronchitis (O'Neil *et al.*, 2006). Interestingly, it has been reported that acid etching using highly toxic HF may be substituted by grit-blasting using Al_2O_3 powder, followed by so-called modified silanization which employes an idea using hot air to cure the silane film. This might lead *in vitro* to durable and reliable resin ceramic bonding because the mean tensile bond strength is similar to that after hydrofluoric acid etching of the ceramic surface (Hooshmand *et al.*, 2002). It may be concluded, however, that there are still far more studies achieving higher bond strengths between resin and ceramic with hydrofluoric acid etching than without it.

5.2.7 Grit-blasting methods in dentistry

Abrasion and roughening with a bur are clearly inconsistent and arbitrary when modifying a ceramic surface and may initiate cracks and flaws. A suitable treatment with many industrial applications on numerous material surfaces is grit-blasting, also known as air abrasion, sandblasting or airborne particle abrasion. In general, grit-blasting cleans any greasy substances and oxide layers from metal surfaces and allows micromechanical retention (Matinlinna and Mittal, 2009; Lung and Matinlinna, 2012).

In dental laboratories, grit-blasting can be carried out using alumina powder, typically with parameters such as 50 μm average particle diameter, a constant perpendicular distance of the nozzle from the substrate material surface (usually about 10 mm), a fixed, high air pressure (e.g. 380 kPa) and a particular application time such as 10–15 s per an area unit, which may be, for example, 1 cm^2.

The tribochemical silica-coating method conditions the surface by depositing alumina powder particles coated with silica onto the substrate surface, using similar parameters as grit-blasting with alumina powder. During tribochemical silica-coating, the particles hit the surface, causing a momentary local temperature of as high as 1200°C. The fresh silica layer then fuses onto the substrate surface. Finally, a silane coupling agent (Lung and Matinlinna, 2012) is applied to the surface to create hydrogen bonds and covalent bonds between the substrate layer and the resin composite. The patented systems (by 3M ESPE) that are commercially available are the Rocatec® system for dental laboratories and CoJet® for the dentist's surgery (Heikkinen *et al.*, 2007).

In dental technology, tribochemical silica-coating (silicatization) is a widely used conditioning method for ceramic and metal alloy constructions in fabrication, repair and cementation. Silica-coating (followed by silanization) is one key pretreatment method for successful resin bonding and it can also be used at the chair-side in the dentist's surgery (Lung and

Matinlinna, 2012). However, oxide ceramics with a high crystalline content, such as alumina and zirconia, cannot be etched with acid etchants. They should, for example, be silica-coated and silanized prior to bonding, as described in detail below.

It has been recently concluded based on laboratory studies that tribochemical silicatization of oxide ceramics (i.e. alumina and zirconia) may be affected by the operating air pressure, that is the air pressure used has a significant effect on shear bond strength. The silica content at the alumina ceramic surface increases as the operating air pressure increases, whereas results on zirconia surfaces are somewhat controversial. When the air pressure of tribochemical silicatization is increased, the shear bond strength of the resin composite of zirconia and alumina ceramics increases (Heikkinen *et al.*, 2007, 2009).

During this application, silica-coated alumina powder particles hit the surface, causing a momentary local temperature as high as 1200°C. The fresh silica layer fuses onto the substrate surface. A significant consequence of tribochemical silicatization is its effect on the surface roughness of, for example, zirconia (Fig. 5.2). Without air abrasion, the shear bond strength values cannot reach an acceptable bond strength level. This finding indicates and supports the importance of micromechanical linking onto the surface during cementation to oxide ceramics (Heikkinen *et al.*, 2010).

5.3 Silane coupling agents and their chemistry

Silane coupling agents (silanes) are not found in nature but they are always synthetic organic–inorganic hybrid compounds with direct one or more ≡C-Si≡ bonds. They have been extensively studied as coupling agents in industrial applications over the past 50 years. Generally, silanes may or may not contain reactive, functional groups. The organofunctional trialkoxysilane is: (i) monofunctional, when there is one silicon atom with three alkoxy groups in the molecule, for example 3-methacryloxypropyltrimethoxysilane (Fig. 5.3); (ii) bis-functional, when there are two silicon atoms, each with three alkoxy groups, for example bis[3-(triethoxysilyl)propyl] tetrasulfide and a so-called cross-linker silane 1,2-bis-(triethoxysilyl)ethane; and (iii) tris-functional when three silicon atoms exist, for example tris-(3-trimethoxysilylpropyl)isocyanurate. A non-functional silane contains aromatic aryl, or alkyl groups, and it has no reactive double bonds; these silanes are not considered coupling agents, but are used for coating purposes. However, it must be borne in mind that the term dual functionality (bifunctionality) denotes the silane coupling agents' property of promoting adhesion between dissimilar materials (Plueddemann, 1991).

Some bis-functional silanes (*bis* = two), also called dipodal silanes (*bis*-silanes), when used in combination with functional silanes, have a significant

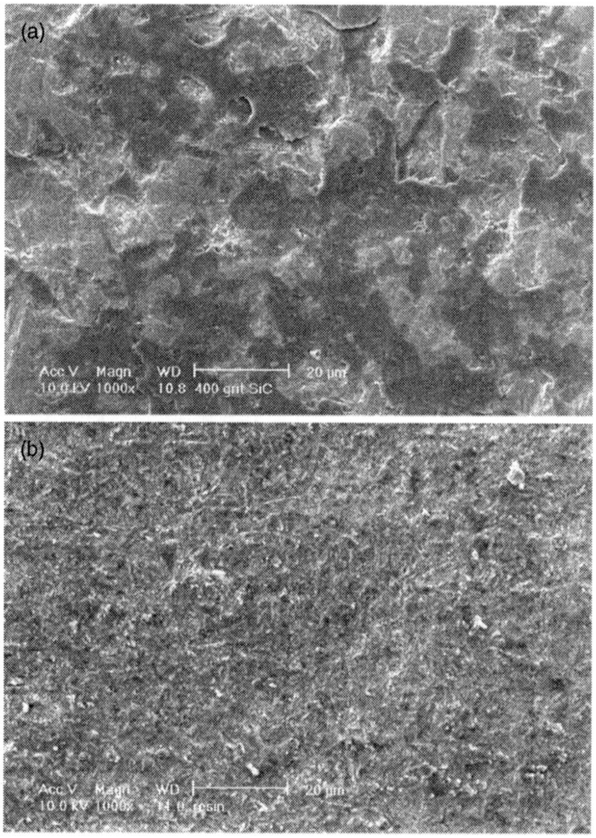

5.2 (a) Polished zirconia surface (SEM image, magnification 1000×). (b) Silica-coated zirconia surface (SEM image, magnification 1000×).

impact on substrate bonding, mechanical strength and hydrolytic stability in many composite systems. In aggressive aqueous environments, dipodal silanes often demonstrate substantial durability performance improvements. 1,2-bis-(triethoxysilyl)ethane is such a dipodal silane, it contains two Si-based groups, and it is widely used as a cross-linker in manufacturing processes (Matinlinna *et al.*, 2006a; Seth *et al.*, 2007).

Most silanes exhibit moderate thermal stability, making them suitable for example for plastics that are processed at below 350°C, or they can even sustain continuous temperature exposure up to 150°C. Selection of the appropriate silane coupling agent is accomplished typically by empirical evaluation of silanes within predicted categories. Organosilanes are either hydrophobic or they can be also hydrophilic; they can also be anionic or cationic. Non-functional silanes are used to alter wetting characteristics of the surface (Plueddemann, 1970, 1991; Rosen, 1978).

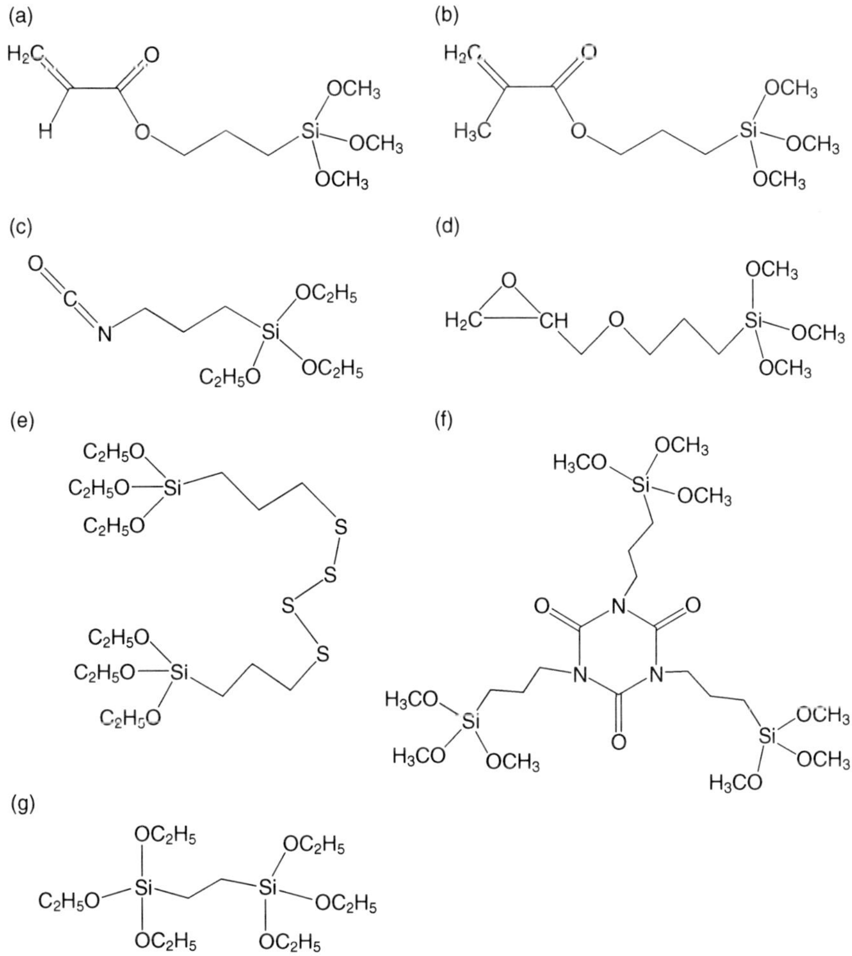

5.3 Silane monomers (courtesy of Dr Christie Lung, 2011)
(a) 3-acryloyloxypropyltrimethoxysilane,
(b) 3-methacryloyloxypropyltrimethoxysilane,
(c) 3-isocyanatopropyltriethoxysilane,
(d) 3-glycidoxypropyltrimethoxysilane,
(e) bis-[3-(triethoxysilyl)propyl]tetrasulfide,
(f) tris-(3-trimethoxysilylpropyl)isocyanurate,
(g) 1,2-bis-(triethoxysilyl)ethane.

Since the 1960s, a plethora of new polymers has been introduced and the number of useful silane coupling agents has risen significantly. Silanes on metal substrates, such as steel and brass, have been studied for over 30 years in industrial applications (Seth *et al.*, 2007). Interestingly, silanes pose neither special safety hazards at the laboratory scale nor cytotoxicological problems (Arkles, 1983).

Silanes can function as mediators and promote adhesion between essentially dissimilar, that is inorganic and organic, matrices through dual reactivity. Silanes used in dentistry are hybrid organic–inorganic trialkoxy ester monomers, which are diluted in an acidified water–ethanol solvent system. Such silane primers are then said to be prehydrolyzed and ready-to-use. As the reactive monomer, they usually contain 3-methacryloxypropyltrimethoxysilane. In dentistry, silanes are used also as coupling agents for resin composites to silica-coated ceramics, acid-etched porcelain, base metal and noble metal alloys, Ti and Ag-amalgams (Matinlinna *et al.*, 2004; Lung and Matinlinna, 2012). A silane coupling agent should be applied to the ceramic surface after silica-coating to achieve chemical bonding and optimal durable bond strength. Moreover, in dentistry, silanes are indicated for veneering, prior to cementation of ceramic, and repairing ceramic/composite veneers (Blatz *et al.*, 2003; Matinlinna and Vallittu, 2007b). There is a plethora of commercially available prehydrolyzed silanes for use in dentistry, but these may demonstrate drastically different bonding properties from their solvent system, pH, silane concentration and so on (Matinlinna *et al.*, 2006b). Even so, silanes are also used when manufacturing resin composites for any dental use, because the fillers have to be silanized to keep them bound in the matrix (Arkles, 1977).

In general, organosilicon compounds are characterized by direct silicon–carbon, ≡Si-C≡, bonds, which are calculated to be as strong as, and in some cases even stronger than analogous C—C bonds. Tetrachlorosilane (silicon tetrachloride), $SiCl_4$, is a convenient precursor for the synthesis of other functional and more advanced, complicated silanes. Elements other than Si or C bonded to Si generally undergo rapid hydrolysis. However, most bonds to Si oxidize slowly, and protecting silanes from moisture is more important than protecting them from O_2. $SiCl_4$ hydrolyzes easily but this reaction, on the other hand, is impossible for carbon tetrachloride:

$$SiCl_4\ (l) + 2H_2O\ (g\ or\ l) \rightarrow SiO_2\ (s) + 4HCl\ (g) \qquad [5.5]$$

$$CCl_4\ (l) + 2H_2O\ (g\ or\ l) \rightarrow \text{no reaction} \qquad [5.6]$$

This reactivity [5.5] is understood to be due to the empty 3d-orbitals of Si atoms. Moreover, —Si-Si— bonds are definitely weaker than analogous —C—C— bonds (Arkles 1977; Rosen, 1978; Plueddemann, 1991).

Interestingly, over 100 identified species may be synthesized using the following general reaction:

$$CH_3Cl + Si(Cu) \rightarrow Me_nSiCl_{4-n} + Me_xSi_wH_yCl_z \qquad [5.7]$$

This reaction may be optimized to produce Me_2SiCl_2 which is a start reagent for silicone synthesis. Silicones have the R—O—(—Si—O—)$_x$—R backbone which typically contains the polydimethylsiloxane repeat unit and end-capping alkyl groups. Vast amount of silicones are used as lubricants, waxes, high boiling oils, flexible polymers, sealants, impression materials in dentistry (Powers and Sakaguchi, 2006) and as biomaterials (Arkles, 1983).

5.3.1 Silanization

In general, silanes used industrially for surface pretreatment in order to promote adhesion between dissimilar materials are usually organofunctional trialkoxy silanes. They are also chemically named as silane esters, with the general formula R-Y-SiX_3, where R is a non-hydrolyzable organic group, Y is a linker, and X is a hydrolyzable group. Silanes are bifunctional: they have dual reactivity. The non-hydrolyzable functional group (e.g. methacrylate, ureido, acrylate, vinyl, allyl, isocyanato) can polymerize with monomers containing double bonds. The hydrolyzable alkoxy groups, such as methoxy -O-CH_3, and ethoxy -O-CH_2CH_3, react with an inorganic substrate rich in hydroxyl groups. Alkoxy groups are intermediates in the formation of silanol groups, ≡Si—OH, for bonding to suitable inorganic surfaces (Plueddemann, 1970; Rosen 1978).

The number of hydrolyzable groups is an important parameter that controls bonding characteristics of silane coupling agents. Trialkoxysilanes (i.e. with three alkoxy groups) have the maximum stability, but they tend to be hygroscopic. Monoalkoxysilanes (with one alkoxy group), form the most hydrophobic siloxane films but have the lowest long-term hydrolytic stability. Dialkoxysilanes, often used as coupling agents for low modulus thermoplastics and elastomers, form less rigid interfaces than trialkoxysilanes (Rosen, 1978).

Activated silane coupling agents with three alkoxy groups tend to deposit as polymeric films, maximizing the appearance of organic functionality. It is generally accepted that hydrophobic silanes must first be hydrolyzed (activated) and then condensed (deposited) onto the inorganic substrate. In aqueous solution, the labile alkoxy groups react with water to form reactive, hydrophilic, acidic silanol groups, ≡Si—OH. Hydrolysis has been suggested as a crucial step in adsorption onto an OH-group covered substrate. In the simplified schematic presentation illustrated in Fig. 5.4, hydrolysis (which takes place in three steps for a trialkoxy silane) is followed by condensation of monomers to dimers and trimers. Finally, they deposit onto the surface and set to a polymer matrix (Plueddemann, 1991).

Silane coupling agents (silanes) act as mediators that bond two dissimilar materials together through a process called silanization. They are structured to have dual-function monomers, consisting of alkoxy groups that when hydrolyzed react with the ceramic surface and are separated by a linker part (usually a hydrocarbon chain). Silanes may have a methacrylate group with reactive vinylic C=C bonds that copolymerize with the monomers of

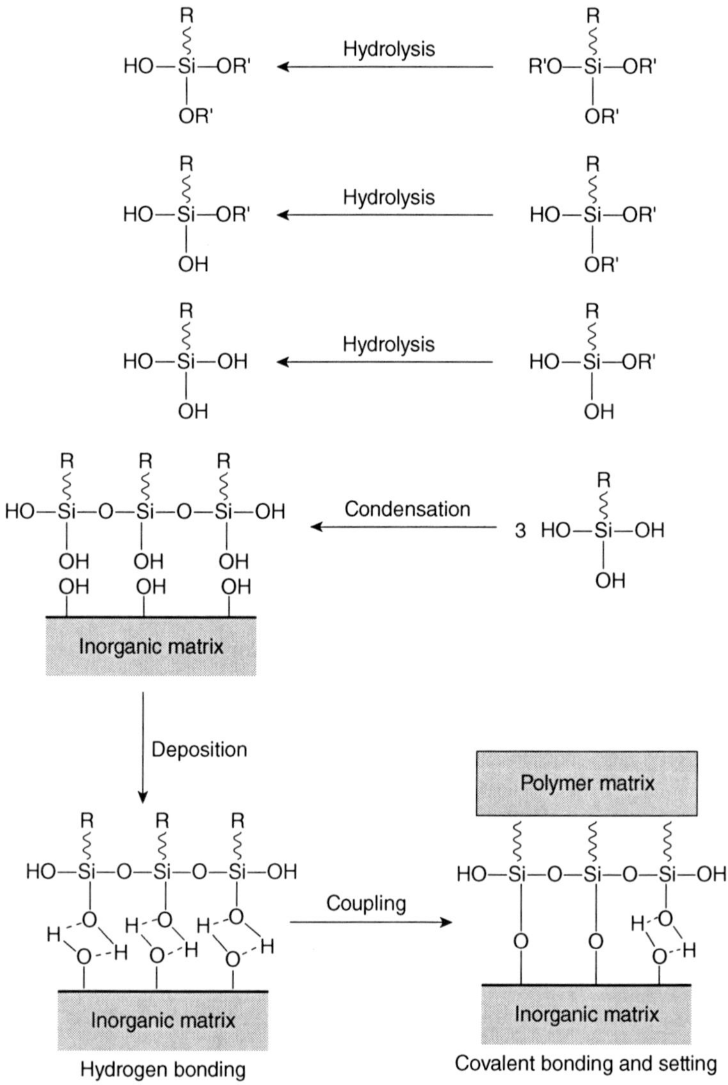

5.4 Silane activation (hydrolysis) and deposition mechanisms (courtesy of Dr Christie Lung, 2011).

the resin composite matrix. Indeed, silanes bond dissimilar materials together, inorganic to organic, by forming a branched, complicated three dimensional (3D) polysiloxane (-Si-O-Si-) film in the interphase between the two materials. The type and topography of the siloxane film depends on several factors, such as silane concentration, functionality, hydrolysis characteristics, reaction time and deposition (Plueddemann, 1970; Seth *et al.*, 2007).

Silanes are used as surface primer agents for adhesion promotion, a process called conditioning or priming. Conditioning may increase the critical surface energy of a surface by wetting the surfaces. High surface energy on the substrate surface and low surface tension of a liquid are desired because liquids then will spread spontaneously and evenly onto the surface. Low energy contaminants such as oil and grease inhibit wetting and prevent adhesion. In order to achieve complete wetting, the adhesive must have a low viscosity and a surface tension that is lower than the critical surface tension (γ_c) of the substrate surface (Rosen 1978; Plueddemann, 1991).

Silane coupling agents for dental use contain silane monomers that are diluted with a solvent, usually ethanol, to produce about 1–2% silane primers. They are used to wet the silica-coated substrate surface of an indirect restoration and reduce the surface tension. For common preactivated dental silane products, the shelf-life of silanes is usually several years (Matinlinna *et al.*, 2006b; Lung and Matinlinna, 2012).

Now, by silanizing the acid etched porcelain surface, the bond strength between the ceramic and the resin can improve significantly (Sorensen *et al.*, 1991). A report assessing the bonding between resin composite cement and Al_2O_3-reinforced feldspar ceramic concluded that Al_2O_3-reinforced ceramics should be silica-coated and silanized to achieve durable bond strength after artificial ageing (thermocycling, water storage). Etching Al_2O_3-reinforced ceramics with 9.5% HF followed by silanization may result in a higher bond strength than silica-coating an Al_2O_3-reinforced ceramic followed by silane application. After dry and long-term water storage at 37°C for 150 days followed by thermocycling for 12 000 cycles, silica-coating with silanization could sustain significantly higher bond strengths than HF treatment combined with silanization (Ozcan *et al.*, 2009).

3-Methacryloxypropyltrimethoxysilane (Fig. 5.3(a)) is a widely used coupling agent for unsaturated polyester–fibreglass composites and it is also the most used functional silane monomer in dental silane products (Plueddemann, 1970). Many other silane monomers may also promote adhesion. Interestingly, some recent *in vitro* studies suggest that resin bonding to silica-coated Ti might be significantly stronger when diluted 3-isocyanatopropyltriethoxysilane was used as a coupling agent (Matinlinna *et al.*, 2005). Reactive 3-acryloxypropyltrimethoxysilane has also exhibited superior adhesion promotion to the same substrate (Matinlinna *et al.*, 2007a). These examples with surprisingly high bonding strength results illustrate the unlimited opportunities what we may have in silane chemistry.

5.4 Resin zirconia bonding

Creating a durable bond between all-ceramic restorations and the tooth structure is a prerequisite for a successful restoration for several reasons:

(i) it will increase fracture resistance of the restoration; (ii) it will prevent microleakage; and (iii) it will enhance the stability and retention of the restoration (Parker, 2007). Turning our thoughts first to alumina, silica-coating may be useful: once the resin composite is bonded to silica-coated and silanized alumina ceramics, shear bond strengths as high as 21.54 ± 1.4 MPa may be obtained after 5000 times thermocycling between +5°C and +55°C. Etching or sandblasting only resulted in shear bond strengths of 5.5 ± 0.7 MPa or 12.9 ± 2.0 MPa, respectively (Ozcan *et al.*, 2001). Dental ceramics with a high crystalline content such as alumina and zirconia may be silica-coated prior to silanization because they do not contain a large amount of glassy phase for etching (Matinlinna *et al.*, 2006c; Heikkinen *et al.*, 2009).

The literature contains numerous laboratory investigations that have evaluated the effect of different surface treatments on the established bond strength in the laboratory. Methods such as acid etching by hydrofluoric acid, sand blasting using alumina powder with various particle sizes, sand-blasting with silica-coated alumina powder particles and, more recently, application of laser irradiation, have been reported to improve the bond strength significantly (Atsu *et al.*, 2006; Matinlinna *et al.*, 2006c; Cavalcanti *et al.*, 2009; Kern *et al.*, 2009; Heikkinen *et al.*, 2009). On the other hand, without proper surface treatment or application of a suitable priming agent, the shear bond strength between luting cements and zirconia has been reported to be only a minimal about 1.5 MPa (Derand *et al.*, 2005). We may surmise that a major concern while performing the required surface treatment and bonding procedure is the possibility of surface contamination during handling. Slight surface contamination, even in the form of adsorption of atmospheric gases – let alone, an innocent fingerprint – could result in a significant drop in bond strength. Under clinical conditions, salivary contamination presents a major risk of surface contamination (Yang *et al.*, 2007).

5.4.1 Approaches to resin zirconia bonding

Establishing a strong durable bond strength to zirconia is further complicated by the problem of polymerization stresses of the adhesive resin (Kleverlaan and Feilzer, 2005) and the influence of water absorption (Feilzer *et al.*, 1995), which could significantly deteriorate the established bond. For a stiff material like zirconia, any sort of deformation and compliance must be compensated by the weaker adhesive resin. Additionally, the established bond must resist the alternating chemical environment of the oral cavity and hydrolytic enzymes present in saliva.

In summary, approaches to promote resin zirconia bonding promotion produce mainly physical changes on the surface topography of zirconia

Table 5.2 Some alternative *in vitro* approaches to resin zirconia bonding

Method description	Year	Reported by
Resin composites alone	1998	Wegner and Kern (2000)
MDP monomer-based resin composite cements alone	2007	Blatz *et al.* (2003)
Combination of sand blasting and MDP monomer the most recommended method for bonding zirconia restorations	2007	Quaas *et al.* (2007)
Selective infiltration etching (SIE)	2007	Aboushelib *et al.* (2007)
Zirconia + zirconia coating	2009	Phark *et al.* (2009)
Alumina particles + metal primers	2009	Cavalcanti *et al.* (2009)
New etching approaches	2009	Casucci *et al.* (2009)
SIE + silane primers + organophosphate cement	2009	Aboushelib *et al.* (2009)
An impact method	2010	Papia *et al.* (2012)
Surface modifications and silane monomers	2010	Lung *et al.* (2010)
Silica-coating + a universal primer	2011	Attia *et al.* (2011)
Nanostructured alumina coating	2011	Jevnikar *et al.* (2010)
Silica-coating and various silane monomers	2011	Matinlinna and Lassila (2011)

(Table 5.2). After application of the surface treatment of choice, the surface roughness and, as a result, the surface energy is increased, which results in better wetting of the bonding agent on zirconia restorations. Direct chemical treatment of the zirconia surface by reaction with concentrated mineral acids and bases might be a surface pretreatment. However, zirconia remains more resistant to strong acids like hydrofluoric acid than other glass ceramics (Lohbauer *et al.*, 2008). Silica-coating combined with etching acids has been proposed as a potential approach for resin zirconia adhesion promotion owing to the dramatic changes it may cause to the surface topography and texture (Lung *et al.*, 2010). It is noteworthy that any fingerprint on zirconia before its cementation may compromise resin zirconia bonding efforts.

Approaches such as micromechanical retention, chemical bonding, or a combination of both have been suggested as prerequisites for a durable bond between the resin composite cement and the cementation surface of zirconia restorations. It is frequently advised that before bonding resin to zirconia ceramics, zirconia should be treated either by air abrading the surface with alumina particles or silica-coating before silanization to achieve adequate bond strengths. Zirconia that had no surface treatments before silanization resulted in low bond strength of 7.6 ± 3.0 MPa, but after 30 μm alumina powder air abrasion followed by silanization, a bond strength as high as 18.6 ± 5.9 MPa was obtained (Yoshida *et al.*, 2006). However, alumina cannot be as readily silanized as zirconia, because the forming =Al-O-Si≡ bonds are hydrolytically weaker, that is less stable and durable, than ≡Si-O-Si≡ bonds (Plueddemann, 1991).

Silanes cannot react chemically directly with zirconia, that is they are not known directly to form strong, durable ≡Si-O-Zr≡ bonds. Some other reactive functional silane monomers other than 3-methacryloxypropyltrimethoxysilane have been recently evaluated in laboratory studies using different bonding resins and luting cements to silica-coated zirconia: following silica-coating, they may significantly enhance resin zirconia bonding because, in principle, silica-coating may provide a large number of ≡Si-OH groups on the zirconia surface, as suggested in Fig. 5.5 (Feilzer *et al.*, 1995; Yoshida *et al.*, 2006; Matinlinna *et al.*, 2006c, 2007b; Lung *et al.*, 2010; Matinlinna and Lassila, 2011).

Today, different forms of organophosphate monomers are available from various dental product manufacturers. These monomers differ in structure and the number of active sites in the molecular structure of the monomer. Three different phosphate monomer agents were previously assessed and differences in bond strength values were observed, indicating different reactivity of these monomers (Mirmohammadi *et al.*, 2010a).

The combination of acidic organophosphate monomers like 10-methacryloyloxydecyldihydrogenphosphate (MDP, 10-MDP) monomers with airborne particle abrasion application (i.e. that are not silica-coated) is currently considered the gold standard method of cementation for zirconia restorations. Organophosphate primers contain an organofunctional part that contains a methacrylate group that copolymerizes with resin composite. The phosphate monomers bond with some transition metal oxides on zirconia that derive from dyeing agents with which zirconia is treated before firing (Fig. 5.6).

Bond strength stability (durability) up to 150 days has been reported for this bonding concept (Mirmohammadi *et al.*, 2010a). However, there is a lack of understanding of the details of the mechanism of the chemical reaction between organophosphate monomers and zirconia (Yoshida *et al.*, 2006). On the other hand, in a comparison of bond strengths of different combinations of bonding agents, silane coupling agents and resin cements to zirconia, it was concluded that conditioning with a bonding/silane agent that also contains a phosphate ester monomer, MDP could exhibit superior resin bonding to zirconia which was first sandblasted with Al_2O_3 powder (Blatz *et al.*, 2004).

It has been suggested that MDP-containing dental cement materials could be used with oxide ceramics in order to achieve sufficient long-term bond durability (Blatz *et al.*, 2004; Yang *et al.*, 2010). Given this, it has been shown that even if zirconia is bonded using a 10-MDP-containing

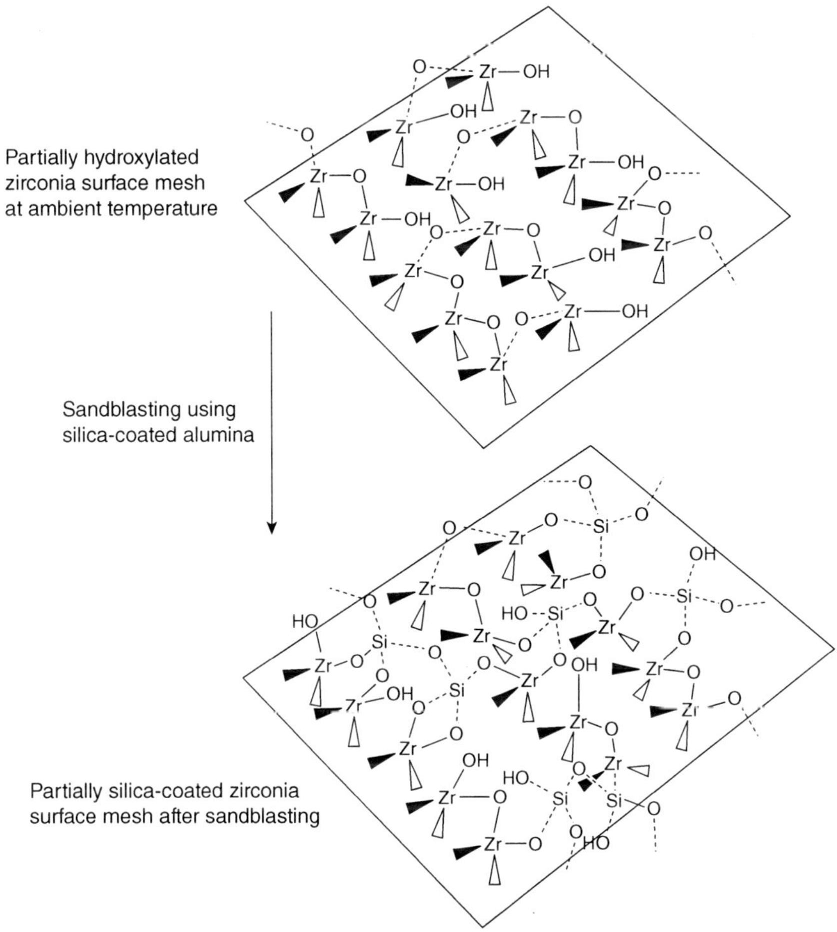

5.5 Silica coating and its effect on the hydroxylation of zirconia surface (courtesy of Dr Christie Lung, 2011).

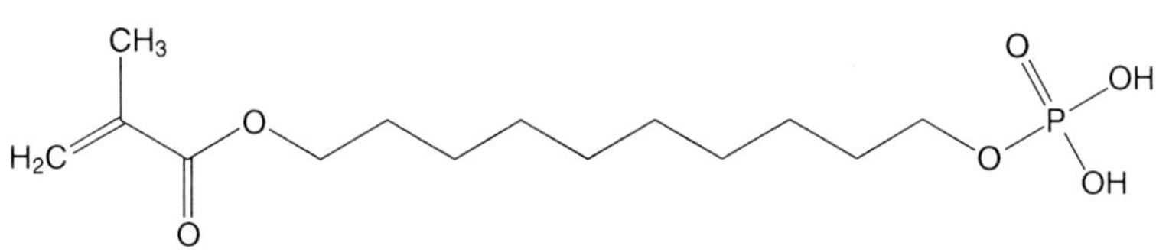

5.6 Molecular structure of 10-methacryloyloxydecyldihydrogenphosphate (MDP) monomer (courtesy of Dr Timo Heikkinen).

organophosphate resin without airborne particle abrasion of the zirconia surface, specimens demonstrate low bond strength values (Aboushelib *et al.*, 2007). This finding might suggest that without Al_2O_3 powder sand-blasting as a pretreatment, no beneficial effect can be attributed to the phosphate monomer alone.

Zirconia-based biomaterials can be described as dynamic materials on a microscopic level: they undergo a tetragonal to monoclinic transformation (Piconi and Maccauro, 1999). The surface and bulk grains may grow in size when allowed sufficient time and an appropriate ambient temperature. The selective infiltration etching (SIE) technique of preparing zirconia utilizes this very dynamic feature to increase surface nanoporosity for the adhesive resin to infiltrate, interlock and finally polymerize. By applying a specific, optimized infiltration glass powder and heating the specimen to the required temperature, the molten infiltration glass forces the surface grains to split and slide over each other to create the required surface porosity. After this infiltration glass is rinsed and washed off, the new nanoscale rough surface becomes ready to establish a durable bond with the adhesive resin of choice (Aboushelib *et al.*, 2007).

Actually, the application of a glassy layer on the fitting surface of zirconia restorations has some drawbacks, as the layer may interfere with the seating accuracy of these restorations. It may also be cumbersome to apply as an even layer, in particular on small-sized zirconia restoration surfaces. The application of phosphate monomer agents on a smooth as-sintered zirconia surface without the application of particle abrasion would result in quick deterioration of the established bond, indicating that micromechanical retention is an indispensable part of the bonding procedure (Mirmohammadi *et al.*, 2010b). Similar observations were reported for the reactivity of different experimental silane primers used to enhance wetting of the nanoporous zirconia surface, as differences in the observed bond strength indicated different reactive capacities of these silane primers (Aboushelib *et al.*, 2009).

Recently, two laboratory study approaches were introduced for enhanced resin zirconia bonding. First, a modified, relatively rough surface can be produced on zirconia after milling and then coating it with a slurry containing zirconia powder and a specific pore-forming agent. The slurry is then sintered. This method produces *in vitro* significantly more durable bonding than airborne-particle abrasion (Phark *et al.*, 2009). Second, a nanostructural sintered alumina coating prepared by the sol–gel technique may also chemically modify the zirconia surface and thus promote resin adhesion onto it (Jevnikar *et al.*, 2010). An impaction method to modify zirconia surface was suggested and reported recently (Papia *et al.*, 2012).

5.4.2 Bond strength testing

Regarding the measurement of bond strength, laboratory approaches are used to evaluate bond strength values by shear, micro-shear, tensile, push-out, pull-out, or micro-tensile bond strength tests, (van Noort, 2007; Matinlinna and Mittal, 2009). In each set-up, the loading forces (caused by a load) are delivered by the universal testing machine and are thus transmitted through the attachment unit to the specimen and then to the bonded interface, which has to resist these forces until failure occurs. Micro-tensile bond strength testing has become popular to evaluate bond strength, since it allows numerous microbars to be obtained from small-sized specimens and it subjects the bonded interface to a direct tensile force. Unfortunately, these *in vitro* tests do not reflect the fact that stresses in the oral cavity are not unidirectional. Interestingly, a new test has been introduced to rotate fatigue and thereby subject the bonded interface to alternating tensile and compressive stresses without the need to load the specimens to failure (Mirmohammadi *et al.*, 2010b).

When comparing bond strengths between different studies, one should be very cautious because dissimilar ceramic types, different bond test methods, varying concentrations of acid etchant, different numbers of specimens (and specimen groups), and different ageing (storage) methods and periods are used. Also, paying too much attention to the absolute numerical bond strength values is misleading and meaningless; the comparison should be made against the control group behaviour in each study. Therefore, a challenge remains: researchers should come up with a standardized method to make studies more comparable.

There is growing evidence that the shear bond test is not adequate to measure bond strength values of resin bonded to ceramic, because the shear test may result in cohesive failure within the ceramic or within the composite. Cohesive failure may end the bond test early, leading to lower, premature bond strength values. The material (either ceramic or resin composite) is the limitation of the test, but this also gives an indication that the material is weak and further improvements in the material may need to be made. The main point of using a bond test is to test bond quality rather than to vet whether the material is strong or not.

Shear bond strength values obtained for resin composite bonded to ceramic are of the magnitude of 5–30 MPa when the ceramic is etched and silanized. However, in a lone experiment, the bond strength reached as high as 46.9 ± 6.6 MPa using the shear bond strength test (Lacy *et al.*, 1988). The shear bond test is 'simple' to set up and is, in principle, good for hard ceramic materials, such as zirconia, that are not reported to fail cohesively. In contrast, micro-tensile bond strength tests produce more consistent and usually higher bond strength values. They may be in the range of 25–55 MPa when the ceramic is etched and silanized prior to bonding with resin and the predominant mode of failure is adhesive. Are we in this case actually testing 'bond' strength? The question remains. One should also note that shear bond values and micro-tensile bond values are not comparable with each other.

As previously mentioned in this chapter, porcelain in the presence of a glassy phase needs to be acid etched and then silanized. We might conclude also that high crystalline content ceramics (zirconia) should be silica-coated followed by silanization, however, only when the restoration wall is not too thin. Perhaps surprisingly, many reported laboratory studies do not test different storage media other than conventional storage conditions such as water storage or thermocycling. Some recent laboratory studies based on experimental silane coupling agents suggest significantly improved bond strengths. Moreover, future laboratory studies should consider the use of artificial saliva or food beverages (Ho and Matinlinna, 2011c) as storage media.

5.5 Future trends

It is apparent that ceramics/porcelain as a material group will continue to play a vital role in dentistry owing to their natural aesthetics and sovereign biocompatibility: no adverse reactions are known. However, there will always remain a compromise between aesthetics and biomechanical strength. Good translucency requires a higher content of the glassy phase and good strength requires a higher content of the crystalline phase. Hence, there needs to be a balance between the two material phases. Even so, hydrofluoric acid etching and silanization can achieve an optimal bond strength in comparison to other etchants if the porcelain etched is feldspar-based. However, a few other laboratory studies presented above demonstrated that other methods can also attain comparable bond strengths.

While on the topic of ceramic dental materials, recent research in contemporary biomaterials science has been heavily focused on resin zirconia bonding and porcelain zirconia bonding. It has become more obvious that the extremely thin bonding interphase is a very complex and dynamic 3D region where different material interfaces meet. There, at the interphase, the interaction of chemical and micromechanical retention, chemical composition, polymerization stresses, surface roughness and porosity, water absorption, degradation and cyclic loading all take place. Thus, we may conclude that surface treatments are vital to achieving durable bonding and high bond strength between resin and ceramics (Ho and Matinlinna, 2011b).

Silane coupling agents (Lung and Matinlinna, 2012) with new formulations and as the reactive monomers may have a huge potential as components in more durable bonding systems.

5.6 Sources of further information and advice

Curtis R V and Watson T F (2008), *Dental Biomaterials: Imaging, Testing and Modelling*, Woodhead Publishing, Cambridge.

Matinlinna J P and Mittal K L (2009), *Adhesion Aspects in Dentistry*, VSP/Brill, Leiden.

Powers J M and Sakaguchi R L (2006), *Craig's Restorative Dental Materials*, Elsevier, St Louis.

Powers J M and Wataha J C (2008), *Dental Materials: Properties and Manipulation*, Elsevier, St Louis.

van Noort R (2007), *Introduction to Dental Materials*, Elsevier, Philadelphia.

ADM The Academy of Dental Materials: *www.academydentalmaterials.org*

FDI World Dental Federation: *www.fdiworldental.org*

HKU The University of Hong Kong, Faculty of Dentistry: *facdent.hku.hk*

IADR International Association for Dental Research: *www.iadr.org*

NIOM Nordic Institute of Dental Materials: *www.niom.no*

5.7 References

Aboushelib M N, Kleverlaan C J and Feilzer A J (2007), 'Selective infiltration-etching technique for a strong and durable bond of resin cements to zirconia-based materials', *J Prosthet Dent*, **98**, 379–88.

Aboushelib M N, Mirmohamadi H, Matinlinna J P, Kukk E, Ounsi H and Salameh Z (2009), 'Innovations in bonding to zirconia based materials. Part II: Focusing on chemical interactions', *Dent Mater*, **25**, 989–93.

Arkles B (1977), 'Tailoring surfaces with silanes', *CHEMTECH*, **7**, 766–78.

Arkles B (1983), 'Look what you can make out of silicones', *CHEMTECH*, **13**, 542–55.

Atsu S S, Kilicarslan M A, Kucukesmen H C and Aka P S (2006), 'Effect of zirconium–oxide ceramic surface treatments on the ond strength to adhesive resin', *J Prosthet Dent*, **95**, 430–36.

Attia A, Lehmann F and Kern M (2011), 'Influence of surface conditioning and cleaning methods on resin bonding to zirconia ceramic'. *Dent Mater*, **27**, 207–13.

Blatz M B, Sadan A and Kern M (2003), 'Resin–ceramic bonding: a review of the literature', *J Prosthet Dent*, **89**, 268–74.

Blatz M B, Sadan A, Martin J and Lang B (2004), '*In vitro* evaluation of shear bond strengths of resin to densely sintered high-purity zirconium-oxide ceramic after long-term storage and thermal cycling', *J Prosthet Dent*, **91**, 356–62.

Canay S, Hersek N, and Ertan A (2001), 'Effect of different acid treatments on a porcelain surface', *J Oral Rehabil*, **28**, 95–101.

Canullo L (2007), 'Clinical outcome study of customized zirconia abutments for single-implant restorations', *Int J Prosthodont*, **20**, 489–93.

Cappelli D P and Mobley C C (2008), *Prevention in Clinical Oral Health Care*, Elsevier, St Louis, 199.

Casucci A, Osorio E, Osorio R, Monticelli F, Toledano M, Mazzitelli C and Ferrari M (2009), 'Influence of different surface treatments on surface zirconia frameworks'. *J Dent*, **37**, 891–7.

Cavalcanti A N, Foxton R M, Watson T F, Oliveira M T, Giannini M and Marchi G M (2009), 'Bond strength of resin cements to a zirconia ceramic with different surface treatments', *Oper Dent*, **34**, 280–87.

Chen T M and Brauer G M (1982), 'Solvent effects on bonding organo-silane to silica surfaces', *J Dent Res*, **61**, 1439–43.

Chevalier J (2006), 'What future for zirconia as a biomaterial?', *Biomaterials*, **27**, 535–43.

Choi B K, Han J S, Yang J H, Lee J B and Kim S H (2009), 'Shear bond strength of veneering porcelain to zirconia and metal cores', *J Adv Prosthodont*, **1**, 129–35.

Claussen N (1976), 'Fracture Toughness of Al_2O_3 with an Unstabilized ZrO_2 Dispersed Phase', *J Am Ceram Soc*, **59**, 49–51.

Clelland N L, Ramirez A, Katsube N and Seghi R R (2007), 'Influence of bond quality on failure of leucite- and lithia disilicate-based ceramics'. *J Prosthet Dent*, **97**, 18–24.

Della Bona A, Anusavice K J and Shen C (2000), 'Microtensile strength of composite bonded to hot-pressed ceramics', *J Adhes Dent*, **2**, 305–13.

Della Bona A, Anusavice K J and Hood J A (2002), 'Effect of ceramic surface treatment on tensile bond strength to a resin cement', *Int J Prosthet*, **15**, 248–53.

Della Bona A, Anusavice K J and Mecholsky J J (2003), 'Failure analysis of resin composite bonded to ceramic', *Dent Mater*, **19**, 693–9.

Derand T, Molin M and Kvam K (2005), 'Bond strength of composite luting cement to zirconia ceramic surfaces', *Dent Mater*, **21**, 1158–62.

Feilzer A J, Kakaboura A I, de Gee A J and Davidson C L (1995), 'The influence of water sorption on the development of setting shrinkage stress in traditional and resin-modified glass ionomer cements', *Dent Mater*, **11**, 186–90.

Garber D A and Goldstein R E (1994), *Porcelain and Composite Inlays and Onlays: Esthetic Posterior Restorations*, Quintessence, Chicago.

Hämmerle C, Sailer I, Thoma A, Hälg G, Suter A, and Ramel C (2008), *Dental Ceramics: Essential Aspects for Clinical Practice*, Quintessence, Surrey.

Hefferman M J, Aquilino S A, Diaz-Arnold A M, Haselton D R, Stanford C M and Vargas M A (2002), 'Relative translucency of six all-ceramic systems. Part I: core materials', *J Prosthet Dent*, **88**, 4–9.

Heikkinen T T, Lassila L V J, Matinlinna J P and Vallittu P K (2007), 'Effect of operating air pressure on tribochemical silica-coating', *Acta Odontol Scand*, **65**, 241–8.

Heikkinen T T, Lassila L V J, Matinlinna J P and Vallittu P K (2009), 'Dental zirconia adhesion with silicon compounds using some experimental and conventional surface conditioning methods', *Silicon*, **1**, 199–201.

Heikkinen T T, Lassila L V J, Matinlinna J P and Vallittu P K (2010), 'Effect of primers and resins on the shear bond strength of resin composite to zirconia', *SRX Dentistry*, Article ID 295137.

Heslop R B and Robinson P L (1967), *Inorganic Chemistry – A Guide to Advanced Study*, Elsevier, Amsterdam, 363–78.

Hjerppe J, Närhi T, Fröberg K, Vallittu P K and Lassila L V (2008), 'Effect of shading the zirconia framework on biaxial strength and surface microhardness', *Acta Odontol Scand*, **66**, 262–7.

Ho G W and Matinlinna J P (2011a), 'Insights on porcelain as a dental material. Part I: ceramic material types in dentistry', *Silicon*, **3**, 109–15.

Ho G W and Matinlinna J P (2011b), 'Insights on porcelain as a dental material. Part II: chemical surface treatments', *Silicon*, **3**, 117–123.

Ho G W and Matinlinna J P (2011c), 'Evaluation of the microtensile bond strength between resin composite and hydrofluoric acid etched ceramic in different storage media', *J Adhes Sci Technol*, **25**, 2671–2685.

Hooshmand T, van Noort R and Keshvad A (2002), 'Bond durability of the resin-bonded and silane treated ceramic surface', *Dent Mater*, **18**, 179–188.

Jevnikar P, Krnel K, Kocjan A, Funduk N and Kosmač T (2010), 'The effect of nano-structured alumina coating on resin-bond strength to zirconia ceramics', *Dent Mater*, **26**, 688–96.

Kaminski H D and Easton A D (2009), *Dental Materials Research*, Nova Science, New York, 1–21.

Keith O, Kusy R P and Whitley J Q (1994), 'Zirconia brackets: an evaluation of morphology and coefficients of friction', *Am J Orthod Dentofac Orthoped*, **106**, 605–14.

Kern M, Barloi A and Yang A B (2009), 'Surface conditioning influences zirconia ceramic bonding', *J Dent Res*, **88**, 817–22.

Kleverlaan C J and Feilzer A J (2005), 'Polymerization shrinkage and contraction stress of dental resin composites', *Dent Mater*, **21**, 1150–7.

Kukiattrakoon B and Thammasitboon K (2007), 'The effect of different etching times of acidulated phosphate fluoride gel on the shear bond strength of high leucite ceramics bonded to composite resin', *J Prosthet Dent*, **98**, 7–23.

Lacy A M, Laluz J, Watanabe L G and Dellinges M (1988), 'Effect of porcelain surface treatments on the bond to composite', *J Prosthet Dent*, **60**, 288–91.

Liu D, Matinlinna J P and Pow E H N (2012), 'Insights into porcelain zirconia bonding', *J Adhes Sci Technol*, **26**, 1249–65.

Lohbauer U, Zipperle M, Rischka K, Petschelt A and Müller F A (2008), 'Hydroxylation of dental zirconia surfaces: Characterization and bonding potential', *J Biomed Mater Res B*, **87**, 461–7.

Lung C Y K and Matinlinna J P (2012), 'Aspects of silane coupling agents and surface conditioning in dentistry: An overview', *Dent Mater*, **28**, 467–77.

Lung C Y K, Kukk E, Hagerth T, Matinlinna J P (2010), 'Surface hydroxylation of silica-coated zirconia by various chemical treatments', *Appl Surf Sci*, **257**, 1228–35.

Matinlinna J P and Lassila L V J (2011), 'Enhanced resin-composite bonding to zirconia framework after pretreatment with selected silane monomers', *Dent Mater*, **27**, 273–80.

Matinlinna J P and Mittal K L (2009), *Adhesion Aspects in Dentistry*, VSP/Brill, Leiden.

Matinlinna J P and Vallittu P K (2007a), 'Bonding of resin composites to etchable ceramic surfaces – an insight review to the chemical aspects on surface conditioning', *J Oral Rehabil*, **34**, 622–30.

Matinlinna J P and Vallittu P K (2007b), 'Silane based concepts on bonding resin composite to metals', *J Contemp Dent Pract*, **8**, 1–8.

Matinlinna J P, Lassila L V J, Özcan M, Yli-Urpo A and Vallittu P K (2004), 'An introduction to silanes and their clinical applications in dentistry', *Int J Prosthodont*, **17**, 155–64.

Matinlinna J P, Lassila L V J, Kangasniemi I and Vallittu P K (2005), 'Isocyanato- and methacryloxysilanes promote bis-GMA adhesion to titanium', *J Dental Res*, **84**, 360–4.

Matinlinna J P, Lassila L V J and Vallittu P K (2006a), 'The effect of a novel silane blend system on resin bond strength to silica-coated Ti substrate', *J Dent*, **34**, 436–43.

Matinlinna J P, Lassila L V J, and Vallittu P K (2006b), 'Evaluation of five dental silanes on bonding a luting cement onto silica-coated titanium', *J Dent*, **34**, 721–6.

Matinlinna J P, Heikkinen T, Özcan M, Lassila L V J and Vallittu P K (2006c), 'Evaluation of resin adhesion to zirconia ceramic using some organosilanes', *Dent Mater*, **22**, 824–31.

Matinlinna J P, Lassila L V J, and Vallittu P K (2007a), 'The Effect of Five Silane Coupling Agents on the Bond Strength of a Luting Cement to a Silica-coated Titanium', *Dent Mater*, **23**, 1173–80.

Matinlinna J P, Lassila L V J, Vallittu P K (2007b), 'Pilot evaluation of resin composite cement adhesion to zirconia using a novel silane system', *Acta Odontol Scand*, **65**, 44–51.

McLean J W (2001), 'Evolution of dental ceramics in the twentieth century', *J Prosthet Dent*, **85**, 61–6.

Meyenberg K H, Luthy H and Schärer P (1995), 'Zirconia posts: a new all-ceramic concept for nonvital abutment teeth', *J Esthet Dent*, **7**, 73–9.

Mirmohammadi H, Aboushelib M N, Salameh Z, Feilzer A J and Kleverlaan C J (2010a), 'Innovations in bonding to zirconia based ceramics: Part III. Phosphate monomer resin cements', *Dent Mater*, **26**, 786–92.

Mirmohammadi H, Aboushelib M N, Kleverlaan C J, de Jager N and Feilzer A J (2010b), 'The influence of rotating fatigue on the bond strength of zirconia-composite interfaces', *Dent Mater*, **26**, 627–33.

O'Neil M J, Heckelman P E, Koch C B, Roman K J, Kenny, C M and D'Arecca M R (2006), *The Merck Index*, Merck, Whitehouse Station.

Ozcan M, Alkumru H N, Gemalmas D (2001), 'The effect of surface treatment on shear bond strength of luting cement to glass-infiltrated alumina ceramic', *Int J Prosthodont*, **14**, 335–9.

Ozcan M, Valandro L F, Amaral R, Leite F and Bottino M (2009), 'Bond strength durability of a resin composite on a reinforced ceramic using various repair systems', *Dent Mater*, **25**, 1477–83.

Papia E, Zethraeus J, Ransbäck P-Å, Wennerberg A and Vult von Steyern P (2012), 'Impaction-modified densely sintered yttria-stabilized tetragonal zirconium dioxide: Methodology, surface structure, and bond strength', *J Biomed Mater Res B*, **100**, 677–84.

Parker R M (2007), 'Use of zirconia in restorative dentistry', *Dentistry Today,* March, 114–19.

Phark J H, Duarte Jr S, Blatz M and Sadan A (2009), 'An in vitro evaluation of the long-term resin bond to a new densely sintered high-purity zirconium oxide ceramic surface', *J Prosthet Dent*, **101**, 29–38.

Piconi C and Maccauro G (1999), 'Zirconia as a ceramic biomaterial', *Biomaterials*, **20**, 1–25.

Plueddemann E P (1970), 'Adhesion through silane coupling agents', *J Adhes*, **2**, 184–201.

Plueddemann E P (1991), *Silane Coupling Agents*, Plenum Press, New York.

Powers J M and Sakaguchi R L (2006), *Craig's Restorative Dental Materials*, Elsevier, St Louis.

Powers J M and Wataha J C (2008), *Dental Materials: Properties and Manipulation*, Elsevier, St. Louis.

Quaas A C, Yang B and Kern M P (2007), 'F 2.0 bonding to contaminated zirconia ceramic after different cleaning procedures'. *Dent Mater*, **23**, 506–12.

Raigrodski A J (2004), 'Contemporary materials and technologies for all-ceramic fixed partial dentures: a review of the literature', *J Prosthet Dent*, **92**, 557–62.

Rosen M R (1978), 'From treating solution to filler surface and beyond: the life history of a silane coupling agent', *J Coat Technol*, **50**, 70–82.

Rosentritt M, Kolbeck C, Ries S, Gross M, Behr M and Handel G (2008), 'Zirconia resin-bonded fixed partial dentures in the anterior maxilla', *Quintessence Int*, **39**, 313–19.

Schmalz G and Arenholt-Bindslev D (2009), *Biocompatibility of Dental Materials*, Springer, Berlin.

Seth A, van Ooij W J, Puomi P, Yin Z, Ashirgade A, Bafna, S and Shivane C (2007), 'Novel, one-step, chromatfree coatings containing anticorrosion pigments for metals – An overview and mechanistic study', *Progr Org Coat*, **58**, 136–45.

Shriver D F and Atkins P W (2001), *Inorganic Chemistry*, Oxford University Press, Oxford, 364–9.

Sorensen J A, Engelman M J, Torres T J and Avera S P (1991), 'Shear bond strength of composite resin to porcelain', *Int J Prosthodont*, **4**, 17–23.

Stangel I, Nathanon D, and Hsu C S (1987), 'Shear strength of composite bond to etched porcelain', *J Dent Res*, **66**, 1460–5.

Tete S, Mastrangelo F, Bianchi A, Zizzari V and Scarano A (2009), 'Collagen fiber orientation around machined titanium and zirconia dental implant necks: an animal study', *Int J Oral Max Impl*, **24**, 52–8.

Touati B, Miara P and Nathanson D (1999), *Esthetic Dentistry and Ceramic Restorations*, Martin Dunitz, London.

Tylka D F and Stewart G P (1994), 'Comparison of acidulated phosphate fluoride gel and hydrofluoric acid etchants for porcelain-composite repair', *J Prosthet Dent*, **72**, 121–7.

Ubassy G (1993), *Shape and Color: the Key to Successful Ceramic Restorations*, Quintessence, Chicago.

van Noort R (2007), *Introduction to Dental Materials*, Elsevier, Philadelphia.

Wegner S M and Kern M (2000), 'Long-term resin bond strength to zirconia ceramic'. *J Adhes Dent*, **2**, 139–47.

Yang B, Scharnberg M, Wolfart S, Quaas A C, Ludwig K, Adelung R and Kern M (2007), 'Influence of contamination on bonding to zirconia ceramic', *J Biomed Mater Res B*, **81**, 283–90.

Yang B, Barloi A and Kern M (2010), 'Influence of air-abrasion on zirconia ceramic bonding using an adhesive composite resin', *Dent Mater*, **26**, 44–50.

Yen T Y, Blackman R B and Baez R J (1993), 'Effect of acid etching on the flexural strength of a feldspathic porcelain and a castable glass ceramic', *J Prosthet Dent*, **70**, 224–33.

Yoshida K, Tsuo Y, Atsuta M (2006), 'Bonding of dual-cured resin cement to zirconia ceramic using phosphate acidic ester monomer and zirconate coupler', *J Biomed Mater Res B*, **77**, 28–33.

6 Wear properties of dental ceramics

M. K. ETMAN, Division of Prosthodontics, College of Dentistry, University of Saskatchewan, Canada

DOI: 10.1533/9780857096432.2.161

Abstract: Relatively little is known about the clinical performance of the newly developed all-ceramic systems on the posterior teeth and the mechanism of failure. Surface roughness, wear and cracks are considered to be problems for all ceramic restorations. Newly developed all-ceramic restorations are promising and their wear behavior depends on a few factors such as microstructures, hardness, surface finishes and other clinically related factors. *In vivo* and *in vitro* studies showed that change in surface roughness is the first indication of wear. Accurate validation of wear measurement instruments and techniques are problematic for *in vivo* and *in vitro* wear measurements. Descriptions of instrument capability have rarely distinguished between precision and accuracy.

Key words: ceramic wear, confocal microscopy, sub-surface cracking, surface modeling, tooth wear.

6.1 Introduction

Relatively little is known about the clinical performance of newly developed all-ceramic systems on the posterior teeth and the mechanism of failure. Surface roughness, wear and cracks are considered to be problems for all ceramic restorations. Newly developed all-ceramic restorations are promising and their wear behavior depends on a few factors such as microstructures, hardness, surface finishes and other clinically related factors. *In vivo* and *in vitro* studies showed that change in surface roughness is the first indication of wear.

6.2 Clinical performance and wear of all-ceramic restorations

6.2.1 Clinical performance of all-ceramic crowns

The clinical performance and failure mechanisms of recently introduced ceramic crown systems, used to restore posterior teeth, have not been adequately examined (Etman and Woolford, 2010). Dental ceramic materials have demonstrated desirable properties, including biocompatibility, good esthetics, chemical resistance and diminished plaque accumulation

(Chan and Weber, 1986; Anusavice, 1992). Ceramic crowns are thought to be more esthetic and more biocompatible than metal-ceramic crowns. Unfortunately, ceramics are brittle, have low tensile strength, and are prone to have less strength in a moist environment (Yoshinari and Dérand, 1994; Sobrinho *et al.*, 1998). In a traditional metal-ceramic crown, the metal sub-structure provides strength and a porcelain veneer provides esthetics. Since opaque metal substrates adversely affect translucency, the current trend is to develop ceramic systems that eliminate metal sub-structures and provide optical characteristics similar to natural teeth. Early clinical outcomes for these systems have not compared favorably with those for metal-ceramic restorations (Josephson *et al.*, 1991). High failure rates caused by fracture have stimulated the development of ceramic systems with greater strength as well as better esthetics (Josephson *et al.*, 1991).

Recent advances in dental ceramics include the introduction of a promising, high-strength, high-purity alumina core material for coping-based ceramic anterior and posterior complete crown restorations (Scotti *et al.*, 1995; Odén *et al.*, 1998). A technique for manufacturing individual crowns has been described and marketed as the Procera AllCeram System (Nobel Biocare AB, Göteborg, Sweden) (Andersson and Odén, 1993). Procera technology uses computer-aided design and computer-aided manufacturing (CAD/CAM) methods to fabricate dental restorations (Andersson *et al.*, 1998; Russell *et al.*, 1995). The manufacturer claims that the alumina coping material has the potential, in terms of strength, to replace metal copings and substitute for a metal framework (Hegenbarth, 1996). Compressive strength values of about 600 MPa have been reported for this material (Andersson and Odén, 1993). A low-fusing feldspathic porcelain (All-Ceram; DeguDent GmbH, HanauWolfgang, Germany) with a compatible thermal expansion coefficient is used to veneer copings and produce definitive restorations (Andersson and Odén, 1993).

Generally, the fit of Procera crowns is acceptable, but variations in fitting accuracy have been reported for these restorations, possibly owing to scanning, die milling errors, or firing shrinkage (May *et al.*, 1998; Naert *et al.*, 2005). However, a study of controlled marginal fit reported a mean (SD) marginal gap value of 62 (49) μm, which is considered to be within the clinically acceptable range (80–100 μm) (May *et al.*, 1998). A 5-year clinical success rate of 96.9% has been reported for the Procera AllCeram crown, and it appears to offer clinicians a practical, durable ceramic crown for both anterior and posterior teeth (Oden *et al.*, 1998). Other clinical studies of Procera AllCeram crowns have shown variable success rates; one study (Walter *et al.*, 2006) reported a survival rate of 96.7% for anterior crowns and 91.3% for posterior crowns, while another study (Zitzmann *et al.*, 2007) reported a survival rate of 100% in the anterior region and 98.8% in the posterior region after seven years. However, Procera AllCeram crowns, in a recent clinical study (Etman *et al.*, 2008) showed less wear resistance and caused more wear on the opposing tooth enamel compared with an experimental ceramic crown (later identified as IPS e.max Press; Ivoclar Vivadent AG, Schaan, Liechtenstein) and metal-ceramic crowns.

The IPS e.max Press castable glass ceramic is composed primarily of a modified lithium disilicate glass ceramic that forms the primary components of IPS Empress 2 (Ivoclar Vivadent AG). In both IPS Empress 2 and the IPS e.max Press, the glass matrix consists of micrometer-sized lithium disilicate crystals, between which are sub-micrometer lithium orthophosphate crystals (Etman, 2009). A porcelain consisting of fluorapatite crystals in an aluminosilicate glass is used to veneer the IPS Empress 2 core and create the crown morphology and shade. The IPS e.max Press material can be used to form a core or an entire crown. Flexural strength values for the IPS Empress 2 core are reported to be approximately 329 MPa (Nakamura *et al.*, 2002). A two-year clinical evaluation (Taskonak and Sertgöz, 2006) of IPS Empress restorations showed a 100% success rate for crowns and a 50% success rate for fixed partial dentures. An additional study (Marquardt and Strub, 2006) reported survival rates of 100% for crowns and 70% for fixed partial dentures over a five-year period. However, restorations made with this material in another study (Toksavul and Toman, 2007) demonstrated a 95.24% success rate after five years.

The IPS e.max Press is based on the same strengthening mode as IPS Empress 2, but with higher translucency; it was introduced commercially and allows ceramic crowns to be fabricated on the anterior and posterior teeth without the need for veneering (Heintze *et al.*, 2008). The chemical basis of this material is the same as IPS Empress 2, but the mechanical properties changed using a different firing process during laboratory processing. In comparison with IPS Empress 2, the IPS e.max Press material exhibits substantially improved physical properties and greater translucency (Stappert *et al.*, 2005).

A recent study reported that the IPS e.max Press ceramic showed higher resistance to crack formation (Etman, 2009) and this may make it more reliable for crowns placed in stress-bearing areas. An *in vitro* study showed that fracture resistance of crowns made of IPS e.max Press on molar teeth was comparable to the fracture resistance of natural unprepared teeth (Stappert *et al.*, 2006). At the present time, there is little clinical performance data to confirm the use of this material on posterior teeth.

The durability of ceramic crowns should be compared to metal-ceramic crowns, which have become the standard for durability for esthetic crowns (Etman *et al.*, 2008). Metal-ceramic crowns have been shown to have a survival rate of 100%, 99% and 95% after 3, 5 and 11 years, respectively (Leempoel *et al.*, 1985) but long-term studies have suggested that dental caries is the primary cause of failure (Schwartz *et al.*, 1970; Walton *et al.*,

1986). Long-term clinical studies are needed to determine if this is also the major cause of failure in ceramic crowns.

A benefit of both Procera AllCeram and the IPS e.max Press ceramic systems is high strength (Nakamura *et al.*, 2002). However, common ceramic problems, such as surface degradation, cracks, wear and material loss (Etman *et al.*, 2008; Etman, 2009; Etman and Woolford, 2010) still exist and uncertainties remain concerning long-term clinical performance (Haselton *et al.*, 2000; Etman *et al.*, 2008; Etman and Woolford, 2010). The inherent limitations of retrospective studies are well known (Randall and Wilson, 1999).

Prospective clinical study

A prospective clinical study (Etman and Woolford, 2010) evaluated and compared the clinical performance of two new ceramic crown systems with that of metal-ceramic crowns using modified United States Public Health Services (USPHS) criteria. In this study, 90 posterior teeth requiring crown restorations in 48 patients were randomized into three equal groups ($n = 30$) for which different crown systems were used: an experimental hot-pressed glass ceramic based on a modified lithium disilicate ceramic (IPS e.max Press), an alumina-coping-based ceramic (Procera AllCeram) and a metal ceramic (Simidur S 2 veneered with IPS Classic Porcelain). The crowns were assessed over three years using the modified USPHS criteria. Crowns that developed visible cracks were sectioned and removed and the surfaces were analyzed using scanning electron microscopy (SEM). The data were analyzed using the Kruskal–Wallis non-parametric statistical test, followed by the Mann–Whitney test with Bonferroni correction ($\alpha = 0.05$). USPHS evaluation showed that the IPS e.max Press and metal-ceramic crowns experienced fewer clinical changes than Procera AllCeram. Visible roughness, wear and deformity were noticed in occlusal contact areas of Procera AllCeram crowns. SEM images showed well defined wear facets in both ceramic crown systems. Kruskal–Wallis tests showed a significant difference ($P < 0.05$) in alpha scores between the three crown systems. Mann–Whitney tests showed significant differences between groups. IPS e.max Press crowns demonstrated clinical behavior comparable to Procera AllCeram and metal-ceramic crowns, but the wear resistance of this crown type was superior to the Procera AllCeram crowns, according to modified USPHS criteria.

The details of this study as it was reported (Etman and Woolford, 2010) are as follows. A prospective, randomized, controlled clinical trial assessed the clinical performance of crowns made with a castable glass-ceramic material and compared the results with those obtained with Procera AllCeram and metal-ceramic crowns. Modified USPHS criteria (Etman, 2004) were used for evaluation. The USPHS criteria were modified from list of criteria published by Ryge (1980), by adding some criteria and changing the definitions of others. The hypothesis for this study was that castable glass ceramic and alumina coping crowns would perform as well as metal-ceramic crowns when used on premolar and molar teeth.

In this study, three crown systems (IPS e.max Press, metal ceramic and Procera AllCeram) were selected for this study. The study participants were selected from patients attending Guy's and St Thomas' Hospital NHS Foundation Trust. The Research Ethics Committee of King's College London approved the project and all subjects provided informed consent. Patients were screened according to their medical and dental history. The selection of subjects for this clinical study was based on the diagnosed need for a complete crown restoration on a posterior tooth. Individuals falling outside of the conditions stipulated for entry into the study were excluded from participation. The inclusion criteria were: (1) indication for extracoronal single tooth restorations with minimally restored opposing natural teeth; (2) age between 20 and 60 years, with good oral and general health; (3) no history of parafunctional activities; and (4) able to attend a follow-up visit at the hospital every six months for a minimum period of three years. Using a statistical software program (SPSS 11.0; SPSS, Inc, Chicago, IL), the number of restorations required for the necessary statistical power factor was determined to be 30 crowns for each material group; thus, a minimum of 90 crowns was required for the study. The number of patients required depended upon the number of restorations placed in each patient, which was up to three crowns per patient. One operator performed all of the treatment procedures.

Routine treatment procedures were followed for metal-ceramic crowns and Procera AllCeram crowns (Andersson *et al.*, 1998; Rosenstiel *et al.*, 2006). The tooth preparation for castable glass-ceramic crowns was similar to that for Procera AllCeram. A four-point score was used to designate the status for each category assessed. The scoring system was as follows: alpha: excellent result, restorations without changes or clinically ideal; bravo: acceptable result, restorations with changes that are clinically acceptable and do not require replacement; charlie: unacceptable, restorations with major changes that require replacement to prevent further deterioration; delta: unacceptable, immediate replacement necessary. All clinical evaluations were performed using standardized dental diagnostic instruments and visual inspection with the aid of magnification (× 2.5) (ErgoVision HD Telescope; SurgiTel, Ann Arbor, MI) with standard dental unit and overhead lighting. Gingival and plaque indices were recorded using standardized techniques (Löe and Silness, 1963; Silness and Löe, 1964). Thermal testing was performed using a cotton pledget soaked with coolant (Endo-Ice Refrigerant Spray; Coltène/Whaledent, Inc, Cuyahoga Falls, OH) and an electric pulp tester (Vitalometer, model 205MB; Burton Division of Cavitron Corp, Van Nuys, CA).

For a period of three years after placement, patients were recalled at six-month intervals for evaluation, following the protocol described above. The data collected from this clinical trial were analyzed with both descriptive statistics and using analysis of variance (ANOVA) with non-parametric statistical tests. All alpha scores were analyzed using non-parametric statistical tests (SPSS, version 15.0.1; SPSS, Inc) to compare rank sum values of each criterion among all materials and among time periods. The data were analyzed using the Kruskal–Wallis non-parametric statistical test and subsidiary follow up using the Mann–Whitney test was performed with Bonferroni correction ($\alpha = 0.05$). Any crowns that developed cracks rendering them irreparable were removed carefully to avoid destroying occlusal surfaces that contained both contact and non-contact areas.

USPHS evaluation showed that the IPS e.max Press and metal-ceramic crowns experienced fewer clinical changes than Procera AllCeram. The IPS emax Press showed visible cracks in two crowns (Fig. 6.1) and a metal-ceramic crown showed fracture and chipping of the porcelain facing

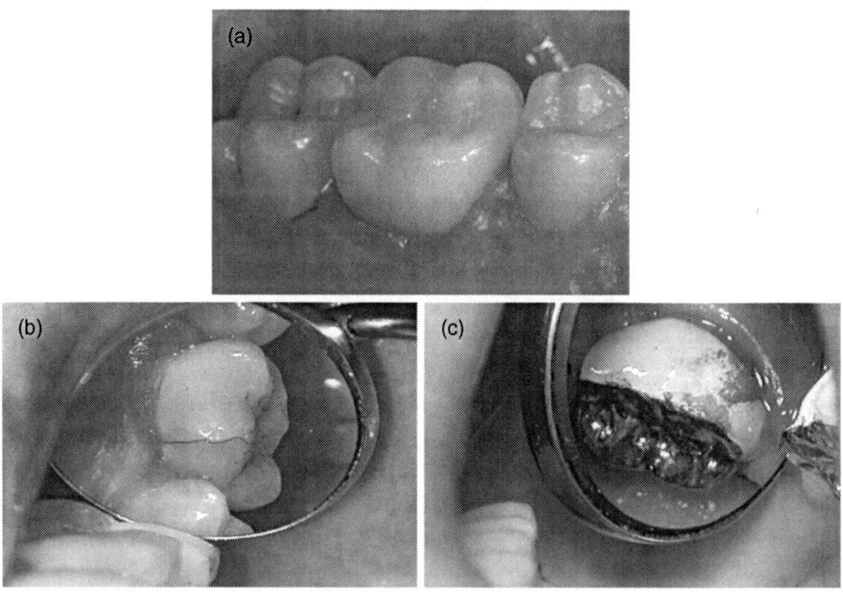

6.1 (a) Experimental ceramic crown (IPS e-max Press) on maxillary right first molar immediately after cementation. (b) The same crown after 36 months; note crack line. (c) Metal ceramic crown on lower left second molar; note fracture and chipping of porcelain facing, suggesting cohesive and adhesive fracture.

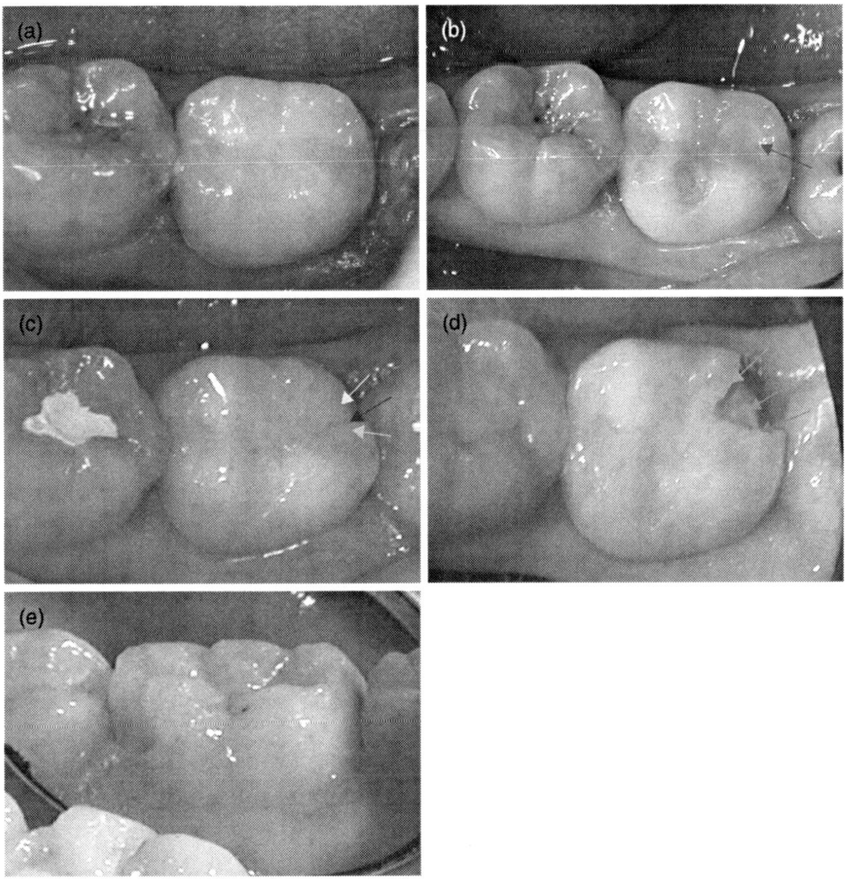

6.2 Procera AllCeram crown on mandibular right second molar. (a) Immediately after placement; note traces of bonding material and anatomic form. (b) After 18 months; note wear facets (arrow) and chipping of veneering material on buccal surface. (c) Fracture of veneering material in distal marginal ridge. (d) Fracture of veneering material and alumina coping in same area as in (c). Fracture is through crown to tooth preparation (arrows are pointing to same locations, respectively, in images (c) and (d). (e) Fracture of veneering material in distolingual angle of Procera crown on mandibular first molar.

(Fig. 6.1) Visible roughness, wear and deformity were noticed in occlusal contact areas of the Procera AllCeram crowns (Fig. 6.2). SEM images showed well defined wear facets in both ceramic crown systems (Figs 6.3 and 6.4). Kruskal–Wallis tests showed a significant difference ($P < 0.05$) in alpha scores among the three crown systems. Mann–Whitney tests showed significant differences between groups.

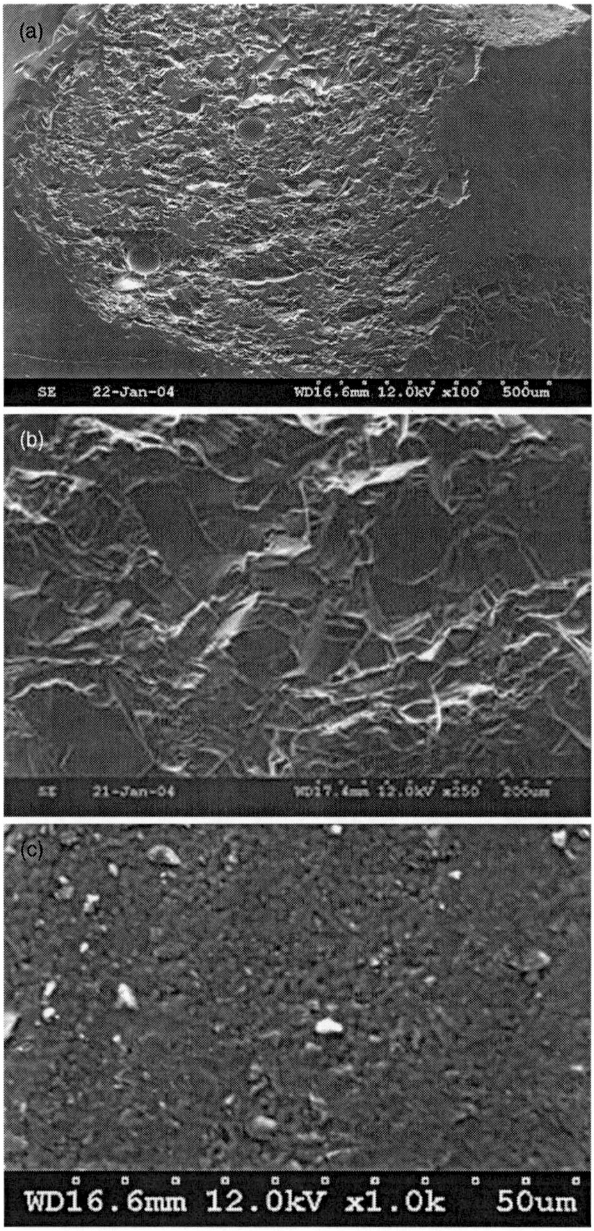

6.3 SEM photomicrographs. (a) Wear facet in Procera AllCeram material after 36 months (original magnification, ×100). (b) Higher magnification of wear facet shows Procera veneering material at 36 months (original magnification, ×250). (c) Exposed Procera alumina coping in center of deep wear facet after 36 months (original magnification, ×1000).

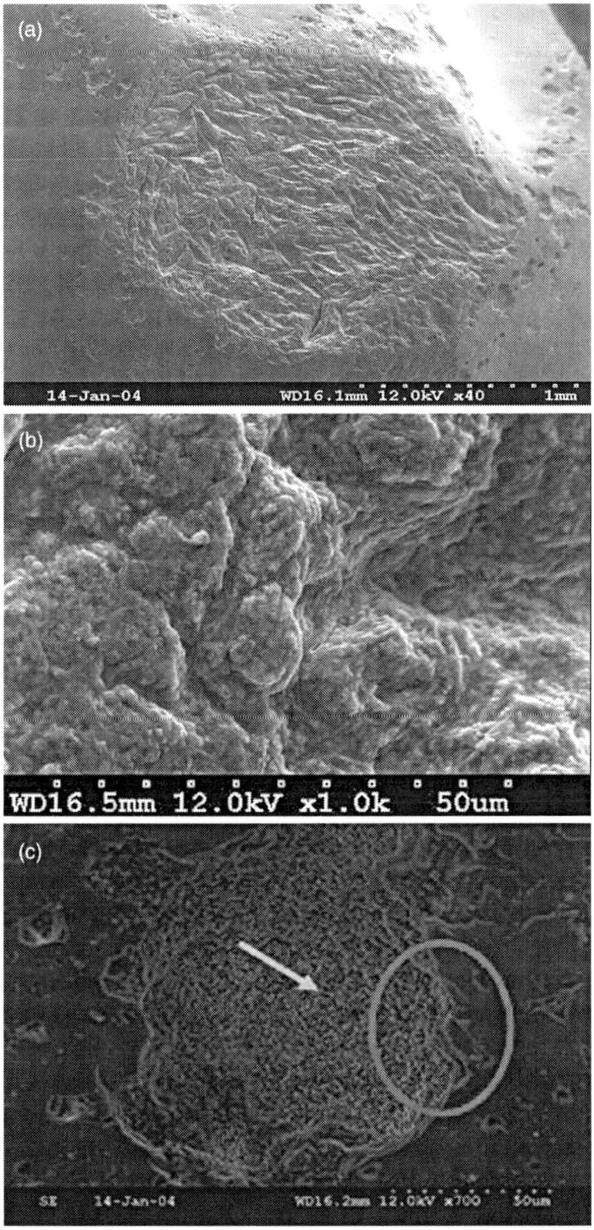

6.4 SEM photomicrographs show wear facet in IPS e.max Press at 36 months on occlusal contact area. (a) Original magnification, ×40. (b) Original magnification, ×1000. (c) Original magnification, ×700. Note surface defect found on buccal surface of experimental crown placed on maxillary left first molar, showing microstructure of experimental ceramic (arrow and circle).

The data from this study support the research hypothesis that ceramic crown systems will demonstrate clinical behavior similar to metal-ceramic crowns over a test period of three years. In particular, evaluation using the modified USPHS criteria revealed that clinical performance of IPS e.max Press ceramic crowns was similar to Procera AllCeram and metal-ceramic crowns. Although not always feasible, a prospective, randomized, controlled study is considered the design of choice for a clinical investigation (Randall and Wilson, 1999). However, an important limitation is that a significant difference can only be generalized for the population segment participating in the study. Forty-eight patients participated in this prospective study, providing 90 crown restorations for evaluation and, considering the statistical power factor used, the results apply to an estimated 100% of the population. The results presented show few clinical changes over three years of study and the statistical model assumed no hazard function during the entire period. This may not be realistic, but an adequate approximation of the true hazard function of the first three years is provided, because the proportion of patients who experienced failure during this time was extremely low.

With a longer observation period, a more complicated failure-time model, such as Weibull, that allows the hazard function to change over time, could be estimated. However, the low failure numbers do not support the meaningful fitting of models that have more parameters at this time. The results of this three-year investigation suggest that acceptable clinical performance can be expected for complete crown restorations made with the experimental IPS e.max Press ceramic material. The three-year follow up of Procera AllCeram crowns showed changes in the surface texture, particularly in areas of occlusal contact, noticeable as early as six months. The early changes in surface texture indicate the beginning of wear, which may be an inherent weakness of the Procera system veneering material (Etman *et al.*, 2008; Etman, 2009).

Apart from the surface texture changes, no other significant changes occurred in crowns made using this system over the three-year period. The Procera AllCeram crown is made with a densely sintered alumina coping veneered with conventional feldspathic dental porcelain (AllCeram; DeguDent GmbH). The coping strength, as claimed by the manufacturer, is amongst the highest for ceramic materials used in dentistry, but the results of this trial have shown that this material can fracture. SEM photomicrographs (Fig. 6.3) showed changes in surface topography that included the alumina core material. This may be due to interaction with the oral environment. These surface changes have the potential to affect the mechanical properties of this material. The clinical behavior results of Procera AllCeram crowns in the present study were similar to the results of another clinical study that evaluated Procera crowns over a five-year period, (Odén *et al.*, 1998) wherein a fracture rate of 7% for molars and 4% for premolars was observed. Vitadur Alpha (VITA Zahnfabrik, Bad Säckingen, Germany) was used for the veneering ceramic in that study, whereas in this study, AllCeram (DeguDent GmbH), a ceramic material specially developed for the alumina copings, was selected. The IPS e.max Press crowns demonstrated clinical performance comparable to Procera AllCeram and metal ceramic crowns over a three-year period of study. The results of this study indicate that, with regard to crack propagation and wear resistance, IPS e.max Press ceramic crowns are likely to perform better than Procera AllCeram crowns on posterior teeth for the first three years.

6.2.2 Measurement of clinical wear

For more than 100 years, dental ceramics have been widely used as esthetic restorative materials. These materials offer a natural tooth appearance and very good mechanical properties. Ceramics are wear resistant, brittle, technique sensitive to polish, and abrasive to the opposing dentition (McLean, 1979; Craig, 1997). This abrasion of opposing natural teeth may be rapid, producing sensitivity and occlusal imbalance, especially when functional paths are generated by the ceramic surface (Jacobi *et al.*, 1991). It has been suggested that ceramic should not be placed on occlusal surfaces because of the wear effect of ceramic on enamel (Wiley, 1989). As a consequence, several modified ceramic materials have been developed in an attempt to decrease antagonistic tooth wear. New ceramic restorative systems and adhesive restorations have greatly contributed to the increased interest in esthetic dentistry (Mahalick *et al.*, 1971).

The wear effects of currently accepted dental ceramic materials have been studied extensively under laboratory conditions. Unfortunately, laboratory studies that evaluate abrasion resistance may produce entirely different results from clinical studies of the same materials. Despite recently developed technologies, no sufficiently valid *in vivo* evaluation method of clinical wear for dental ceramic and opposing enamel has been published. There is a distinct need for controlled clinical studies of wear, since laboratory studies do not accurately simulate clinical performance in a harsh oral environment and the final test will always be clinical success. A new experimental glass ceramic has been produced to be used as a non-layered (non-veneered) crown system and is expected to show favorable wear behavior against tooth enamel. This glass-ceramic material was tested in a clinical trial (Etman and Woolford, 2010).

Prospective clinical study: wear measurement

A clinical study by Etman *et al.* (2008) evaluated qualitatively and measured quantitatively tooth and ceramic wear. This prospective clinical study reports the wear behavior of the IPS e-max Press experimental glass-ceramic crown system against tooth enamel and *vice versa* compared with two commercially available crown systems over a two-year period. Also in this clinical study by Etman *et al.* (2008), ceramic materials with significantly different microstructures were selected for inclusion: a modified lithium disilicate hot-pressed ceramic (IPS e.max Press), alumina-based ceramic veneered with low fusing feldspathic porcelain (Procera AllCeram) and metal ceramic were used. Patients were selected from the normal pool of patients attending a dental hospital for routine dental care. Posterior teeth that required crowns were selected in an otherwise intact dentition without a history of erosion. Patients with reported parafunctional habits were excluded from this study. The study tooth to be crowned had to be opposed by a sound natural tooth or at least the majority of the occlusal surface that includes the occlusal contact areas was enamel.

A novel superimposition technique was used to measure wear of tooth and ceramic quantitatively over a two-year period. Three ceramic systems experimental hot-pressed ceramic (EC), Procera AllCeram (PA) and metal ceramic were used. In this study, a total of 90 posterior crowns in 48 patients were randomized into three groups, and impressions were made at baseline and at six-month intervals for two years. Clinical images were taken after using a dye to highlight surface changes. The impressions were digitized and modeled as superimposable three-dimensional colored surface images. The depth of wear at the occlusal contact areas was quantitatively measured at 6, 12, 18 and 24 months. The quantitative evaluation showed more wear in Procera AllCeram at the occlusal contact areas, whereas the experimental and metal-ceramic systems showed less wear. There was a significant difference in the amount of enamel worn between all types of restorations ($P < 0.05$). There was a statistically significant difference ($P < 0.05$) in the mean depth of wear between all systems. The metal-ceramic and experimental systems showed less change, indicating improved wear resistance compared with Procera AllCeram. In addition, enamel opposing metal-ceramic and experimental crowns showed less wear compared to enamel opposed by Procera AllCeram crowns.

The general clinical procedures for each patient followed a standardized and predetermined protocol. One operator performed all treatment procedures. Metal ceramic (porcelain-fused-to-metal with the occlusal surface in metal) and Procera AllCeram crowns were inserted on suitably prepared abutment teeth and cemented using an appropriate resin luting agent (Panavia F, Kuraray). Routine treatment procedures were followed for metal-ceramic crowns and Procera AllCeram crowns (Andersson *et al.*, 1998; Rosenstiel *et al.*, 2006). The clinical procedures for IPS e-max Press ceramic crowns were the same as for the Procera crowns. The laboratory fabrication of the experimental crowns followed the same technique as for

IPS-Empress ceramic in the surface coloration technique (Dong *et al.*, 1992). Baseline assessment took place when the patient was recalled one week after fitting the definitive restoration. At this visit, an oral examination was conducted, patient concerns were addressed, independent assessors completed the case report form and crown adjustments were made, finished and polished. Clinical photographs were also taken of each restoration. Full-arch polyvinyl siloxane impressions were made of both dental arches to provide accurate baseline records of the morphology of the restored teeth and their antagonists. Impressions were made at baseline and at each six-month interval. Initially, scavenger alginate impressions were made, immediately followed by polyvinyl siloxane impressions using either a stock or custom-made tray depending on the shape and size of the dental arch. All impressions followed the same protocol, which was defined from a pilot study: (1) the same impression material was used for the whole period of study; (2) the impressions for the crowns and their antagonist teeth had to be of the same color and viscosity; (3) the same impression technique was used for the whole period of study. It was determined from a pilot study that there was no difference in the recorded data between impressions made using stock trays or custom-made trays. The former are less time consuming and less expensive, but in some patients, the stock tray did not match the size of the dental arch and thus impressions had to be made using a custom-made tray.

6.2.3 Quantitative wear measurement

The quantitative measurement of wear was conducted by digitizing accurate impressions of the restored teeth and their antagonist teeth. Measurements of wear were made at tooth–restoration contact points that were identified before baseline recording using articulating paper, bite registration material and clinical photographs taken using an intraoral digital camera (Fig. 6.5) Articulating paper (Surgident, Mile Dental Products) was used to identify tooth–restoration contact points by asking the patient to bring the maxillary and mandibular teeth into maximum intercuspation, tapping lightly and then taking photographs of these highlighted contact areas. At the baseline measurement recording, the articulated contacts were used to identify selected measurement points for each subsequent recall visit. Areas selected for measurement were based on articulated points and points that were likely to become contact points. Up to four points were measured on the occlusal surface of each crown and its enamel antagonist. Reference points were selected in non-contacting areas of the tooth surface that were more likely to be stable over the course of the study, for example the occlusal fossa.

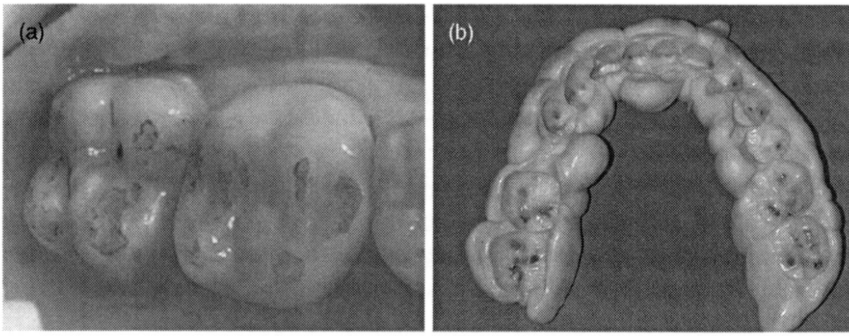

6.5 Articulating paper (a) and occlusal bite registration (b) were used to locate the occlusal contact points and areas that were likely to become contact points.

A computerized non-contact coordinate measurement system was used to digitize the impressions used for wear measurement. All impressions were scanned with a non-contacting laser profilometer (Keyence LC- 2400 series laser displacement meter). Data acquisition and analysis was performed with UBSoft (UBM Messtechnik) and three-dimensional surface modeling software (Fig. 6.6). Scan-Surf mathematical fitting software was used to analyze the occlusal surfaces. In this method, a large number of profiles were assembled into an image of the tooth surface. Data collected from a longitudinal series of impressions of the same tooth surface were analyzed by superimposing the images of anatomically stable occusal areas using the Scan-Surf software. Restoration surfaces and occlusal areas without anatomic changes were used as reference points in the fitting procedures (Fig. 6.6).

The material loss and changes in the occlusal contact areas of the restoration surfaces were measured and analyzed statistically. The data obtained were used to establish linear, area and depth assessments of wear processes occurring on the restored teeth and their antagonists. The amount of material loss was analyzed statistically using the SPSS statistical program (SPSS). A variety of general linear modeling descriptive statistics and comparison of means were used to analyze and compare mean values of the continuously distributed data from the various groups and time periods in the study.

Ceramic wear

The three crown systems showed steadily increasing loss of material and were worn to different extents in the regions of the occlusal contact areas. All showed changes in the amount of material loss over the two-year period. The statistical analysis using Scheffé multiple comparisons of means showed

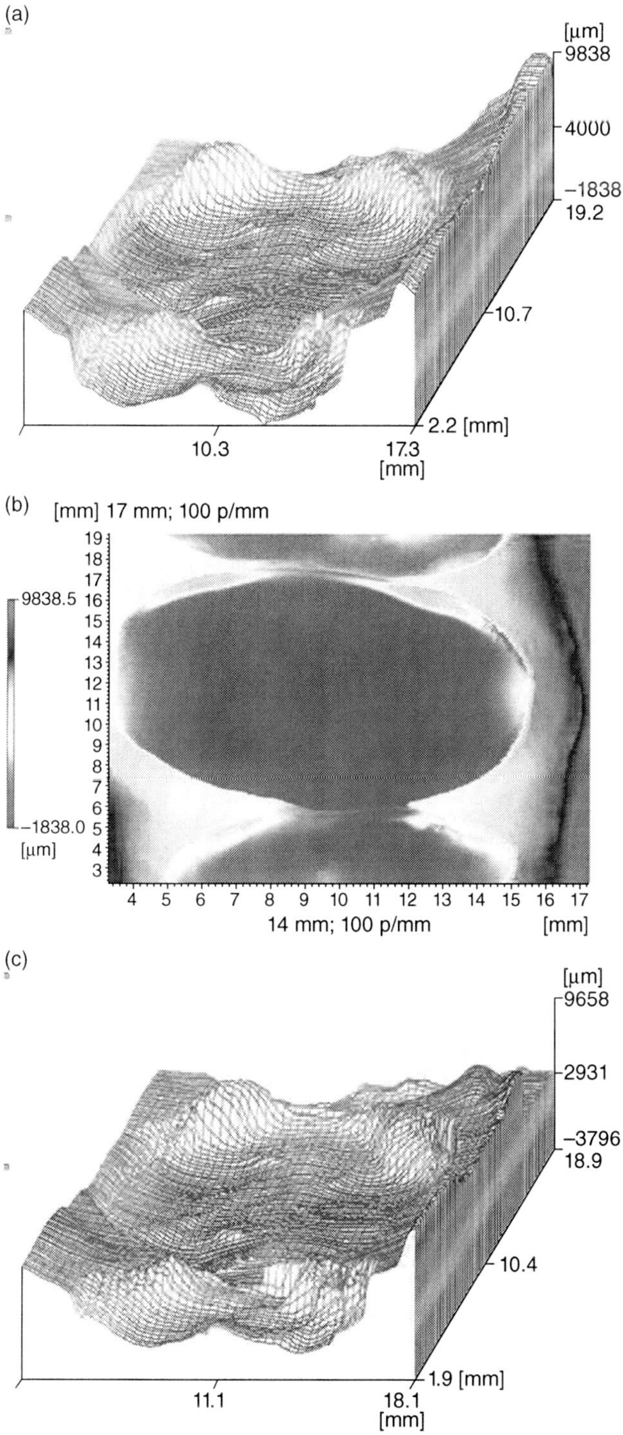

6.6 Measurements of the depth of material loss. (a) Wireframe digital image representing baseline. (b) Contour map. (c) Wireframe digital image for the same crown after 24 months.

(*Continued*)

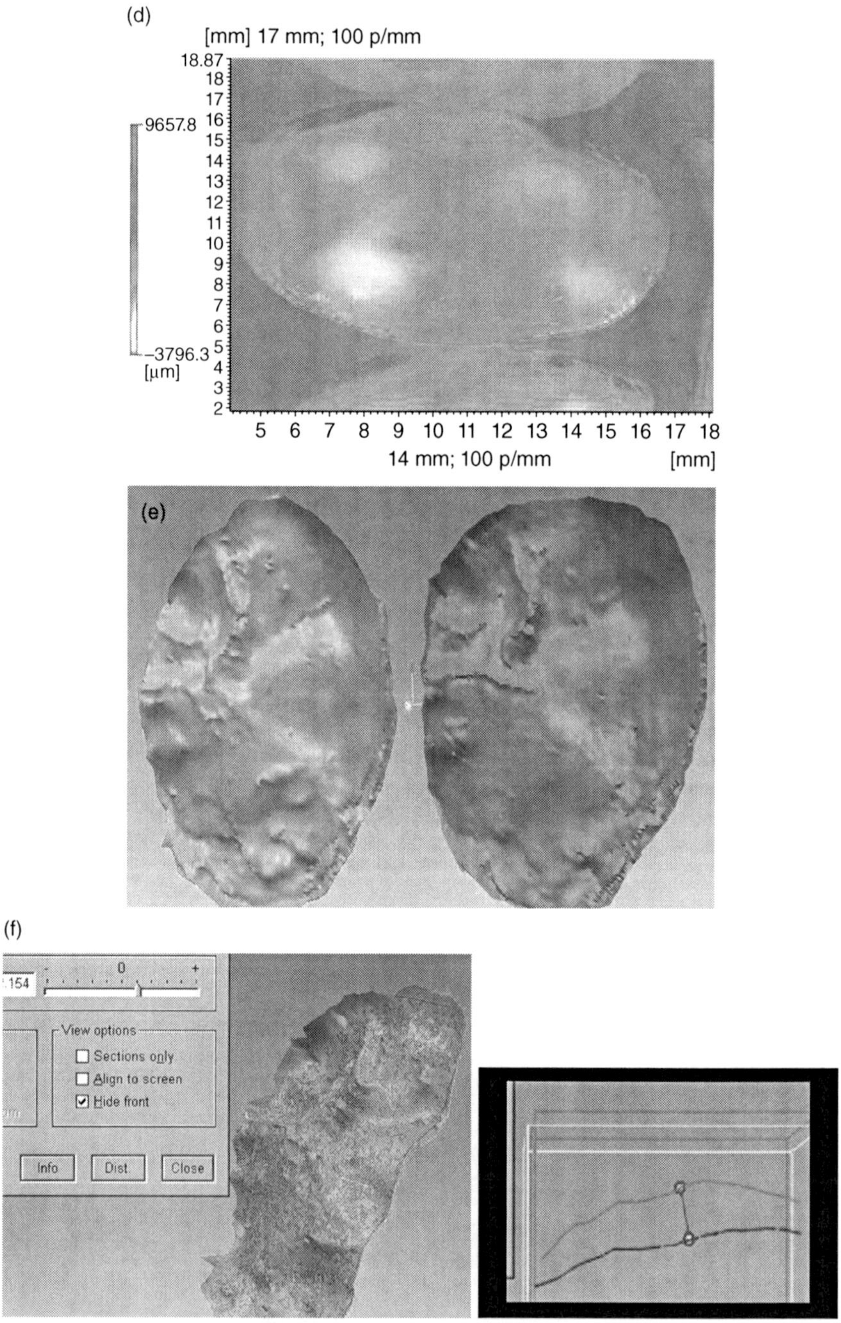

6.6 (d) Contour map. (e) Left-shell modeled surface for image in (a), while the right shell represents the image in (c); arrows in both images show the worn areas after 24 months. (f1) Cross-section of superimposed shells; distance between the two lines (f2) represents the depth of wear in the measured area.

(*Continued*)

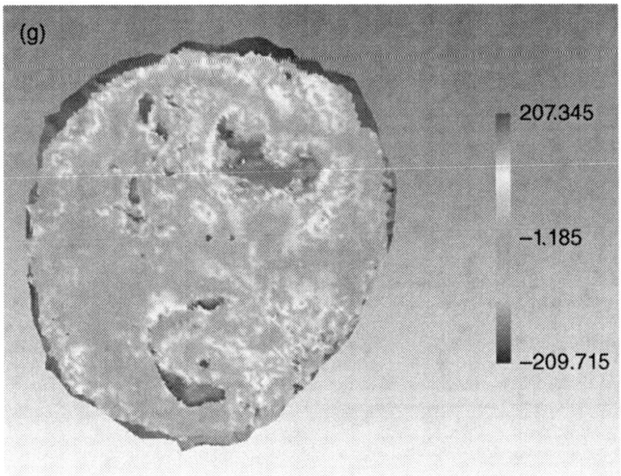

6.6 (g) Globally registered model; red areas represent the pattern and locations of wear.

that there were significant differences ($P < 0.05$) in the amount of ceramic and metallic material worn away by the opposing tooth structure. Statistically, there were significant differences in the amount the restorations had worn between the three restoration systems after a two-year period. There were significant differences in the mean amount of material loss between the three systems at 6, 12, 18 and 24 months. The mean values showed significant differences in loss of depth for each material over the four-time intervals. The mean depths of wear over 24 months for different crown systems are plotted in the graph in Fig. 6.7.

Tooth wear

The results showed that the opposing tooth enamel wore at all contact areas with the three crown systems. These materials also caused reciprocal enamel wear in the occlusal contact areas. Different amounts of enamel were worn away by the three types of restorations. The contact areas of all teeth showed a circular defect of approximately 1–2 mm in diameter in the occlusal contact areas. The metal-ceramic crowns produced the least tooth wear and the least loss of material. Procera AllCeram was the most abrasive ceramic and was responsible for more tooth loss than the metal ceramic and the experimental ceramic. It also suffered the greatest loss of test material. The experimental ceramic caused less enamel wear than Procera AllCeram but more than the metal ceramic. Statistically, one-way analysis of variance confirmed that there was a significant difference in the degree

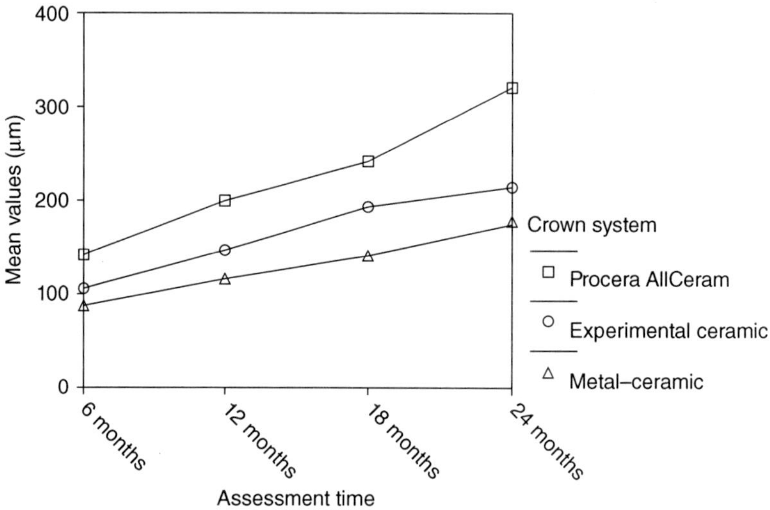

6.7 Mean wear of restorations over 24 months.

of enamel loss between the three materials ($P < 0.05$). This also confirmed that the type of ceramic system opposing enamel influenced enamel wear. The Scheffé test showed that enamel wear opposing the ceramic systems was significantly different from one material to another. However, metal-ceramic crowns demonstrated the least wear in the opposing enamel and the Procera AllCeram system exhibited the greatest effect on the opposing enamel.

Although there was a significant difference from one material to another in terms of causing wear to the opposing tooth enamel, the three materials caused a dramatic increase in tooth wear in the first six months in the occlusal contact areas. After six months, the three materials showed slower rates of wear, but even so, a steady increase in tooth wear in the same areas was evident. Figure 6.8 shows that the mean wear differed significantly from one material to another; further, the mean wear differed significantly over each time period for the same material.

The aim of this investigation was to examine the wear of tooth enamel that may be caused by two commercially available crown systems and one experimental ceramic. The wear effect of the tooth enamel on these crown systems was measured. The measurements of wear were conducted from a clinical perspective. Impressions were examined to obtain coherent data that could describe what was happening on the surface of the restorations and the opposing tooth enamel. All impressions made in this study were digitized. The scanning parameters, area to be scanned, scanning technique and data analysis determined the accuracy and reproducibility of this

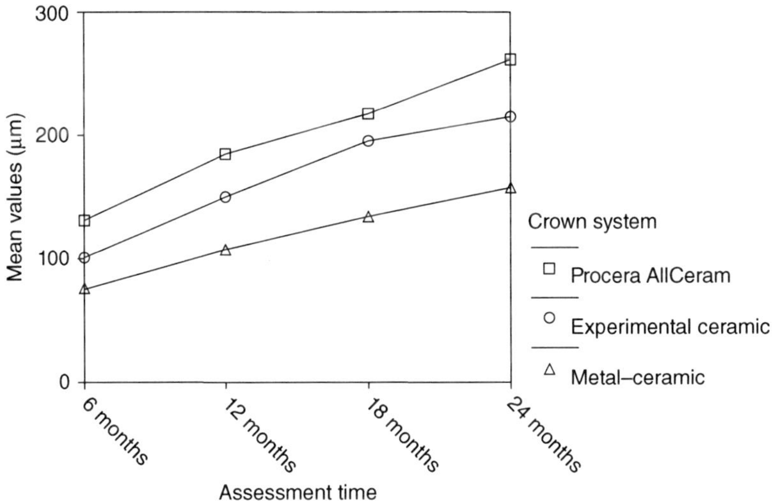

6.8 Mean values of tooth wear over 24 months.

technique. The amount of material loss from both sides was high in the first six months. This may relate to loss of the glaze layer from the ceramic materials and/or undetectable premature contacts during fitting of the crowns. After six months, the amount of material loss decreased but was still higher than physiological tooth loss. This may be related to the abrasive nature of the restorative materials resulting from factors such as differences in hardness and microstructures. Wear of the restorative materials and opposing enamel is a factor in the selection of a restorative material, whereas wear of the restorative material is a predictor of the clinical longevity of a restoration.

This *in vivo* investigation used various methods to rank wear of two dental crown systems and one experimental ceramic opposing enamel and each method showed a different 'best' material for clinical use. Thus, the type of wear evaluation should be considered when interpreting dental literature. The vertical height loss components in enamel wear, material wear and total wear are important factors in wear assessment. Distinct occlusal wear can be determined by both direct and indirect methods. However, general wear of the restorative material caused by other factors, such as fracture, was not detected in this study when it was located outside the occlusal contact areas. However, material loss outside the occlusal contact areas caused by bulk chipping or fracture of the surface layer influences the assessment, resulting in values that are lower or higher than the actual loss of material caused by wear. With the technique employed in this study, not only was the depth at a specific location measured, but also the respective area of wear was determined. Using these two parameters, the overall volume loss of the materials can be calculated mathematically.

New low-fusing ceramic materials have been developed to minimize wear damage. The manufacturers claim that these ceramics are wear friendly because of their lower hardness, lower concentration of crystal phase and smaller crystal sizes. Two all-ceramic systems with different microstructures were used in this study, together with a metal ceramic. Procera AllCeram caused more wear to the opposing tooth enamel and showed more wear itself compared with the other materials, in spite of its low hardness and lower concentration of crystal phase. This finding agreed with evidence suggesting that the hardness of a restorative material alone is not a reliable predictor of the wear of opposing enamel (Seghi *et al.*, 1991; Dahl and Oilo 1994; Callister 1997). In particular, the relationship of wear to hardness is not valid for materials that are brittle in nature. When ceramic slides against ceramic or enamel, wear does not occur by plastic deformation, as with metals, but by microfracture. This type of abrasive wear mechanism has been addressed (DeLong *et al.*, 1986).

Miyoshi and Buckley (1979) reported on the relationship between friction and wear of ceramics. They stated that 'ceramics behave much like metals when they are brought into contact with solids'. For example, when a silicon carbide surface is placed in contact with a diamond under relatively low contact pressure, elastic deformation can occur in both the silicone carbide and the diamond. Sliding occurs at the interface. A large increase in applied contact pressure, however, results in a complete reversal of the friction characteristic. Increased pressure causes plastic deformation in the silicon carbide, causing permanent grooves during sliding that lead to very small cracks. When a much higher contact pressure occurs because of the high concentration of stress in the contact area, the sliding action produces gross surface and sub-surface cracking as well as plastic deformation (Miyoshi and Buckley, 1979).

The natural wear that occurs in dental ceramic is adhesive and abrasive. Wear may occur when adhesion takes place across an interface between ceramic and enamel. If tangential motion results in fracture of the ceramic, adhesive wear has taken place. The fracture strength of one of the two surfaces must be less than that of the interfacial junction. The complex wet environment of the oral cavity, which is impossible to reproduce *in vitro*, can impart positive surface charges on glass or ceramic, leading to loss of sodium ions to the interacting aqueous environment and thereby reducing surface hardness (Milleding *et al.*, 1999a, 1999b, 2002). The microstructural components of different dental ceramics interact differently with the oral environment. This interaction may affect the behavior of the ceramics. Some *in vitro* studies questioned the effect of hardness on wear, finding that relatively soft ceramics exhibited more abrasive action against human enamel than harder ceramics (Seghi *et al.*, 1991; Yap *et al.*, 1997; Magne *et al.*, 1999; Clelland *et al.*, 2001).

The results of this study showed that the >70% ratio of crystals included in a glassy matrix does not necessarily have a negative impact on the wear of enamel. Care must be taken when interpreting data from previous *in vitro* tests, because the wear behavior of a ceramic with fine crystal content may be characterized differently by different wear tests. The outer layer and final surface finish of dental ceramic may affect the wear pattern. In this study, the ceramic surface was polished to the finest particle size and then glazed. In the first six months of clinical performance, the surface glazing layer was lost in the occlusal contact area and some visible wear facets became macroscopically visible, especially with Procera AllCeram crowns. The fabrication of the experimental ceramic crown involved the lost wax process, which requires fabrication of a wax pattern and investment of the pattern in glass-casting procedures. During the glass-casting procedure, a distinct surface layer is produced. The newly formed layer consists of crystalline whiskers oriented perpendicular to the external surface of the glass ceramic. This surface layer may cause enamel abrasion and may be more resistant to abrasion itself. The finishing procedures in this study involved polishing and glazing, which eliminates the effect of this layer. The application of shading porcelain, however, reduced the abrasiveness of the surface layer by filling the microscopic surface irregularities. This layer helped reduce initial wear against enamel until it was worn away by the opposing enamel at the occlusal contact areas.

This study did not measure the wear of enamel against enamel. It has been shown that steady state enamel/enamel wear is in the range of 29 μm per year for molars and 15 μm per year for premolars (Lambrechts *et al.*, 1989). In this study, Procera AllCeram wore four times as much as enamel. The experimental ceramic wore 1.25 times as much as enamel and metal ceramic wore at about the same rate as enamel. Each of these comparisons allows for steady-state wear to have been established after the first year. As conclusions, the experimental ceramic material appeared to provide clinical performance that was superior to that of Procera AllCeram in terms of wear behavior. The experimental ceramic showed friendly wear behavior on the opposing tooth enamel and was more wear resistant than the Procera AllCeram system. The wear behavior of the experimental ceramic was comparable to the metal ceramic crown. Therefore, it is suggested that clinicians should consider the type of ceramic restorative materials used to maintain a stable occlusal relation. Further, ceramic restorations should be sufficiently polished after any chairside adjustment of occlusal surface. Modification of ceramic materials is recommended to produce more durable ceramic in terms of wear resistance and to minimize undesired effects such as wear of ceramic materials on antagonistic enamel.

6.3 *In vitro* evaluation of wear and cracks in all-ceramic materials

6.3.1 Confocal examination of sub-surface cracking in ceramic materials using confocal laser scanning microscopy (CLSM)

Etman (2009) reported the relationship between crack propagation and ceramic microstructure following cyclic fatigue loading. Confocal laser scanning microscopy (CLSM) and SEM were used to measure qualitatively the surface and sub-surface crack depths of three types of ceramic restorations with different microstructures. Twenty ($8 \times 4 \times 2$ mm) blocks of three ceramic materials with different microstructures (Fig. 6.9), AllCeram (AC, Ducera, Germany), experimental ceramic (EC, IPS e.max Press, Ivoclar-Vivadent, Liechtenstein) and Sensation SL (SSL, Dilton Com., USA) were prepared, ten glazed and ten polished of each material.

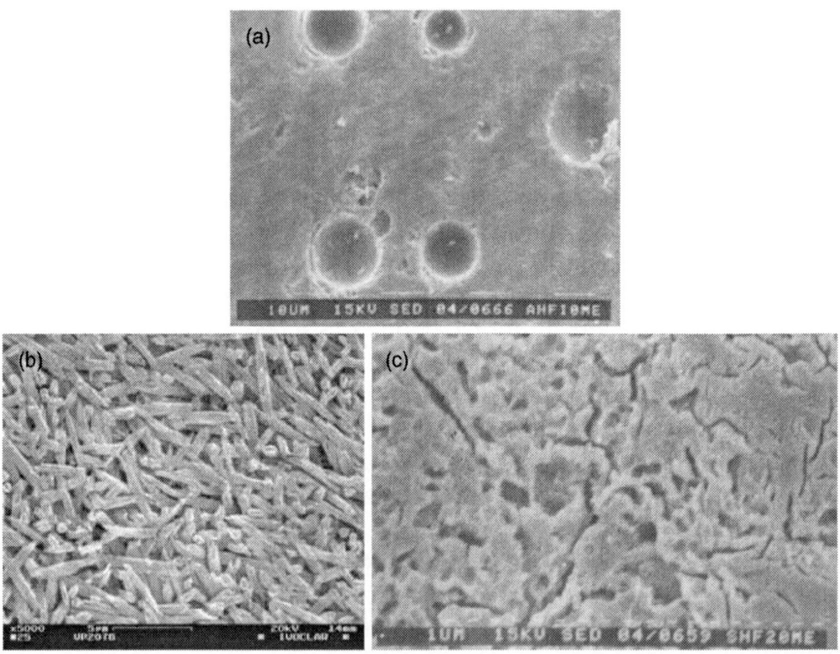

6.9 SEM photomicrographs: (a) Rounded structure in homogeneous glassy matrix in AllCeram. (b) Densely packed rod-like crystals of lithium disilicate crystals in experimental glass ceramic (Courtesy of Ivoclar-Vivadent), from a pilot study. (c) Leucite glass ceramic in Sensation SL.

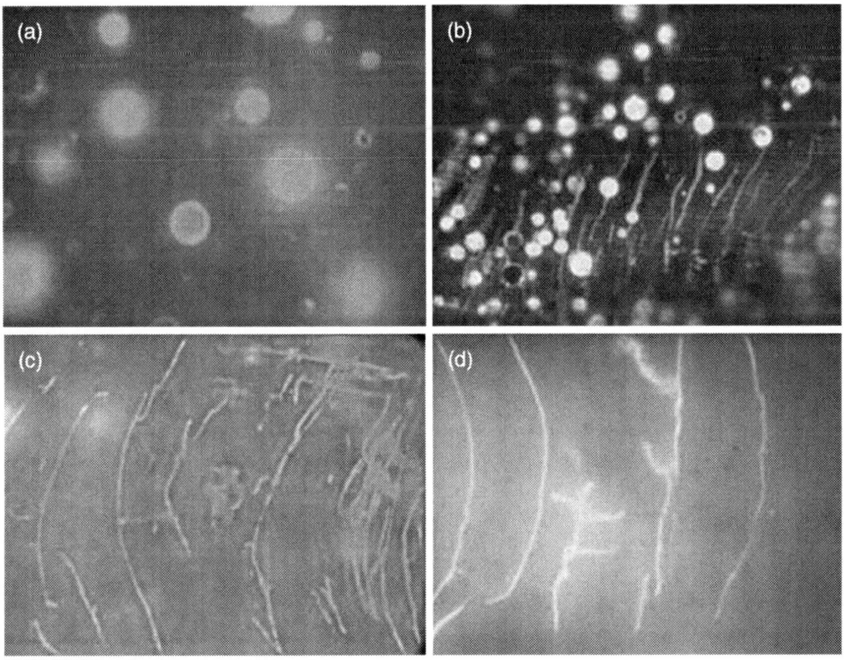

6.10 CLSM images of sub-surface cracks in AllCeram: (a) Baseline 5 μm below the surface; (b) 5-μm sub-surface, note the rounded features and the crack lines; (c) 8–10 μm below the surface, spherical features may be porosity or microstructures; the cracks show up clearly using CLSM in this combined image; and (d) the same field of view, 25 μm below the surface. Perkin-Elmer LSR Ultraview CLSM, ×100/1.3 oil (a, c, d; 102 μm); ×20/0.80 oil (b; 430 μm).

Sixty antagonist enamel specimens were made from the labial surfaces of permanent incisors. The ceramic abraders were attached to a wear machine so that each enamel specimen presented at 45° to the vertical movement of the abraders and immersed in artificial saliva. Wear was induced for 80K cycles at 60 cycles/min with a load of 40 N and 2 mm horizontal deflection. The specimens were examined for cracks at baseline, 5K, 10K, 20K, 40K and 80K cycles. 8–10 μm deep subsurface cracking appeared in AC (Fig. 6.10), with 20–30 μm in SSL (Fig. 6.11) and 7 μm close to the margin of the wear facets in glazed EC after 5K cycles (Fig. 6.12). The EC showed no cracks with increasing wear cycles. 70 μm deep sub-surface cracks were detected in SSL and 45 μm in AC after 80K cycles. Statistically, there was significant difference between the three materials ($p < 0.05$). The Bonferroni multiple comparison of means test confirmed the ANOVA test and showed that there was no statistical difference ($p > 0.05$) in crack depth

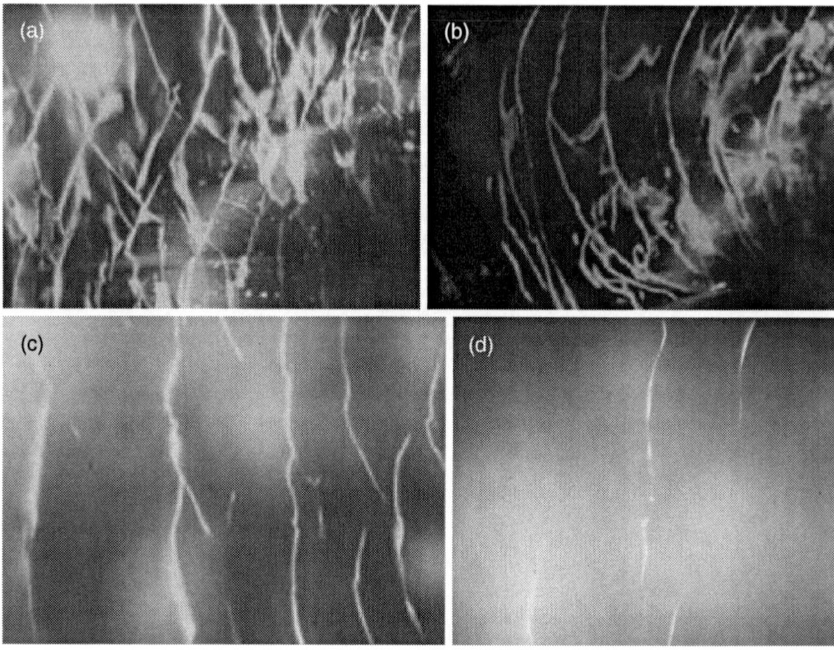

6.11 CLSM images of surface and sub-surface cracks in Sensation SL: (a) Just below the surface, this was a polished surface of Sensation SL; large number of cracks is apparent. (b) Sensation SL near the surface, cracks at 90° to the wear cracks. (c) The same sample as in (d) 20 μm below the surface, the cracks are broadly parallel and at 90° to the wear tracks. (d) The same field of view, 60 μm below the surface. Perkin-Elmer LSR Ultraview CLSM, ×100/1.3 oil. Field width 102 μm.

within the same ceramic material with different surface finishes. SEM photomicrographs showed wear and cracks formation in some materials (Fig. 6.13), (Fig. 6.14) and (Fig. 6.15). The ceramic materials with different microstructures showed different pattern of sub-surface cracking.

The results of this study showed the experimental glass ceramic with its unique microstructures was more crack resistant than other ceramic materials. When grinding forces were measured in alumina and glass ceramics with various microstructures, it was found the microstructures exert a profound influence on the machinability. In particular, the controlling toughness variable pertains to small cracks, not the variable conventionally measured in a large-scale fracture specimen (Marshall *et al.*, 2005). In a clinical study, Etman *et al.*, (2008) reported that the IPS e.max Press ceramic material showed a friendly wear behavior on the opposing tooth enamel and yet was more wear resistant than the Procera AllCeram system.

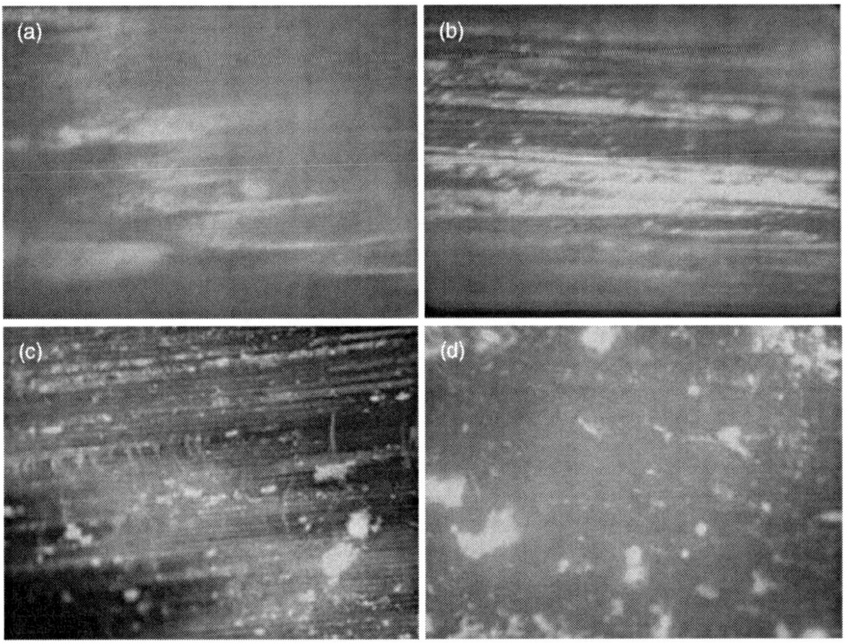

6.12 CLSM image of cracks in experimental ceramic: (a) 10-μm sub-surface view of glazed surface near the margin of a wear facet; note the disappearance of sub-surface cracks. (b) Experimental ceramic, view of the polished surface; note the absence of cracks. (c) Surface view of glazed surface near the margin of a wear facet, cracks at 90° to the wear tracks. (d) The same sample as in (c), 7 μm sub-surface view; note the disappearance of sub-surface cracks. Perkin-Elmer LSR Ultraview CLSM, ×60/1.4NA oil. Field width 170 μm.

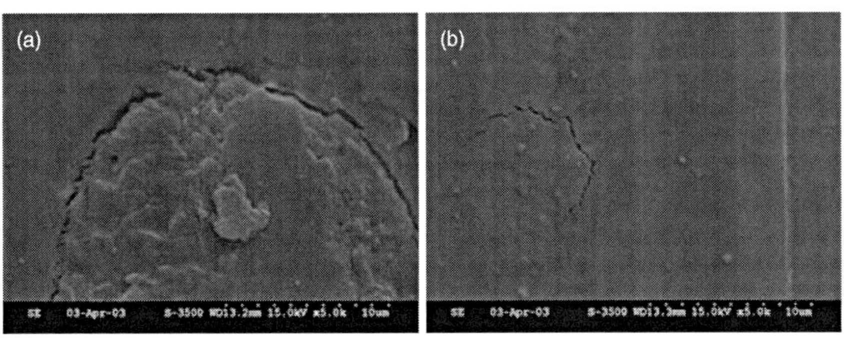

6.13 SEM photomicrographs of the worn Sensation SL ceramic show circular crack lines in both glazed (a) and polished (b) worn surfaces after 80 000 wear cycles (original magnification ×5000).

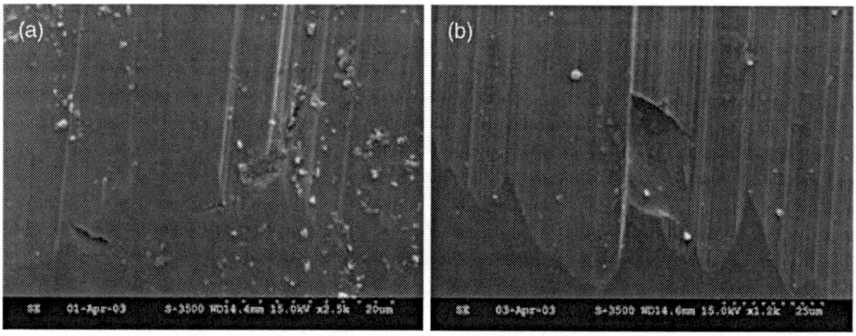

6.14 SEM photomicrographs show bulk fracture of AllCeram in both polished (a) and glazed (b) samples after 80 000 wear cycles. Original magnification, ×2500 (a); ×1200 (b).

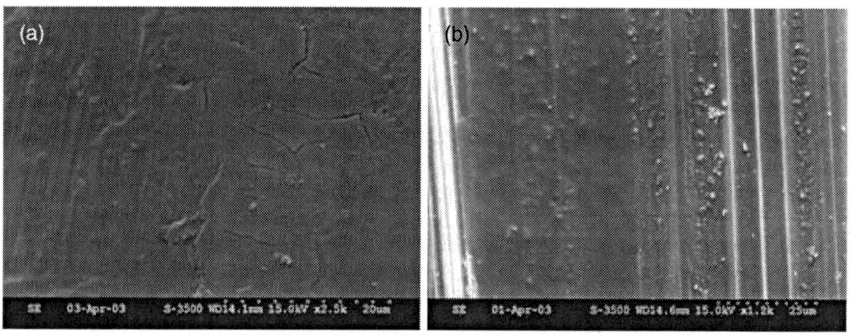

6.15 SEM photomicrographs of the worn experimental ceramic show crack lines located in the glaze layer at 90° to the wear tracks (a); note, no cracks in the polished worn surface after 80 000 wear cycles. Original magnification, ×2500 (a); ×1200 (b).

6.2.2 *In vitro* wear testing of all-ceramic materials

Another study by Etman (2007) reported that the three all-ceramic materials caused enamel wear and were worn by enamel; none retained the final surface finish. The mean depths of wear of the test materials were: AllCeram (polished, 254.17 μm and glazed, 264.48 μm), Sensation SL (polished, 268.09 μm and glazed, 265.69 μm), experimental ceramic (polished, 196.90 μm and glazed, 201.62 μm), tooth enamel (184.48 μm). The antagonist tooth enamel showed wear caused the four test materials. The mean depths of wear in the enamel antagonists were 248.04 μm and 260.34 μm caused by AllCeram polished and glazed, respectively. Sensation SL caused enamel wear (polished, 270.04 μm and glazed, 264.05 μm). The experimental ceramic caused less wear than the other two all-ceramic materials but more wear than tooth enamel. The polished experimental ceramic caused 197.90 μm, while the glazed specimens caused 201.30 μm mean depth of wear. Tooth enamel caused wear on the opposing tooth enamel with a mean depth of wear of 178.36 μm. This appears to confirm the relationship between microstructures, microcracks and wear behavior.

In recent years, many ceramic materials have been developed with different proportions of glassy and crystalline phases with the aim of improving their physical and mechanical properties. Different phases in these multiphase ceramic materials may react in different ways to cyclic fatigue loading and may have an effect on crack initiation and propagation. In this study, surface and sub-surface cracks were investigated, with the results revealing that surface and sub-surface cracks were dependent on the type of ceramic material. The experimental hot pressed lithium disilicate glass-ceramic material showed the highest resistance to crack formation and propagation. This may be due to the crystalline phases in this material. It has been reported that the crystalline phases in ceramic materials may act as crack stoppers to prevent crack propagation (Shareef *et al.*, 1994). However, with Sensation SL, this was not the case in this study. The high leucite crystalline structure showed the least resistance to crack propagation. This may be attributed to phase interaction and separation. Promotion of interaction between fatigue crack and microstructure, such as micro-cracking and phase transformation and separation in the process zone, has been reported (Okabe *et al.*, 1994). AllCeram showed less crack propagation than Sensation SL, even though it is considered to be a single-phase low fusing feldspathic porcelain. Crack initiation and propagation in this material may be explained by correlation between the microcracks, porosity and microstructures. It has been reported that the equilibrium between the external and internal forces inside the damage zone correlates with microstructural features, such as grain size distribution (Buresch, 1985). Crack propagation may depend on the compatibility between the phases in each material and some other microstructural factors, such as density of the material and porosity.

In the first 5000 cycles, AllCeram, Sensation SL and the experimental ceramic all showed multiple crack lines on the glazed surface. With increasing numbers of wear cycles, the glaze layer was removed from the surface of the experimental ceramic leaving a crack free surface. On the other hand, Sensation SL developed more cracks that propagated deeper into the material once the glaze layer was worn away. This may be explained as the driving force required for crack propagation supplied continuously by external stress caused phase separation at a low energy level. These external stresses can provide sufficient energy for crack formation, especially as the crack becomes larger at constant load (Beall *et al.*, 1986). Upon loading the material and inducing stresses, phase separation may occur. This would explain the irregular pattern of cracks in some samples of this material, which are similar to the shape and distribution of the leucite phase. However, another study reported that the crystalline inclusion was thought to help blunt fracture progression and improve fracture resistance (Beham, 1990). Another possible cause of Sensation SL cracks might be thermal mismatch between the leucite phase and the glassy matrix. Also the inclusion of large particle sizes of crystalline phases into a glassy matrix may have a direct correlation to crack formation (Binns, 1962; Frey and MacKenzie, 1967). A smaller crystal size could be beneficial to the strength properties of the experimental ceramic.

AllCeram is considered to be a low fusing feldspathic porcelain. CLSM showed two phases in AllCeram, one a glassy matrix and the other a sparse rounded structure that may represent a crystalline phase or porosity. SEM photomicrographs showed pores on the surface. Both AllCeram and Sensation SL were made using a powder and condensing liquid and repeated firing. This method has inherent problems, such as porosity, which may cause internal microcracks and phase separation from the use of physical mixtures of the glass powder (Piddock *et al.*, 1984.). Whilst the inclusion of phases of different refractive index is believed to be beneficial in terms of light scattering within porcelain (McLean, 1980), problems may ensue owing to incompatibility of thermal expansion of the various phases present (Mackert, 1988; Fairhurst *et al.*, 1992). Imaging of AllCeram worn surfaces showed a high proportion of spherical type pores that may cause further cracking. Small cracks around the periphery of a void have been cited as causing failure owing to the stress concentration at the void (Evans *et al.*, 1979). In this study, the catastrophic effect of cracking is more evident around the larger sized voids in the AllCeram samples. Pores arresting cracks have been described (Nadeau and Bennett, 1978). The crack awaits a load rise to break away or requires extra energy to curve out of the main crack plane because of the pore stress field. This theory was based on evenly spaced-sized pores and does not totally equate to the differing pore size and distribution in AllCeram. Nevertheless, there is an obvious crack–pore interaction.

The experimental ceramic is composed mainly of an interlocking pattern of many elongated lithium disilicate crystals (length up to 6 μm, diameter up to 1 μm) and secondary lithium orthophosphate crystals (0.1 to 0.3 μm) (Höland, 1998). Hot-pressing and continuous growth in the dimensions of these crystals upon heating may create a more dense structure. This may explain the crack resistance of this material. The SEM examination confirmed the CLSM finding, but only on the worn surfaces. This showed that the shape, distribution and location of the microcracks are different from one material to another. The microcracks in Sensation SL related to the wear facets and were perpendicular to the wear tracks. Cracks in this material are semicircular and are distributed all over the wear facets. Also, this material showed considerably more uniform distribution of crack lines, with evidence of microcracking in the semicircular crack patterns. This crack pattern may be related the shape of the leucite-shaped crystals that form the main component of this material. AllCeram was quite different in that there is uniform distribution of a few large crystals. Although there are small cracks within the crystals, these do not extend into the glass matrix. There was also evidence of microcracking within the crystals and, in some instances, cracks ran from the glassy matrix into and through the large crystalline structures. These round structures may have stopped crack propagation.

The presence of microcracks around the clusters of leucite crystal may suggest that non-uniform shrinkage of the glassy matrix and crystalline phases had occurred on cooling caused by differences in their thermal expansion behavior and the cubic to tetragonal leucite transformation (Mackert, 1988). If this is the case, microcracks would have to be found in the polished surface of these materials, which was not the case. These microcracks can also occur around individual leucite crystals but only when these are exceptionally large (Fairhurst *et al.*, 1992). Microcracks combined with the non-uniform distribution of the crystalline phase will severely limit the mechanical properties of these materials because they increase the inherent flaw size and may act as fracture-initiating flaws (Jones and Wilson, 1975), increasing the chances of catastrophic crack propagation. These flaws depend upon the size of the starting particles and distribution of the crystalline phase in the fired ceramics.

Crack formation may serve as a mechanism to relieve the residual stresses (Beall *et al.*, 1986). In this manner, the final size of the crack corresponds to the condition of crack arrest. It is speculated that under these conditions the force derived from relaxation of the residual stress field just suffices to supply the energy required to propagate the crack along a single crack front with little or no probability of secondary cracks or microcrack formation. The deriving force required for crack propagation is supplied continuously by the external stress field, which can provide sufficient energy for microcrack formation, especially as the crack becomes larger at constant load (Beall *et al.*, 1986).

The combination of high strength and fine crystalline structure may have an effect on the long-term performance of all-ceramic restorations, especially in stress-bearing areas. Although no fixed values of masticatory stress could be found in the literature for posterior crowns, using 40 N loads, surface cracks started to develop in the glaze layer as early as 5000 wear cycles. This study showed that these cracks in the glaze layer have no correlation with the underlying ceramic. On the other hand, the sub-surface cracks that occurred in the main bulk of the material have a strong correlation with the microstructure of such material. In conclusion, the microstructure and the technique of build up of ceramic restorations may have an effect on crack initiation and propagation. An overall view of the data from this investigation suggests that Sensation SL is not much more resistant to crack initiation and propagation than AllCeram. The higher sub-surface crack depth of Sensation SL and AllCeram demonstrates the potential unreliability of these materials in stress-bearing areas. High values of sub-surface cracks were recorded as early as 5000 loading cycles. The experimental ceramic showed higher resistance to crack formation and this may make it more reliable for stress-bearing areas. The surface finish has no effect on crack propagation. Knowing the potential for developing cracks in these materials may aid selection in various clinical applications. The CLSM is a useful instrument for detecting sub-surface cracks in ceramics.

6.4 Conclusion

The newly produced all ceramic material, IPS e-max Press showed a comparable clinical performance to Procera AllCeram crowns, but improved durability according to the modified USPHS criteria. All-ceramic materials caused enamel wear and were worn by enamel; none retained the final surface finish. The microstructure has an effect on ceramic and tooth wear. IPS e-max Press ceramic wore less and caused less wear to the opposing enamel. Enamel against enamel showed the least loss. Ceramic materials and tooth enamel showed changes in surface roughness in an *in vitro* study. Neither glazed nor polished ceramic surfaces remained intact. The microstructures of ceramic materials have an effect on surface roughness, wear and crack propagation.

6.5 References

Andersson M. and Odén A. (1993). 'A new all-ceramic crown. A dense-sintered, high-purity alumina coping with porcelain'. *Acta Odontol Scand*, **51**, 59–64.

Andersson M., Razzoog M.E., Odén A., Hegenbarth E.A. and Lang B.R. (1998). 'Procera: a new way to achieve an all-ceramic crown'. *Quintessence Int*, **29**, 285–96.

Anusavice K.J. (1992). 'Degradability of dental ceramics'. *Adv Dent Res*, **6**, 82–9.

Beall G.H., Chyung K. and Stewart R.L. (1986). 'Effect of test method and crack size on the fracture toughness of chain-silicate glass-ceramic'. *J Mater Sci*, **21**, 2365–72.

Beham G. (1990). 'IPS Empress; a new ceramic technology'. *Ivociar-Vivadent Report*, **6**, 1–15.

Binns D.B. (1962). 'Some physical properties of two-phase crystal glass solids. In *Science of Ceramics*', G. H. Stewart (ed.). Academic Press, London, Vol. 1, 315–34.

Buresch F.E. (1985). 'Relations between the damage in and microstructure of ceramics'. *Materi Sci Eng*, **71**, 187–94.

Callister W.D. Jr. (1997). *Material Science and Engineering: An Introduction*, 4th edn, John Wiley & Sons, New York, 179–95.

Chan C. and Weber H. (1986). 'Plaque retention on teeth restored with full-ceramic crowns: a comparative study'. *J Prosthet Dent*, **56**, 666–71.

Clelland N.L., Agarwala V., Knobloch L.A. and Seghi R.R. (2001). 'Wear of enamel opposing low-fusing and conventional ceramic restorative materials'. *J Prosthodont*, **10**, 8–15.

Craig G.R. (1997). *Restorative Dental Materials*, 10th edn, Mosby, St Louis, 91–2, 467–96.

Dahl B.L. and Oilo G. (1994). '*In vivo* wear ranking of some restorative materials'. *Quintessence Int*, **25**, 561–5.

DeLong R., Douglas W.H. and Sakaguchi R.L. (1986). 'The wear of dental porcelain in an artificial mouth'. *Dent Mater*, **2**, 214–19.

Dong J.K., Luthy H., Wohlwend A. and Schärer P. (1992). 'Heat pressed ceramics: technology and strength'. *Int J Prosthodont*, **5**, 9–16.

Etman M.K. (2004). *Clinical and Laboratory Evaluation of Advanced All-ceramic Restorations*. PhD Thesis, University of London.

Etman M.K. (2007). 'Wear of experimental ceramic and human enamel: An *in-vitro* study'. *J.Dent Res*. (IADR, Abstract No. 0183).

Etman M.K. (2009). Confocal examination of subsurface cracking in ceramic materials. *J Prosthodont*, **18**, 550–9.

Etman M.K. and Woolford M.J. (2010). 'Three-year clinical evaluation of two ceramic crown systems: A preliminary study'. *J Prosthet Dent*, **103**(2), 80–90.

Etman M.K., Northeast S.E. and van Noort R. (1999). 'A comparative study of the etched and polished surfaces of two dental and an experimental ceramic'. *J.Dent Res*. (IADR Abstract No. 1614).

Etman M.K., Woolford M.J. and Dunne S. (2008). 'Quantitative measurement of tooth and ceramic wear: *in vivo* study'. *Int J Prosthodont*, **21**, 245–52.

Evans A.G., Biswas D.S. and Fulrath R.M. (1979). 'Some effects of cavities on the fracture of ceramic materials: II: spherical cavities'. *J Am Ceram Soc*, **62**, 101–6.

Fairhurst C.W., Lockwood P.E., Ringle R.D. and Thompson W.O. (1992). 'The effect of glaze on porcelain strength'. *Dent Mater*, **8**, 203–7.

Frey W.J. and MacKenzie J.D. (1967). 'Mechanical properties of selected glass crystal composites'. *J Mater Sci*, **2**, 124–30.

Hegenbarth E.A. (1996). 'Procera aluminum oxide ceramics: a new way to achieve stability, precision, and esthetics in all-ceramic restorations'. *Quintessence Dent Technol*, **19**, 21–34.

Heintze S.D., Cavalleri A., Zellweger G., Büchler A. and Zappini G. (2008). 'Fracture frequency of all-ceramic crowns during dynamic loading in chewing simulator using different loading and luting protocols'. *Dent Mater*, **24**, 1352–61.

Höland W. (1998). 'Materials science fundamentals of the IPS Empress 2 glass-ceramic'. *Ivoclar-Vivadent Rep*, **12**, 3–10.

Haselton D.R., Diaz-Arnold A.M. and Hillis S.L. (2000). 'Clinical assessment of high-strength all-ceramic crowns'. *J Prosthet Dent*, **83**, 396–401.

Jacobi R., Shillingburg H.T. and Duncanson M.G. (1991). 'A comparison of the abrasiveness of six ceramic surfaces and gold'. *J Prosthet Dent*, **66**, 303–9.

Josephson B.A., Schulman A., Dunn Z.A. and Hurwitz W. (1991). 'A compressive strength study of complete ceramic crowns. Part II'. *J Prosthet Dent*, **65**, 388–91.

Jones D.W. and Wilson H.J. (1975). 'Some properties of dental ceramics'. *J Oral Rehabil*, **2**, 379.

Lambrechts P., Braem M., Vuylsteke-Wauters M. and Vanherle G. (1989). 'Quantitative *in vivo* wear of human enamel'. *J Dent Res*, **68**, 1752–4.
Leempoel P.J., Eschen S., De Haan A.F. and Van't Hof M.A. (1985). 'An evaluation of crowns and bridges in a general dental practice'. *J Oral Rehabil*, **12**, 515–28.
Löe H. and Silness J. (1963). 'Periodontal disease in pregnancy. I. Prevalence and severity'. *Acta Odontol Scand*, **21**, 533–51.
Mackert J.R., Jr (1988). 'Effect of thermally induced changes on porcelain-metal compatibility'. In *Perspectives in Dental Ceramics, Proceedings of the Fourth International Symposium on Ceramics*, Preston, J.D. (ed), Quintessence Publishing, Chicago, IL, USA, 53–64.
Magne P., Oh W.S., Pintado M.R. and Delong R. (1999). 'Wear of enamel and veneering ceramics after laboratory and chairside finishing procedures'. *J Prosthet Dent*, **82**, 669–79.
Mahalick J.A., Knap F.J. and Weiter E.J. (1971). 'Occlusal wear in prosthodontics'. *J Am Dent Assoc*, **82**, 154–9.
Marquardt P. and Strub J.R. (2006). 'Survival rates of IPS Empress 2 all-ceramic crowns and fixed partial dentures: results of a 5-year prospective clinical study'. *Quintessence Int*, **37**, 253–9.
Marshall D.B., Lawn B.R. and Cook R.F. (2005). 'Microstructural effects on grinding of alumina and glass-ceramics'. *J Am Ceram Soc*, **70**, 139–40.
May K.B., Russell M.M., Razzoog M.E. and Lang B.R. (1998). 'Precision of fit: the Procera AllCeram crown'. *J Prosthet Dent*, **80**, 394–404.
McLean J.W. (1979). *The Science and Art of Dental Ceramics*, Quintessence, Chicago.
McLean J.W. (1980). 'Aesthetics in restorative dentistry: the challenge for the future'. *Br Dent J*, **149**(12), 368–74.
Milleding P., Gerdes S., Holmberg K. and Karlsson S. (1999a). 'Surface energy of non-corroded and corroded dental ceramic materials before and after contact with salivary proteins'. *Eur J Oral Sci*, **107**, 384–92.
Milleding P., Wennerberg A., Alaeddin S., Karlsson S. and Simon E. (1999b). 'Surface corrosion of dental ceramics *in vitro*'. *Biomaterials*, **20**, 733–46.
Milleding P., Haraldsson C. and Karlsson S. (2002). 'Ion leaching from dental ceramics during static *in vitro* corrosion testing'. *J Biomed Mater Res*, **61**, 541–50.
Miyoshi K. and Buckley D.H. (1979). 'Friction, deformation and fracture of single-crystal silicon carbide'. *ASLE Trans*, **22**, 79–90.
Nadeau J.S. and Bennett R.C. (1978). 'Some effects of dispersed phases on the fracture behaviour of glass'. In *Fracture Mechanics of Ceramics*, Vol. IV, R.C. Bradt D.P.H. Hasselman and F.F. Lang (eds), Plenum Press, New York, 961–2.
Naert I., Van der Donck A. and Beckers L. (2005). 'Precision of fit and clinical evaluation of all-ceramic full restorations followed between 0.5 and 5 years'. *J Oral Rehabil*, **32**, 51–7.
Nakamura T., Ohyama T., Imanishi A., Nakamura T. and Ishigaki S. (2002). 'Fracture resistance of pressable glass-ceramic fixed partial dentures'. *J Oral Rehabil*, **29**, 951–5.
Odén A., Anderson M. and Krystek-Ondracek I. (1998). 'Magnusson D. Five-year clinical evaluation of Procera AllCeram crowns'. *J Prosthet Dent*, **80**, 450–6.
Okabe T., Kido M. and Miyahara T. (1994). 'Fatigue fracture behavior of oxide ceramics in water'. *Engineering Fracture Mechanics*, **48**, 137–46.
Piddock V., Marquis P.M. and Wilson H.J. (1984). 'Structure–property relationships of dental porcelains used in jacket crowns'. *Br Dent J*, **156**(11), 395–8.

Randall R.C. and Wilson N.H. (1999). 'Clinical testing of restorative materials: some historical landmarks'. *J Dent*, **27**, 543–50.
Rosenstiel S.F., Land F.M. and Fujimoto J. (2006). *Contemporary Fixed Prosthodontics*, 4th edn, Elsevier, St Louis, 272–85.
Russell M.M., Andersson M., Dahlmo K., Razzoog M.E. and Lang B.R. (1995). 'A new computer-assisted method for fabrication of crowns and fixed partial dentures'. *Quintessence Int*, **26**, 757–63.
Ryge G. (1980). 'Clinical criteria'. *Int Dent J*, **30**, 347–58.
Schwartz N.L., Whitsett L.D., Berry T.G. and Stewart J.L. (1970). 'Unserviceable crowns and fixed partial dentures: life span and causes for loss of serviceability'. *J Am Dent Assoc*, **81**, 1395–401.
Scotti R., Catapano S. and D'Elia A. (1995). 'A clinical evaluation of In-Ceram crowns'. *Int J Prosthodont*, **8**, 320–3.
Seghi R.R., Rosenstiel S.F. and Bauer P. (1991). 'Abrasion of human enamel by different dental ceramics *in vitro*'. *J Dental Res*, **70**, 221–5.
Shareef M.Y., Van Noort R., Messer P.F. and Piddock V. (1994). 'The effect of microstructural features on the biaxial flexural strength of leucite reinforced glass ceramics'. *J Mater Sci: Mater Med*, **5**, 113–18.
Silness J. and Löe H. (1964). 'Periodontal disease in pregnancy. II. Correlation between oral hygiene and periodontal condition'. *Acta Odontol Scand*, **22**, 121–35.
Sobrinho L.C., Cattel M.J., Glover R.H. and Knowles J.C. (1998). 'Investigation of the dry and wet fatigue properties of three all-ceramic crown systems'. *Int J Posthodont*, **11**, 255–62.
Stappert C.F., Stathopoulou N., Gerds T. and Srub J.R. (2005). 'Survival rate and fracture strength of maxillary incisors, restored with different kinds of full veneers'. *J Oral Rehabil*, **32**, 266–72.
Stappert C.F., Att W., Gerds T. and Strub J.R. (2006). 'Fracture resistance of different partial- coverage ceramic molar restorations: an *in vitro* investigation'. *J Am Dent Assoc*, **137**, 514–22.
Taskonak B. and Sertgöz A. (2006). 'Two-year clinical evaluation of lithia-disilicate-based all-ceramic crowns and fixed partial dentures'. *Dent Mater*, **22**, 1008–13.
Toksavul S. and Toman M. (2007). 'A short-term clinical evaluation of IPS Empress 2 crowns'. *Int J Prosthodont*, **20**, 168–72.
Walter M.H., Wolf B.H., Wolf A.E. and Boening K.W. (2006). 'Six-year clinical performance of all ceramic crowns with alumina cores'. *Int J Prosthodont*, **19**, 162–3.
Walton J.N., Gardner F.M. and Agar J.R. (1986). 'A survey of crown and fixed partial denture failures: length of service and reasons for replacement'. *J Prosthet Dent*, **56**, 416–21.
Wiley M.G. (1989). 'Effects of porcelain on occluding surfaces of restored teeth'. *J Prosthet Dent*, **61**, 133–7.
Yap A.U., Teoh S.H., Histings G.W. and Lu C.S. (1997). 'Comparative wear ranking of dental restorative materials utilizing different wear simulation modes'. *J Oral Rehabil*, **24**, 574–80.
Yoshinari M. and Dérand T. (1994). 'Fracture strength of all-ceramic crowns'. *Int J Prosthodont*, **7**, 329–38.
Zitzmann N.U., Galindo M.L., Hagmann E. and Marinello C.P. (2007). 'Clinical evaluation of Procera AllCeram crowns in the anterior and posterior regions'. *Int J Prosthodont*, **20**, 239–41.

7
Sol-gel derived bioactive glass ceramics for dental applications

X. CHATZISTAVROU, University of Michigan, USA, E. KONTONASAKI, K. M. PARASKEVOPOULOS, P. KOIDIS, Aristotle University of Thessaloniki, Greece and A. R. BOCCACCINI, University of Erlangen-Nuremberg, Germany

DOI: 10.1533/9780857096432.2.194

Abstract: Sol-gel derived silica-based bioactive glasses and ceramics attain many advantages owing to silicon which has a beneficial role in bone formation *in vivo*. They exhibit mesoporous architecture with interconnected pore structure and a high specific surface area that positively affects their bioactivity. Their compositions of up to 100 mol% SiO_2 in binary, ternary or quaternary systems, the potential for varying the microstructure in the same composition by controlling the chemical reactions and their ability to form scaffolds are some of the unique properties that distinguish them from their melt-derived counterparts. In the field of dental restoration and regeneration, sol-gel silica-based bioactive composites have started to emerge in various applications including coatings, scaffolds and dental tissue regeneration.

Key words: bioactivity, silica-based ceramics, silica-based glasses, sol-gel coatings, sol-gel dental composites, sol-gel synthesis.

7.1 Introduction

Glasses, ceramics and glass ceramics are considered 'bioactive' when the material surface is able to bond to bone or soft tissues via specific biological reactions that occur at the interface with tissues (Hench, 1991, 1998). The creation of this bond is the result of a series of reactions that occur at the surface in contact with the tissues, starting with surface dissolution and the breakdown of the silica network, forming silanol bonds (Si-OH) that repolymerize to form a hydrated, high surface-area, silica-rich layer. This silica-rich surface enhances the migration of Ca^{2+} and PO_4^{3-} groups to the surface forming an amorphous CaP layer, which is further crystallized in a hydroxycarbonate apatite (HCAp) layer.

Silica-based bioactive glasses and ceramics may offer advantages over calcium phosphates such as hydroxyapatite or tricalcium phosphate owing to the presence of silicon which appears to have a beneficial role in bone formation *in vivo* (Jugdaohsingh, 2007). The increased release rate of silicon has been reported to be the reason for the support of osteoblastic cell attachment and proliferation, the up-regulation of the expression of major bone markers and of a number of genes including IGF-I, gpl30 or MAPK3/ERK1 (Christodoulou *et al.*, 2006) as well as the formation of mineralized bone nodules on sol-gel SiO_2-P_2O_5-CaO glasses (Gough *et al.*, 2004; Hattar *et al.*, 2006; Gerhardt and Boccaccini, 2010). *In vivo* studies using rabbit models have shown that these sol-gel glasses showed an excellent degree of biocompatibility, a very low inflammatory response, full osteointegration with direct apposition of the newly formed bone and no fibrous tissue around the implants (Hamadouche *et al.*, 2001; Gil-Albarova *et al.*, 2004, 2005; Meseguer-Olmo *et al.*, 2006). Factors such as pore size and distribution are strongly related to both the rate of ion release and biodegradability, and affect the *in vitro* and *in vivo* biocompatibility (Yun *et al.*, 2011). The first and well-studied composition of bioactive glass is 45S5 Bioglass®, in the system SiO_2 45–Na_2O 24.5–CaO 24.5 and P_2O_5 6 in wt%. The low silica content and the presence of sodium ions in the glass result in very rapid ion exchange with physiological solutions and an alkaline pH (>7) at the implant interface with body fluids leading to the nucleation and crystallization of a carbonated apatite layer that is equivalent chemically and structurally to the biological bone mineral (Hench, 1998). 45S5 Bioglass® is usually synthesized by conventional glass melting technology. The glass components in the form of oxides or carbonates are mixed, melted and homogenized at high temperatures, 1250–1400°C, and then quenched to room temperature in order to form the amorphous melt-derived glass. There are some potential disadvantages of these melt-derived methods for the fabrication of bioactive glasses, including low purity levels, due to the high temperatures associated with melting and homogenization, but also due to the low silica and the high alkali content which is characteristic for the most traditional bioactive glass compositions (Li *et al.*, 1991).

It is widely accepted that increasing the silica content of a melt-derived glass decreases its bioactivity leading to complete elimination of bioactive behavior as the silica content approaches 60%. This is the result of decreased dissolution of the high silica containing surfaces which reduces the exchange of cations such as Ca^{2+} from the glass with H^+ and H_3O^+ from the solution, inhibiting subsequent silica-gel layer formation on the surface. Li *et al.* (1991) were the first to apply the sol-gel process in order to create bioactive glasses of various compositions, taking full advantage of the technique's benefits such as homogeneity and high surface area, as well as the presence of a silica-rich layer, which are the critical elements for the formation of the hydroxycarbonate bonding layer.

The sol-gel process is considered to be a chemical synthesis technique for the preparation of advanced glasses and ceramics. The process consists of the transition of a liquid state system (sol) into a wet solid (gel) state, which can subsequently be dried and sintered forming inorganic materials with various properties. The chemistry involved in the process is based on inorganic polymerization reactions of metal alkoxide precursors M(OR)*n*, where M represents a network forming element such as Si, Ti, Zr, Al and so on, and R stands for an alkyl group C_xH_{2x+1} (Brinker and Scherer, 1990; Tanaka and Yamashita, 2008). In the case of silicate-based bioactive glasses, the silicate precursor is usually an alkoxide such as tetraethyl orthosilicate (TEOS) or tetramethyl orthosilicate (TMOS). If other components, apart from silica, are required in the glass composition they are added to the sol either as other alkoxides or as salts.

Sol-gel-derived glasses with SiO_2 in the range 58–100 mol% have been studied for a number of applications. Sol-gel-derived bioactive glasses are reported to exhibit mesoporous architecture with interconnected pore structure and a high specific surface area. The pore sizes, as well as the porosity and the surface area, are linearly dependent on the composition of the glasses (Li *et al.*, 1991; Sepulveda *et al.*, 2001; Saravanapavan and Hench, 2003). The bioactivity of sol-gel glasses and glass ceramics is affected by their composition as well as their textural characteristics, including porosity and surface area and the number of silanol groups that serve as sites for HCAp nucleation (Cho *et al.*, 1998; Radin *et al.*, 1997). Negatively charged pores larger than 2 nm in radius provide favorable conditions for the apatite nucleation and hence act as nucleation sites (Pereira *et al.*, 1995; Pereira and Hench, 1996), while the ratio between network formers (SiO_2 and P_2O_5) and network modifiers (Na_2O and CaO) is a very important parameter for Si-OH formation (Arcos *et al.*, 2003).

The main advantages of the sol-gel derived materials over their melt-derived counterparts are lower processing temperatures and easy powder technology production (Hench and West, 1990), improved homogeneity and purity of the products and their increased bioactivity (Li *et al.*, 1991). Furthermore, the synthesis of a wider range of bioactive compositions with up to 100 mol% SiO_2 (Cho *et al.*, 1998), the potential to vary the microstructure in the same composition by control of hydrolysis and polycondensation reactions, their interconnected porosity and their ability to form macroporous structures by foaming (scaffolds) are some of their unique properties that distinguish them from the melt-derived bioactive glasses. Moreover, sol-gel processing can be applied to thin film fabrication, for example to develop thin layers of sol-gel derived glasses of few μm with high homogeneity and mechanical and chemical stability which can be deposited on bulk materials in a wide range of applications.

Since 1991, when Li *et al.* (1991) used the sol-gel process to synthesize bioactive glasses of various compositions with an initial high-specific surface area, binary, ternary and quaternary systems have been systematically investigated as promising candidates for bone graft applications (Zhong and Greenspan, 2000), while a variety of sol-gel coatings and composites have been synthesized for different biomedical applications. To improve certain properties such as the bioactivity of sol-gel glasses, additives can be easily introduced during the sol-gel synthesis. Doping elements are generally chosen either because of their existence as trace elements in the human body or for their biological activity. These ions include mainly Sr, Zn, Mg and B and their specific role in *in vitro* and *in vivo* conditions is reported in detail in a recent review by Hoppe *et al.* (2011).

7.2 Sol-gel-derived glasses and glass ceramics

7.2.1 In binary systems

SiO_2–CaO

Binary calcium silicate ceramics were introduced as potential biomaterials in 1990 when it was demonstrated that melt-derived P_2O_5-free wollastonite ceramics (SiO_2–CaO) showed *in vitro* (Ebisawa *et al.*, 1990) and *in vivo* (Ohura *et al.*, 1991) bioactivity. However owing to the high melting temperatures applied to their synthesis and their inferior bioactivity compared to other available quaternary bioactive glass compositions, little interest was attracted by these ceramics. On the other hand, use of the sol-gel method provided evidence that highly bioactive compositions can be synthesized in the binary SiO_2–CaO system. Hayashi and Saito (1980) were the first to prepare gels in the binary SiO_2–CaO system, while many other research groups have synthesized bioactive binary sol-gel glasses of varying Ca/Si molar ratios (0–1.5) (Catauro *et al.*, 1997; Martínez *et al.*, 2000; Saravanapavan and Hench, 2000; Salinas *et al.*, 2001; Iimori *et al.*, 2004; Chrysafi *et al.*, 2007; Meiszterics *et al.*, 2010) (Table 7.1).

The sol-gel synthesis of CaO–SiO_2 glasses is generally based on the polycondensation of metal alkoxides (e.g. $Si(OR)_4$, $Ca(OR)_4$) or inorganic precursors (e.g. $Ca(NO_3)_2$) using hydrolysis and condensation processes that require either acid or base catalysis. These catalysts may be strong acids (e.g. nitric acid) (Salinas *et al.*, 2001), acetic acid (Meiszterics *et al.*, 2010; Chrysafi *et al.*, 2007) or base (e.g. ammonia (Iimori *et al.*, 2004), sodium hydroxide (Siriphannon *et al.*, 2002)). Meiszterics *et al.* (2010) synthesized materials in the SiO_2–CaO system using both acidic and basic catalysts and concluded that the acid-catalyzed reactions produced a less compact and randomly branched three-dimensional (3D) network compared to a denser network produced by basic catalysts, owing to faster hydrolysis.

The bioactivity of these binary systems depends on a complex relationship between composition, surface area and porosity. A larger surface area and smaller pore size are obtained for higher SiO_2 contents and lower CaO contents (Saravanapavan and Hench, 2000). According to Saravanapavan

Table 7.1 Sol-gel-derived silica-based glasses and glass ceramics in binary systems

System (%mol)	Stabilization temperature	Heat treatment	Crystal phases		Surface area ($m^2 g^{-1}$)	Total pore volume ($cm^3 g^{-1}$)	Averge pore size (nm)	Reference
			Before heat treatment	After heat treatment				
$CaO–SiO_2$								
99–90 SiO_2	600–970°C	1300°C	Amorphous, wollastonite	α-quartz, wollastonite and cristobalite	184.63–186	0.342	6–7.42	Catauro and Laudisio (1998); Martínez *et al.* (2000); Saravanapavan and Hench (2000, 2003)
89–80 SiO_2	300–970°C	800–1000°C	Amorphous, wollastonite	wollastonite and cristobalite	154–172.3	0.498	11.64–12	Hayashi and Saito (1980); Martínez *et al.* (2000); Saravanapavan and Hench (2000, 2003); Salinas *et al.* (2001)
79–70 SiO_2	700–1400°C		Amorphous, wollastonite, pseudowollastonite and cristobalite		126–135.87	0.713	15–20.99	Martínez *et al.* (2000); Róman *et al.* (2003); Saravanapavan and Hench (2000, 2003)
69–60 SiO_2	800–970°C		wollastonite and cristobalite		41–87.01	0.742	24–34.13	Martínez *et al.* (2000); Saravanapavan and Hench (2000, 2003); Catauro *et al.* (1997)

and Hench (2003), the mean surface area of binary SiO_2–CaO sol-gel glasses is reported to increase from 40–180 $m^2 g^{-1}$ as the silicon content is increased from 50–90 %wt, while the total pore volume and the average pore diameter are reported to decrease as the silicon content increases. The pore system consists of a 3D network of cavities (pores) interconnected by constrictions (throats) (Saravanapavan and Hench, 2003). These differences in textural and compositional properties give rise to important variations in their *in vitro* behavior. In general, glasses with lower SiO_2 content and higher CaO content exhibit higher apatite layer growth rates and *vice versa* when immersed in simulated body fluid (SBF) (Martínez *et al.*, 2000). A high amount of CaO results in a higher proportion of silanol groups following the release of calcium ions to the SBF. This fact, in combination with their smaller pore size, can explain the lower growth rate of the apatite-like layer on these glasses.

In order to improve the mechanical properties of the bioactive glasses and to make them suitable materials for load-bearing applications, efforts have been made to sinter bioactive glasses at their crystallization temperatures (Chu and Liu, 2008). However, it was reported that crystallization of bioactive glasses could decrease the level of bioactivity (Peitl *et al.*, 1996) and even turn a bioactive glass into an inert material (P. Li *et al.*, 1992).

Upon heat treatment, sol-gel derived SiO_2–CaO glasses are crystallized to $CaSiO_3$ ceramics and in most cases to α-$CaSiO_3$ (wollastonite; the low temperature phase) and β-$CaSiO_3$ (pseudowollastonite; the high temperature phase of $CaSiO_3$) with various densities and porosities depending on the applied heat treatment (Table 7.1). Wollastonite and pseudowollastonite ceramics are bioactive, showing a fast and high growth rate formation of apatite layer after immersion in SBF, which was observed to be faster than than on many other ceramics in SBF (De Aza *et al.*, 1994; Siriphanon *et al.*, 2002; Iimori *et al.*, 2004). This apatite formation behavior, however, varies greatly with the chemical composition, porosity and microstructure of the $CaSiO_3$ ceramics.

SiO_2–SrO

Another important bioactive binary system is the SiO_2–SrO system, which is expected to present a similar behavior to that of the binary system SiO_2–CaO, as strontium and calcium ions are comparatively similar in size, while strontium ions are additionally known to stimulate osteoblast cells. Strontium has been used in bone substitution biomaterials owing to its great affinity for bone tissue. Incorporation of Sr in bioactive glasses has been proposed (Lao *et al.*, 2008; Gorustovich *et al.*, 2007; Isaac *et al.*, 2011), based on the natural occurrence of strontium as a trace element in the human body and the reduction of incidence of fractures in osteoporotic patients treated with strontium renalate (Meunier *et al.*, 2004; Reginster *et al.*, 2008). Both *in vitro* and *in vivo* studies have demonstrated the stimulatory effects of Sr on osteoblasts and an inhibitory effect on osteoclasts, associated with an increase in bone density and resistance (Marie *et al.*, 1993; Bonnelye *et al.*, 2008).

Non-crystalline solids within the liquid–liquid immiscibility region in the system SiO_2–SrO have been prepared using the sol-gel method (Yamane and Kojima, 1981). The received pore-free, clear glassy solids attained a density and refractive index similar to melt-derived SiO_2–SrO glasses with high SrO content. As the amount of Sr^{2+} increased above a maximum number of Sr^{2+} ions in the aqueous solution of SrO 10–SiO_2 90 wt%, the increase was accompanied by crystal growth of $Sr(NO_3)_2$. In a recent study, Wu *et al.* (2011) incorporated Sr into mesoporous SiO_2 in an effort to develop a bioactive mesoporous SiO_2–SrO (Si–Sr) glass with the capacity to deliver Sr^{2+} ions, as well as a drug, for bone repair. The prepared mesoporous Si–Sr glass was found to release bioactive Sr^{2+} ions and dexamethasone (DEX) and the incorporation of Sr^{2+} improved structural properties, such as mesopore size, pore volume and specific surface area, as well as the rate of dissolution and protein adsorption. The mesoporous Si–Sr glass had no cytotoxic effects and the release of Sr^{2+} and SiO_4^{4-} ions enhanced alkaline phosphatase (ALP) activity – a marker of osteogenic cell differentiation – in human bone mesenchymal stem cells (BMSCs).

7.2.2 In ternary systems

In order to mimic the nature and replicate more complex natural systems, the development of more complicated systems was considered important. Ternary and quaternary systems were fabricated (see Table 7.2).

SiO_2–CaO–P_2O_5

The most studied sol-gel-derived glasses are those of the ternary SiO_2–CaO–P_2O_5 system (Table 7.2). Li *et al.* (1991) obtained bioactive powders of the SiO_2–CaO–P_2O_5 system with bioactivity considerably higher than that of melt-derived glasses. Sol-gel-derived glasses of the SiO_2–CaO–P_2O_5 system were also obtained by Pereira *et al.* (1994) using the alternative calcium methoxyethoxide instead of calcium nitrate that was previously applied. Pereira *et al.* (1994) reported that the use of calcium nitrate resulted in non-homogeneous glasses that varied in their bioactivity. The lack of homogeneity was attributed either to Ca^{2+} ions migrating out of the pores during processing of the gel forming regions with a high Ca^{2+} concentration or to uncontrolled crystallization due to calcium nitrate. Although calcium methoxide improved the homogeneity of these sol-gel glasses, the rapid hydrolysis of calcium methoxide made it difficult to prepare large batches of homogeneous sol-gel bioactive glasses. Zhong and Greenspan (2000) reported that the use of a high relative-humidity environment during the drying stages of the process produces homogeneous glass with high bioactivity and resorbability *in vitro*, while ethanol treatment prior to humidity drying results in crack-free, monolithic structures with a yield of over 80%. However, even though they succeeded in synthesizing microporous, high surface-area bioactive materials by sol-gel processing, they could not prevent the presence of a small amount of a crystalline phase.

Many compositions of sol-gel ternary glass ceramics of the system SiO_2–CaO–P_2O_5 have been synthesized with varying degrees of *in vitro* apatite forming ability. Gel powders, which have a lower SiO_2 content and higher CaO and P_2O_5 content, exhibit higher rates of HCAp formation (Li *et al.*, 1991; Sepulveda *et al.*, 2001; Chen *et al.*, 2008). Chen *et al.* synthesized ternary SiO_2–CaO–P_2O_5 glasses with high specific surface areas, mainly composed of amorphous silicate phases. They further reported not only that the rate is different but that the morphology of the precipitates also follows a different pattern.

Mesoporous and hierarchically porous sol-gel-derived SiO_2–CaO–P_2O_5 balls with pores ranging in size from nanometer to micrometer exhibit good biocompatibility with attractive bone forming ability. However, large sized pores in the range of several tens of micrometers have been reported to cause an abrupt change in pH and rapid biodegradation (Yun *et al.*, 2011). Recently, sol-gel-derived SiO_2–CaO–P_2O_5 xerogels were proposed as promising candidates for the controlled release of metronidazole in periodontal disease treatment (Czarnobaj and Sawicki, 2011). The most characteristic sol-gel derived bioactive glass is 58S, containing SiO_2 60–CaO 36–P_2O_5 4 mol% (Chen *et al.*, 2008), which has been released in the market as a component of a bone-filling bioactive glass. Thermal treatment of the SiO_2–CaO–P_2O_5 sol-gel glasses under different conditions can affect their microstructure and thus influence their bioactivity (Laczka *et al.*, 1997; Goudouri *et al.*, 2009). Generally, the sol-gel systems SiO_2–CaO–P_2O_5 are prone to form various Ca–P or Ca–Si phases under specific conditions, such as excessive stirring or sintering (Goudouri *et al.*, 2009).

SiO_2–CaO–SrO

The advantages of the incorporation of SrO in to the silicate network of the binary system SiO_2–SrO have been discussed earlier in Section 7.2.1. Studies on the sol-gel-derived Sr-doped glasses in the system SiO_2–CaO (with SrO in the range 1 and 5 wt%) performed by Lao *et al.* and Isaac *et al.* have shown both faster apatite formation and enhanced osteoblast

Table 7.2 Sol-gel-derived silica-based glasses and glass ceramics in ternary systems

System (%mol)	Stabilization temperatures	Heat treatment	Crystal phases	
			Before heat treatment	After heat treatment
SiO_2–CaO–P_2O_5				
49–40 SiO_2	700–800°C	450–1300°C	Amorphous, wollastonite	Apatite, Ca_2SiO_4 and wollastonite
59–50 SiO_2	580–700°C		Amorphous, $Ca_3(PO_4)_2 \cdot 2H_2O$ and apatite	Pseudowollastonite, tricalcium phosphate (TCP), wollastonite and cristobalite
69–60 SiO_2	500–959°C	450–1025°C	Amorphous, Ca_2SiO_4 and apatite	Wollastonite, apatite, pseudowollastonite, quartz
79–70 SiO_2	600–959°C		Amorphous and apatite Amorphous	
89–80 SiO_2	600–700°C	450°C	Amorphous	
99–90 SiO_2	600°C		N/A	
SiO_2–CaO–ZnO				
79–70SiO_2	650–850°C		N/A	
SiO_2–CaO–SrO				
79–70SiO_2	700°C		N/A	
CaO–MgO–SiO_2				
49–40 SiO_2	1000–1400°C			Merwinite, diopside akermanite, bredigite, Ca_2SiO_4 and wollastonite

differentiation compared to a non-doped binary SiO_2–CaO glass (Lao *et al.*, 2008; Isaac *et al.*, 2011). In particular, gene expression of Runx2, Osx, Dlx5, Collagen I, ALP, BSP and OC was up-regulated on day 12 of calvarial bone cells culture and ALP activity was increased on day 6. The authors suggested a strontium dose-dependent effect on osteoblast differentiation. Sr^{2+} is incorporated into the bone matrix by two mechanisms: (i) surface exchange involving the incorporation of Sr^{2+} into the crystal lattice of the

Surface area ($m^2 g^{-1}$)	Total pore volume ($cm^3 g^{-1}$)	Average pore size (nm)	Reference
18.23–29.02	0.097–0.101	13.29–24.3	Łączka *et al*, (1997, 2000); Hesaraki *et al.* (2010)
<2.0–236.96	0.26–0.57	5.0–5.7	Li *et al.* (1991); Róman *et al.* (2003); Vulpoi *et al.* (2012); Balas *et al.* (2001); Ma *et al.* (2010)
71–324	0.11–0.534	2.7–19.6	Li *et al.* (1991); Pereira *et al.* (1994); Łączka *et al.* (1997); Balas *et al.* (2001); Sepulveda *et al.* (2002); Bini *et al.* (2009); Chen *et al.* (2008); Arcos *et al.* (2002); Pérez-Pariente *et al.* (1999); Goudouri *et al.* (2009); Zhong and Greenspan (2000)
141–380	0.10–0.53	2.0–8,7	Li *et al.* (1991); Pereira *et al.* (1994); Bini *et al.* (2009); Salinas *et al.* (2001); Arcos *et al.* (2002); Pérez-Pariente *et al.* (1999); Balas *et al.* (2001)
136.69–627	0.104–0.63	1.4–4.0	Li *et al.* (1991); Pereira *et al.* (1994); Łączka *et al.* (1997); Vallet-Regí *et al.* (1999); Balas *et al.* (2001); Bini *et al.* (2009); Chen *et al.* (2008); Zhong and Greenspan (2000)
–	0.45	1.4	Li *et al.* (1991)
21–179.1	0.067–0.445	5.12–11.77	Jaroch and Clupper (2007); Courtéoux *et al.* (2008)
24–28	0.066–0.069	9.3–11.8	Isaac *et al.* (2011)
			Wu and Chang (2004); Wu *et al.* (2005, 2006); Ou *et al.* (2008); Chen *et al.* (2008); Huang *et al.* (2009)

bone mineral, and (ii) ionic substitution whereby Sr^{2+} is taken up by ionic exchange with Ca^{2+}. In the *in vitro* studies by Lao *et al.* (2008) and *in vivo* studies by Gorustovich *et al.* (2007) strontium was substituted for calcium on a weight basis. As strontium, which is a heavier ion, is substituted for calcium, the silica content in terms of molecular percentage or silicon content in atomic percentage actually increases (1% wt Sr^{2+} substitution corresponds to 0.36% mol increase and 5% wt Sr^{2+} substitution corresponds to 1.83% mol increase) (O'Donnell and Hill, 2010). As the silica content increases, the fraction of cross-linked Q^3 $[SiO_4]^{4-}$ units in the glass increases at the expense of the more soluble Q^2 chains. This will have the effect of decreasing glass solubility, slowing degradation and hence reducing bioactivity. This was clearly seen in the studies by Lao *et al.* (2008) where faster apatite formation was recorded for the 1 wt% Sr^{2+} substitution. However an increase of Sr^{2+} release from the 5 wt% doped glasses led to enhanced osteoblast differentiation.

SiO_2–CaO–ZnO

Zinc (Zn) is the second most abundant trace element in the human body and is reported to promote bone mineralization (Radin *et al.*, 2005), improve the healing of bony tissues (Zhang *et al.*, 2005), inhibit osteoclastic bone resorption and prevent osteoporosis (Yamaguchi, 2010). Zinc is an effective antibacterial agent to strains commonly associated with orthopedic surgeries' infections (R. Li *et al.*, 1992). Severe zinc deficiency is characterized by growth retardation, skin lesions, impaired wound healing and depression of the immune system (Haase and Rink, 2009; Maggini *et al.*, 2010).

Glasses in the SiO_2–CaO–ZnO system have been synthesized by the sol-gel method. Jaroch and Clupper (2007) investigated the microstructure and release profile of the ternary 70 SiO_2/(18 + x) CaO/(12 − x) ZnO system (where x = 0, 4 or 8 mol%) and showed that the addition of ZnO decreased the pore diameter and volume and altered the pore shape from predominantly cylindrical to quasi ink bottle shaped. Upon heat treatment, crystalline phases $CaSiO_3$ and $Ca_2ZnSi_2O_7$ developed at 850°C. A dose/temperature dependent inhibitory effect of Zn on rapid crystalline HCAp formation was demonstrated. Furthermore, despite the relatively large concentration of zinc in the glasses, zinc release into SBF was limited to relatively low levels (<1.2 $\mu g\,ml^{-1}$), partly because of its incorporation into the forming calcium phosphate surface layer preventing potentially toxic levels.

The inhibiting effect of Zn on *in vitro* apatite formation was also reported by Courthéoux *et al.* (2008) and was attributed to a delayed breakdown of the glass silicate network in biological fluids. The reason is that Zn adopts a tetrahedral coordination in the glassy network and copolymerizes with $[SiO_4]$ tetrahedra (Linati *et al.*, 2005). This results in a complex glassy network that leads to an increase in its chemical durability.

SiO_2–CaO–MgO

Mg is the fourth highest concentrated cation in the human body after calcium, potassium and sodium, showing beneficial effects on the physicochemical properties of minerals and on bone metabolism (Creedon *et al.*, 1999; Maguire and Cowan, 2002). Bone minerals contain various amounts of magnesium, either adsorbed at the surface of hydroxyapatite crystals or incorporated inside its crystallographic structure (Aoba *et al.*, 1992; Bigi *et al.*, 1993). Glass ceramics of the ternary SiO_2–CaO–MgO-system have attracted interest in recent years because of their good mechanical and chemical properties. Novel single-phase or multi-phase sol-gel-derived glass ceramics in the system SiO_2–CaO–MgO have been synthesized.

Various crystalline phases such as diopside ($CaMgSi_2O_6$), merwinite ($Ca_3MgSi_2O_8$), akermanite ($Ca_2MgSi_2O_7$), wollastonite ($CaSiO_3$) and dicalcium silicate (Ca_2SiO_4) have been thoroughly investigated, respectively, showing that they possess suitable mechanical and biological properties (Nonami and Tsutsumani, 1999; Liu *et al.*, 2004; Wu *et al.*, 2005; Wu and Chang, 2006; Wu *et al.*, 2006; Ou *et al.*, 2008). Diopside ceramics release ions at a definite concentration which helps osteoblasts to grow and differentiate and provide the ability to induce apatite formation *in vitro* in SBF and bone formation *in vivo* (Nakajima *et al.*, 1989; Nonami and Tsutsumani, 1999). Sol-gel-derived glass ceramics composed of akermanite, wollastonite and dicalcium silicate crystalline phases possess appropriate mechanical properties, good bioactivity and biocompatibility *in vitro*, as well as antibacterial activity (Hu *et al.*, 2011) and can be used as promising bioactive glass ceramics for bone regeneration and tissue engineering applications.

Chen *et al.* (2010) reported that a glass ceramic with a molar composition of 45.98% SiO_2–43.3% CaO–10.72% MgO presented increased viability and proliferation of osteoblast and increased ALP activity after 7 days' culturing, while its bending strength was 87.62 MPa and its Young's modulus was 29.73 GPa, similar to that of cortical bone. Furthermore, sol-gel-derived akermanite can promote osteoblastic differentiation of hBMSC (human bone marrow stromal cells) (Huang *et al.*, 2009) and has the potential to stimulate angiogenesis, which contributes to its ability to enhance bone regeneration. Bredigite ceramics prepared by sintering sol-gel-derived bredigite powder compacts at 1350°C for 8 h resulted in ceramics with a high bending strength, fracture toughness and Young's modulus, apatite-forming ability in SBF and promotion of osteoblasts growth (Wu *et al.*, 2005). Zhai *et al.* (2012) reported that akermanite ion extracts up-regulated the expression of genes encoding the receptors of proangiogenic cytokines *in vitro*, while when implanted in rabbit femoral condyle model they promoted neovascularization after 8 and 16 weeks of implantation, which further confirmed the stimulation effect on angiogenesis *in vivo*.

7.2.3 In quaternary systems

Bioactive glass-ceramic materials of the system SiO_2-CaO-P_2O_5 modified by adding various elements such as magnesium, zinc, strontium, silver, etc., have been obtained using the sol-gel method with different effects on their microstructural properties and bioactivity (Table 7.3.). Factors such as type of doping element, surface area, porosity, calcium solubility and the crystallization of particular phases on their surface have been involved in the apatite forming ability and the biocompatibility of these glass-ceramics.

SiO_2–CaO–P_2O_5–MgO

The incorporation of MgO has been extensively examined in quaternary compositions of the system SiO_2–CaO–P_2O_5–MgO in concentrations varying in the range 2.9–13 mol% with varying bioactivity and good biocompatibility (Vallet-Regí *et al.*, 1999; Pérez-Pariente *et al.*, 1999, 2000; Laczka *et al.*, 2000; Abiraman *et al.*, 2002; Balamurugan *et al.*, 2007b; Radev *et al.*, 2009; Erol *et al.*, 2010). New studies have shown that sol-gel-derived bioactive glass in the system SiO_2–CaO–P_2O_5–MgO has the ability to support the growth of human fetal osteoblastic cells (hFOB 1.19). This material has also proved to be non-toxic and compatible in segmental defects in the goat model *in vivo* (Saboori *et al.*, 2009).

Perez-Pariente *et al.* (1999) applied the sol-gel method to obtain glasses with four different compositions in the system SiO_2–CaO–P_2O_5–MgO [SiO_2 (60–80%)–CaO (12.8–28.8%)–P_2O_5 (4%)–MgO(3.2–7.2%) mol%] showing high values of porosity and surface area. In lower SiO_2 content glasses the surface decreased and a faster growth rate of the calcium phosphate–rich layer was recorded, while in cases with lower CaO content the lower porosity delayed the apatite nucleation. In a further study by the same group (Pérez-Pariente *et al.*, 2000), sol-gel derived glasses in the system SiO_2–CaO–P_2O_5–MgO with 65 and 75 mol% SiO_2 presented lower apatite formation compared to respective glasses without 4.2 mol% MgO content. Although MgO increased the surface area of the glasses that would lead to increased apatite forming ability, the inhibitory effect of MgO was attributed to the lack of calcium phosphate domains which are present in the MgO-free glasses and act as preferential nucleation centers for the crystallization of apatite in SBF. The inhibitory effect of MgO was also verified by Lazcka *et al.* (2000), who reported that although MgO did not reduce Ca solubility and resulted in SBF pH values similar to those of the amorphous SiO_2–CaO–P_2O_5, the surface crystallization of the calcium phosphate layer was significantly restricted.

Balamurugan *et al.* (2007b) synthesized a sol-gel glass in the system SiO_2–CaO–P_2O_5–MgO with a high MgO content (SiO_2 55%, CaO 26%, P_2O_5

Table 7.3 Sol-gel derived silica-based glasses and glass-ceramics in quaternary systems

System (%mol)	Stabilization temperatures	Heat treatment	Crystal phases		Surface area ($m^2 g^{-1}$)	Total pore volume ($cm^3 g^{-1}$)	Average pore size (nm)	Reference
			Before heat treatment	After heat treatment				
$CaO–SiO_2–P_2O_5–MgO$								
89–80 SiO_2	700°C		Amorphous		319	0.2	–	Vallet-Regí *et al.* (1999); Pérez-Pariente *et al.* (1999)
79–70 SiO_2	700°C		Amorphous		303	0.22		Pérez-Pariente *et al.* (1999)
69–60 SiO_2	700–950°C		Amorphous, christobalite and wollastonite		151–222.66	0.349–0.41	5.51	Pérez-Pariente *et al.* (1999); Erol *et al.* (2010); Saboori *et al.* (2009); Ma *et al.* (2010)
59–50 SiO_2	800–1100°C		Amorphous, wollastonite $(CaMg)_3PO_4$, Mg_2SiO_4		145	0.22	9	Balamurugan *et al.* (2007b)
39–30 SiO_2	800–1200°C		Apatite, Ca_2SiO_4, akermanite and hydroxyapatite		16.02	0.099	24.2	Radev *et al.* (2009); Łączka *et al.* (2000)
29–20 SiO_2	1200°C		Mg-substituted β-TCP and silicocarnotite		–	–	–	Radev *et al.* (2009)

Continued

Table 7.3 Continued

System (%mol)	Stabilization temperatures	Heat treatment	Crystal phases		Surface area ($m^2 g^{-1}$)	Total pore volume ($cm^3 g^{-1}$)	Average pore size (nm)	Reference
			Before heat treatment	After heat treatment				
SiO_2–CaO–ZnO–P_2O_5								
69–60 SiO_2	700–1100°C		Amorphous, wollastonite $(CaMg)_3PO_4$, Mg_2SiO_4		145–221	0.22–0.37	3.7–9	Oki *et al.* (2004); Balamurugan *et al.* (2007b); Erol *et al.* (2010); Bini *et al.* (2009)
SiO_2–CaO–P_2O_5-Ag_2O								
79–70 SiO_2	450°C		N/A		72.2	0.502	28.2	Belantone *et al.* (2000)
69–60 SiO_2	700°C		N/A		70	0.495	27.6	Balamurugan *et al.* (2008)
59–50 SiO_2	580°C		Ag, Ag_2O, apatite, $Ca_3(PO_4)_2{\cdot}2H_2O$		16.53–76.16	0.05–0.22	–	Vulpoi *et al.* (2011)
SiO_2–CaO–SrO–P_2O_5								
69–60 SiO_2	800°C	1000°C	Amorphous, pseudowollastonite and apatite	Amorphous Ca_2SiO_4, Sr-doped apatite				Hesaraki *et al.* (2010)

6%, MgO 13%) and lower surface area. After sintering in the range 900–1100°C they reported that the sol-gel-derived glass transformed to a glass ceramic with the formation of crystalline phases [wollastonite, $(CaMg)_3(PO_4)_2$ and Mg_2SiO_4] and a dramatic decrease in its bioactivity. Amorphous calcium phosphate was formed after 21 days of soaking in SBF. This glass ceramic however supported the growth of osteoblast-like cells *in vitro* and promoted osteoblast differentiation by stimulating the expression of major phenotypic markers. Vallet-Regí *et al.* (1999) demonstrated that if the MgO content is above 7 mol%, the formation rate of the apatite layer slows down although the precipitated layer is thicker. Mg^{2+} released from the glass ceramic (together with the Ca^{2+}) is incorporated in the layer formed on the surface of the glasses after immersion in SBF, as proved by the precipitation of a magnesium-substituted whitlockite-like phase (b-$(Ca,Mg)_3(PO_4)_2$).

SiO_2–CaO–P_2O_5–ZnO

Conflicting data exist on both biocompatibility and bioactivity of sol-gel glasses in the system SiO_2–CaO–P_2O_5–ZnO. Sol-gel glasses in the system SiO_2 64–CaO 26–P_2O_5 5–ZnO 5 mol% fabricated by Oki *et al.* (2004) were found to be bioactive, as an apatite layer was precipitated after seven days in SBF. They also established that human fetal osteoblastic cells (hFOB 1.19) underwent increased alkaline phosphatase activity and expression relative to cells cultured on tissue culture polystyrene, which indicates that the zinc-containing composition stimulates bone cells production of APL. These findings are in agreement with the results of Balamurugam *et al.* (2007a) who recently reported similar bioactivity and good biocompatibility of a sol-gel glass with composition SiO_2 64–CaO 26–P_2O_5 5–ZnO 5 mol% towards murine osteoblasts. However Erol *et al.* (2010) reported that the main effect of ZnO in the sol-gel glass of the same system is a decrease in the growth rate of the HCAp layer (after only 28 days in SBF, a HCAp layer was formed). This observation is a significant restriction compared to the sol-gel glass in the system SiO_2 64–CaO 26–MgO 5–P_2O_5 5, where the HCAp layer was precipitated after only 1 day of immersion, in the same study. Sol-gel-derived bioactive glasses in the system SiO_2 60–CaO 36–P_2O_5 4 mol% (58S) with a wide composition range of ZnO (0.4, 2 and 5 wt%) were synthesized by Bini *et al.* (2009). The authors reported that the addition of even small quantities (0.4 wt%) of ZnO at the expenses of both CaO and P_2O_5 in the 58S glass leads to an increase in both formation rate and content of the HCAp after 8 days of treatment in SBF, compared to the 58S sample. However in a preliminary biocompatibility study with SAOS-2 cells they reported that higher amounts of ZnO were toxic and only 0.4 wt% ZnO resulted in good biocompatibility. Despite the fact that *in vitro* studies have shown the osteogenic effect of Zn, definite answers about the osteogenic expression effect of Zn as ionic dissolution product from Zn-doped bioactive silicate glasses are still missing.

SiO_2–CaO–P_2O_5–SrO

Sr has been used to modify the apatite formation of quaternary melt-derived glasses (Fredholm *et al.*, 2012). Sr release increased linearly with Sr substitution and apatite formation was enhanced significantly in the fully Sr-substituted glass. Sr-doped glasses have been shown to exhibit enhanced bioactivity and to release critical concentrations of Sr ions in the range 1–5 ppm into the dissolution medium (Lao *et al.*, 2008, 2009). Substitution of Sr for Ca in the silicophosphate glass composition of the system CaO 22.3–SrO 7.9–SiO_2 58.8–P_2O_5 11 mol% can increase the rate of glass dissolution, the density and glass crystallization temperature and change the type of the crystallized phase. The increased rate of dissolution is related to increased disorder in the glass network induced by substitution of Ca^{2+} ions by larger ions (e.g., Sr^{2+}). The formation of apatite phases on the surface of Sr glass is slightly retarded when it is soaked in SBF solution. According to Hesaraki *et al.* (2010) the produced sol gel glasses increased proliferation of rat calvaria osteoblastic cells and enhanced the ALP activity, after five days of culture. However more studies are necessary to provide definite conclusions about the effect of Sr release from quaternary sol-gel glasses on cell viability and bone formation *in vivo*.

7.3 Sol-gel-derived coatings

Surface coating technology on implants includes a variety of deposition methods such as plasma-spraying, sputter-deposition, sol-gel coating, electrophoretic deposition or biomimetic precipitation. Plasma spray and sol-gel are the most widely used techniques. In plasma spraying, owing to the high temperature process, changes in the layer properties can occur (Radin and Ducheyne, 1992), while considerable cracking and scraping of the coating can cause the delamination of the coating or the release of particles resulting in failure (Wheeler 1996; Chang *et al.*, 1999; Tinsley *et al.*, 2001). Moreover this technique is not suitable for coating porous surfaces; to control exactly the structure and chemistry and to develop a strength bonding is not as greatly desired as it is for some applications. Sol-gel involves a low-temperature heating process with relatively low annealing temperatures and offers the possibility of coating over large areas in a cost effective manner. It allows a better control of the chemical composition of the coating and produces high purity homogeneous films. The critical stage in a sol-gel process is the heat treatment, since it affects the quality, compactness and structure of the surface layer.

The most commonly used sol-gel coating techniques are dip coating, spin coating, spray coating and roll coating. Dip coating (Fig. 7.1(a)) is a process where the material to be coated is immersed in a liquid and then withdrawn at an adjustable predetermined speed under specific conditions (i.e. temperature and atmosphere) (Innocenzi *et al.*, 1992; Balamurugan *et al.*, 2002). The coating thickness depends mainly on the withdrawal speed, the solid content and the viscosity of the immersion liquid (Attia *et al.*, 2002). In spin coating, the coating material is dissolved or dispersed in a solvent and this coating solution is then deposited onto the substrate which is rotating at a specific speed (rpm), leaving a uniform layer (Fig. 7.1(b)) (Ilican *et al.*, 2008). This deposition/rotating procedure is repeated until a layer of the desired thickness has been deposited. Subsequent processing stages such as drying or heating are necessary to stabilize the coating. Spray coating (Suciu *et al.*, 2009) involves dispersion of the synthesized powder in a wet medium (i.e. isopropanol) at a specific concentration. This solution is then sprayed at a specific rate with appropriate spray coating guns (Fig. 7.1(c)). Roll coating is a process by which a thin liquid film is formed on a continuously

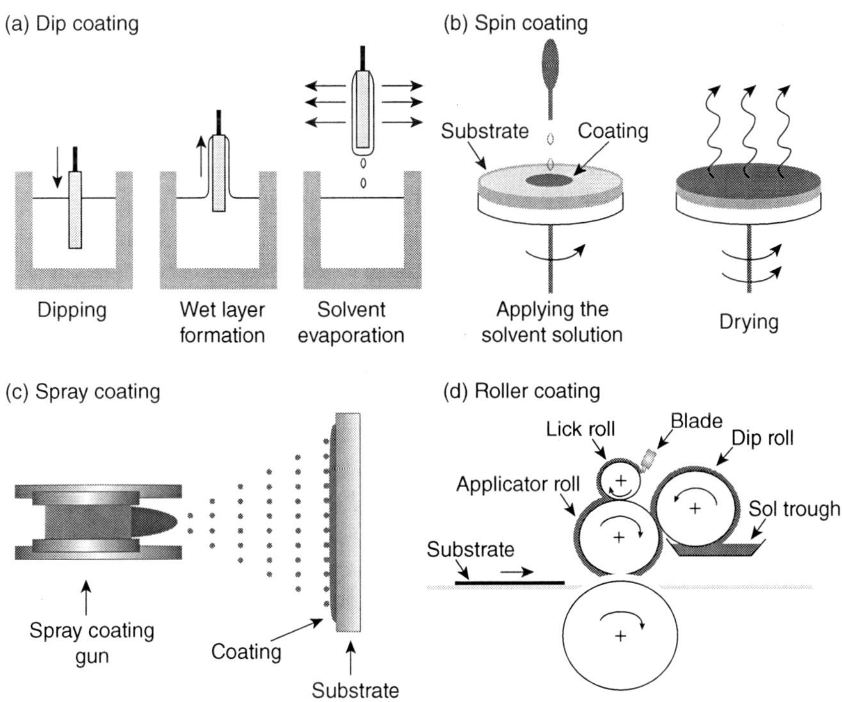

7.1 Different sol-gel coatings fabrication techniques. (a) Dipcoating, (b) spin coating, (c) spray coating and (d) roller coating.

moving web or substrate by using one or more rotating rolls (Fig. 7.1(d)) (Muromachi *et al.*, 2006). The glass substrate is transferred using a table. The coating solution can be supplied by both dip and lick rolls and transferred to the glass substrate on the moving transportation table through the applicator roll.

Sol-gel thin films have been used in dental restoration and repair and especially in titanium and stainless steel implants coatings (Gan and Pillar, 2004; Kim *et al.*, 2003, 2004; Ballarre *et al.*, 2010). These coatings are composed mainly of bioactive calcium phosphates such as hydroxyapatite that have shown promising result (Yamashita *et al.*, 1996). However, delamination of HAp coatings from Ti alloys occurs owing to their poor bond strength and insufficient chemical stability (Bauer *et al.*, 1991; Kweh *et al.*, 2002). Various silicate coatings have been proposed (Table 7.4) for the improvement of different properties such as bioactivity, bone bonding and adhesive bonding ability of certain substrates. Besides their role as barriers against corrosion, they could improve bonding with tissues by developing a bioactive interphase. In Table 7.4 the main sol-gel coatings in silicate systems are presented in relation to their composition and intended applications.

7.3.1 Silicate systems

Unary SiO_2

Yoshida *et al.* (1999 (a) and (b)) reported the formation of silica sol-gel coatings on the surface of dental casting alloys and pure titanium casting via the sol-gel dipping process. The formation of thin SiO_2 and SiO_2/F-hybrid films resulted in a high bond strength to the metal substrate, extremely small amounts of metallic ions being released and high hydrophobicity. The authors suggested that this layer could enhance the bond strength of dental adhesive resin cements to metal ceramic restorations. Bieniaś *et al.* (2009) proposed a thin sol-gel intermediate silicate coating on metal restoration sub-structures that could enhance the bond strength to the veneer ceramic. Although cracking was apparent, the bond strength was significantly higher compared to the bond between the sandblasted sub-structure and the veneer. Xie *et al.* (2009) used the sol-gel coating method to verify the effects of a sol-gel processed silica coating on the bond strength between the resin cement and glass-infiltrated aluminum oxide ceramics. They reported the effectiveness of the process and the significant improvement of the resin bond strength of glass-infiltrated alumina ceramics. They also reported that sol-gel processed silica coating can enhance the fracture strength of In-Ceram alumina ceramic bonded to dentin 24 h and after 20 days of storage in water.

Table 7.4 Sol-gel coatings in silicate systems

System/composition	Substrate	Coating technique	Heat treatment	Crystal phases	Application	Reference
Unary SiO_2						
SiO_2, SiO_2/F-hybrid	Ag-Pd-Cu-Au alloy, CPTi	Dip coating, 2 mm min^{-1}	120°C, 20 min	–	Dental metal–ceramic restorations	Yoshida *et al.* (1999a, 1999b)
SiO_2 and SiO_2–TiO_2	CPTi, Ti-6Al-4V alloy	Dip coating 200 mm min^{-1}	500°C, 0.5 h → 750°C, 0.5 h	–	Dental metal–ceramic restorations	Bieniaś *et al.* (2009)
SiO_2	Glass-infiltrated aluminum oxide ceramic	Dip coating 200 mm min^{-1}		–	Dental all-ceramic restorations	Xie *et al.* (2009)
Binary SiO_2–CaO						
$xSiO_2$–$(1 - x)$ CaO ($x = 0.8$)	Ti-6Al-4V alloy	Dip coating 1.5 mm min^{-1}	500°C, 10 min	Amorphous silica	Biomedical (implant restorations)	Izquierdo-Barba *et al.* (2003a, 2003b, 2006)
SiO_2–CaO	CPTi	Dip coating	900°C, 30 min	Wollastonite, SiO_2, $CaSi_2O_5$	Biomedical (implant restorations)	Bao *et al.* (2010)
Ternary SiO_2–CaO–P_2O_5						
$63SiO_2$–33CaO–$4P_2O_5$ (%mol)	Stainless steel AISI 409	Dip coating, 30–50 mm min^{-1}	200°C → 15–60 min 400°C → 15–60 min	–	Biomedical (implant restorations)	Federman *et al.* (2007)
$58SiO_2$–38CaO–$4P_2O_5$	Dense polycrystalline alumina	Dip coating	900°C, 48 h 1200°C, 1 h	–	Biomedical (implant restorations)	Hamadouche *et al.* (2000)
$77SiO_2$–19CaO–$4P_2O_5$ (%mol)			900°C, 48 h → 700°C, 48 h			Liu *et al.* (2004)

Continued

Table 7.4 Continued

System/ composition	Substrate	Coating technique	Heat treatment	Crystal phases	Application	Reference
Others						
Sphene	Ti-6Al-4V alloy	Spin coating 2000 rpm, 10 s	875°C, 4°C min^{-1}	Sphene ($CaTiSiO_5$), titanium substrate	Biomedical (implant restorations)	Wu *et al.* (2008)
$2SiO_2$–$3Al_2O_3$	Carbon steel (SAE 1020)	Dip coating 0.04 m min^{-1}	5°C min^{-1} to 400°C → 10°C min^{-1} to 600°C, 800°C	–	Biomedical (implant restorations)	Conde *et al.* (1992)
$2Al_2O_3$–SiO_2	a-alumina	Spin coating	700°C, 5°C min^{-1} 1000°C, 2 h	Amorphous Transitional mulite	Biomedical (implant restorations)	Leivo *et al.* (2006)
$xTiO_2$–$(100 - x)$ SiO_2, $x = 0$, 10, 20, 30, 40, 50, 60, 70, 80, 90	Titanium	Dip coating, 0.3 mm s^{-1}	500°C for 10 min	Titanium, anatase	Biomedical (implant restorations)	Ääritalo *et al.* (2007)

Binary SiO_2–CaO

Vitreous non-crystalline coatings in the $x\text{SiO}_2\text{–}(1 - x)\text{CaO}$ ($x = 0.8$) system onto metallic substrates with different textural parameters and thickness were synthesized using the sol-gel method by Izquierdo-Barba *et al.* (2003a, 2003b, 2006). Their work on vitreous coatings of SiO_2–CaO on Ti-6Al-4V alloy substrates revealed that the porosity and roughness of the coatings are determined by the precursor solutions used in the coating procedure. The textural parameters (porosity and roughness) and thickness of the coatings increased when the concentration of the precursor solutions was raised. It was found that the less concentrated the sol, the denser and smoother was the resulting coating. Very concentrated sols produced porous films and, conversely, diluted sols formed dense films, the average pore diameter was seen to decrease by an order of magnitude when the alcohol content increased. Differences in the chemical reactivity of these coatings were evidenced when using SBF or osteoblast-like cells. In SBF, the coatings presented a complete dissolution of the vitreous matrix without forming a bioactive surface. However, in osteoblast-like cell culture, the coatings were more stable and showed biocompatible behavior. Enhancement of cell attachment, proliferation and differentiation was observed as the porosity and roughness of the coatings increased. Bao *et al.* (2010) prepared wollastonite coatings on commercially pure titanium by the sol-gel method and reported the formation of many cracks in the coatings owing to the different coefficients of thermal expansion between coatings and substrate. Differential scanning calorimetry and thermogravimetric analysis results showed that after calcination at 900°C, the crystalline phase of coatings consisted of wollastonite, SiO_2 and $CaSi_2O_5$. Cracks on sol-gel coatings can be formed by shrinking of the gel caused by solvent evaporation, polymerization and crosslinking of the gel matrix, which changes its mechanical properties like brittleness and crack-resistance and formation of tensile stress due to capillary forces, which are determined by the pore-size distribution and the surface tension of the solvent.

Ternary SiO_2–CaO–P_2O_5

Federman *et al.* (2007) reported that a thin, uniform, pore/crack-free ternary biofilm in the ternary SiO_2–CaO–P_2O_5 system can be synthesized using the sol-gel method and a dip coating technique. Furthermore they reported that the formation of different textures and topographies can be tailored by temperature and time of heat treatment. Similarly, Liu and Miao (2004) developed a 58S bioactive glass coating on alumina substrates via a dip coating method. The drying and firing processes at 1200°C led to wollastonite ($CaSiO_3$) platelet development in the bioactive glass coating, with limited densification, decreased bioactivity and increased hardness.

Hamadouche *et al.* (2000) investigated the *in vitro* and *in vivo* osteoconductive properties of sol-gel bioactive glass-coated dense polycrystalline alumina implants. Two sol-gel glass compositions (58S and 77S bioactive glasses) were used as coatings on alumina substrates and implanted in a rabbit model. The percentage of bone in direct contact was greater for coated implants when compared to bulk alumina implants, while the presence of osteoid tissue, related to aluminum release from the alumina substrates, was greatly diminished when compared to melt-derived glass-coated alumina implants.

Other silicate systems

Melt-derived bioactive glasses have been used as coating materials on alumina owing to their enhanced bioactivity. However, the high temperatures applied have been demonstrated to be responsible for a crystallographic change in the alumina substrates, from the α-stable state to a γ-unstable allotropic phase. In addition, the contamination of the glasses by aluminum leaching from the alumina substrates during the coating procedure inhibited the bone interaction (Greenspan and Hench, 1976; Torricelli *et al.*, 2001). Sol-gel coating allows lower temperatures during the thermal process, thus preventing possible damage to the alumina and consequently the leaching of Al. Mechanically stable ceramic coatings of amorphous aluminosilicate have been applied to a carbon steel substrate, using the sol-gel process, by the traditional dipping method. Amorphous thick coatings (>5 μm) were obtained with an acceptable oxidation resistance in air atmosphere at 600°C (Di Gianpaolo Conde *et al.*, 1992). Based on the inhibiting effect of the Al entrapment on a non-leachable crystalline ceramic phase, such as mullite, on its leaching behaviour, sol-gel-derived aluminosilicate coatings on alumina substrates have been proposed by Leivo *et al.* (2006). They reported that nanosized 2/1-mullite sol-gel spin coatings showed *in vitro* osteoblast biocompatibility and being potential candidates for osteoconductive coatings on alumina implants.

A series of sol-gel derived mixed TiO_2–SiO_2 coatings were prepared by Ääritalo *et al.* (2007) consisting of 10–100% SiO_2. With this method homogeneous TiO_2–SiO_2 mixtures could only be obtained at low TiO_2 content, with a maximum TiO_2 concentration of less than 15 wt%. At higher concentrations, some of the Ti atoms do not react with silica and TiO_2 tends to form a separate phase. Silica release from the coatings was analogous to SiO_2 and a Ca-P layer was able to nucleate on their surface. Si release from the TiO_2–SiO_2 (30:70) and (10:90) coatings extended osteoblast proliferation and differentiation (Areva *et al.*, 2007). The potential application for orthopedic implants of sphene ($CaTiSiO_5$) coatings was proposed by Wu *et al.* (2008), who synthesized coatings on Ti–6Al–4V using sol-gel spin coating. Coatings possessed a significantly improved adhesion strength compared to those of HAp and although their chemical stability was higher with minimal release of ions, a layer of apatite formed on their surface after 21 days of soaking in SBF.

Some glass ceramics based on the CaO–MgO–SiO_2 system have also been regarded as potential candidates for biomedical applications in recent years. In this system, crystalline phases such as diopside ($CaMgSi_2O_6$), akermanite ($Ca_2MgSi_2O_7$), wollastonite ($CaSiO_3$), merwinite ($Ca_3MgSi_2O_8$) and dicalcium silicate (Ca_2SiO_4), have been developed, with attractive mechanical and biological properties and the ability to undergo osseointegration (Nonami and Tsutaumi, 1999; Siriphannon *et al.*, 2002; Liu and Ding, 2002; Wu *et al.*, 2006) indicating that they may be suitable for the repair and replacement of living bone, especially for load-bearing situations (Zhang *et al.*, 2011). CaO–MgO–SiO_2 glass-ceramic coatings are currently prepared by plasma spraying. However, owing to the rapid heating/cooling and solidification process, the coatings are usually not homogeneous and have a rough surface. Although they can be effectively synthesized via sol-gel routes, they have not been until now applied as coatings to titanium implants, to the authors' knowledge.

7.4 Sol-gel-derived composites

The development and production of composite materials have mainly occurred in order to achieve a combination of properties which are not achievable with any of the elemental materials alone. Hydroxyapatite in a carbonated form is the major inorganic constituent of natural bone and cementum (Roseberry *et al.*, 1931; Dorozhkin and Epple, 2002). Synthetic HAp has long been used in medicine and dentistry owing to its ability to attach chemically to bone. However other more soluble calcium phosphate phases are preferred as bone-substitute materials in order to combine calcium-ion release properties with chemical stability (Pasteris *et al.*, 2004; Legeros *et al.*, 2003). As an interesting means of tuning the calcium phosphate dissolution kinetics, a combination of these mineral phases with bioactive glasses has been considered applying the sol-gel method which can lead to homogeneous composites at low temperatures (Goller *et al.*, 2003; Zhong *et al.*, 2002). Furthermore, sol-gel-derived bioactive composites incorporating aluminosilicate networks have been synthesized (Kokoti *et al.*, 2001; Papadopoulou *et al.*, 2003; Kontonasaki *et al.*, 2003) that have potential use in dentistry. It has been proposed that the development of dental materials with a cementum-like behavior could provide the biological surface required for selective attachment and spread of specific cell types able to promote tissue regeneration.

7.4.1 Incorporation of calcium phosphate phases

Apatite

A combination of apatite and gel-derived silicate glasses has been applied successfully for fabrication of new composite bioactive materials. Andersson *et al.* (2005) developed a degradable, hierarchically porous silica/apatite composite material applying a simple low-temperature synthesis. The presence of silica was shown to improve the bioactivity of many biocompatible and bioactive materials (Porter *et al.*, 2004) since silanol groups provide suitable nucleation sites (Kokubo *et al.*, 2003). Particularly, crystalline HAp is fabricated at close to room temperature conditions and subsequently it is coated with a mesoporous silica matrix using the same template as was present during apatite mineralization. The resulting composite material exhibits a coralline-like, macroporous crystalline structure with a siliceous mesoporous coating layer suitable as a drug carrier agent that could serve in localized biodegradable therapy and furthermore obviating the need for removal of the implant after the treatment. The silica coating layer induces more rapid *in vitro* and *in vivo* mineralization, with the precipitated apatite layer on the surface of the composite able to block the pore openings and slow down the release of the drug. Otsuka *et al.* (1997) observed changes and a reduction of the release rate of an antibiotic from bioactive glass, while the slowed-down release was found to be caused by geometrical changes due to nucleated HAp on the surface.

Different composite materials incorporating commercial HAp and sol-gel-derived bioactive glasses in the system SiO_2–CaO–P_2O_5 and in different amounts were fabricated by sintering processes (Cholewa-Kowalska *et al.*, 2009), presenting a microporous structure with a density approximately 60% of the theoretical density of the HAp alone and exhibiting better bioactivity and biocompatibility. The incorporation of bioactive glass in the composites seems not to affect the microstructure but leads to faster decomposition of HAp at 1300°C into TCP (tricalcium phosphate). Additionally, a cristobalite phase is formed in composites with a higher content of SiO_2 (80 mol%) or wollastonite and a lower content of SiO_2 (40 mol%). The increased density and the presence of the cristobalite phase are beneficial to the stiffness of the composite structure which is not the same as for the increase in the wollastonite phase. Finally the composite materials promote osteogenic differentiation as the cellular activity of alkaline phosphatase was observed to be higher for the composites compared to the respective pure starting materials.

β-Tricalcium phosphate (β-TCP)

β-Tricalcium phosphate (β-TCP) is another bone substitute osteoinductive material (Kondo *et al.*, 2006) with a higher resorption rate than HAp. It is considered to be a biodegradable material that allows bone growth and replacement. Similarly to the HAp phase, β-TCP presents weak mechanical strength and poor ability to induce calcium phosphate precipitation both *in vitro* and *in vivo*. The use of sol-gel-derived bioactive glasses in composite materials with β-TCP has shown the fabrication of new stronger materials with better biological properties than the pure starting materials. Particularly, the composite material of β-TCP with sol-gel-derived bioactive glass SiO_2–CaO–P_2O_2–MgO has exhibited bioactivity with significantly improved mechanical strength and biological responses to osteoblastic cells compared to pure β-TCP for sintering at 1200°C. The mechanical strength is significantly dependent on the amount of bioactive glass in the composite, while the brittleness does not present any change (Hesaraki *et al.*, 2009).

7.4.2 Incorporating a dental aluminosilicate network

Sol-gel-derived aluminosilicate porcelains have been fabricated. The application of the sol-gel method is expected to lead to good control of composition, microstructure and properties, owing to the provision of intrinsic high homogeneity. Particularly, the sol-gel-derived monophasic mixed potassium–sodium kalsilite ($K_{0.5}Na_{0.5}AlSiO_4$) presents reasonable resistance to different eroding solutions, while the new sol-gel glass ceramic (GC) in the system SiO_2 60%–P_2O_5 3%–Al_2O_3 14%–CaO 6%–Na_2O 7%–K_2O 10% (wt.%) presents microstructural and thermal properties similar to a commercial leucite-based fluorapatite melt-derived dental glass ceramic (Bogdanoviciene *et al.*, 2008). Furthermore, several efforts have been made to synthesize bioactive sol-gel-derived composites incorporating dental aluminosilicate systems for potential use in dentistry. With this aim, Chatzistavrou *et al.* (2010) fabricated a novel bioactive composite material incorporating the new GC glass ceramic into 58S bioactive glass (GC 30 wt%–58S 70 wt%). The new fabricated composite (COMP) was confirmed to exhibit bioactive behavior and microstructural properties similar to those of a commercial dental ceramic. The bioactive behavior of the composite material was confirmed based on the rapid formation of the HCAp layer upon three days' immersion in SBF (Fig. 7.2 (b)–(d)). The feasibility of the new composite for application as coating on base porcelain was confirmed. The observed cross-sections and fracture surfaces of the specimens revealed (qualitatively) good attachment of the coating and strong bonding at the interface (Fig. 7.2 (a)). This new bioactive material

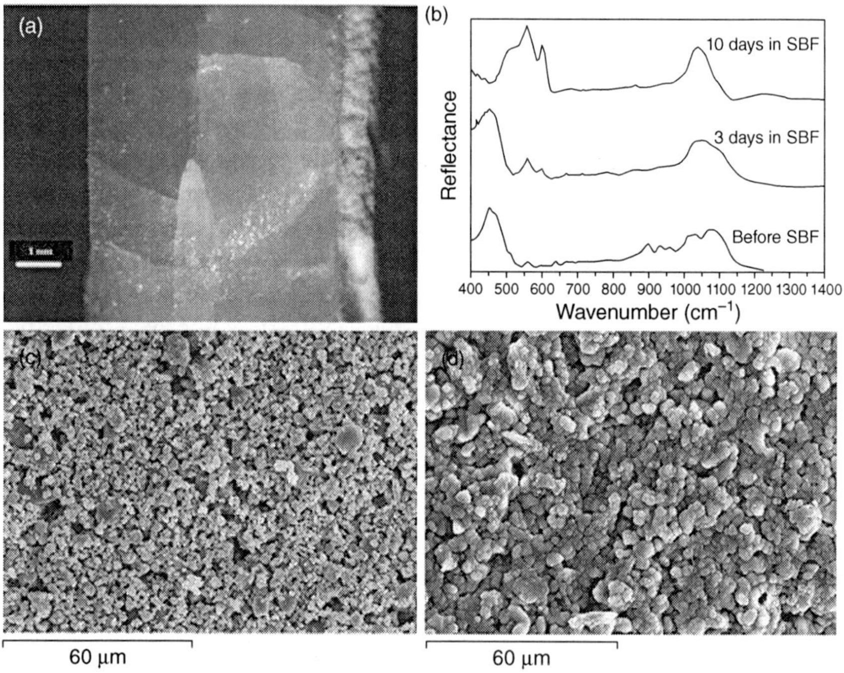

7.2 (a) Fracture surface at the coating/substrate interface, (b) Reflectance infrared spectra from the surface of coated porcelain bases before and after immersion in SBF for 3 and 10 days. SEM images of the surfaces of the coatings before (c) and after (d) the immersion in SBF for 3 days (Chatzistavrou *et al.*, 2010; reproduced with permission of Elsevier).

has potential applications in dental restorations, exhibiting better control of the characteristic properties.

An intermediate silicate composition has been fabricated which is situated between the existing commercial dental ceramics and the bioactive sol-gel glass ceramic composite (COMP) presented above. This new composite material (labeled COMP1) is expected to combine the bioactive behavior of the sol-gel bioactive glass better with the thermal and mechanical properties of a commercial dental ceramic, owing to the incorporation of a commercial ceramic in powder form at the synthesis stage of the sol-gel bioactive glass (Chatzistavrou *et al.*, 2011).

Furthermore, sol-gel-derived bioactive glass/dental ceramic composites with various concentrations of the leucite-based dental ceramic have been synthesized (Goudouri *et al.*, 2009, 2011a, 2011b) resulting in composite systems with enhanced bioactivity but low mechanical integrity. Recently Goudouri *et al.* (2011c, 2011d), evaluated the textural characteristics and the flexural strength of a new glass-ceramic composite synthesized via the incorporation of high percentage (80 wt%) of a commercial dental ceramic in a sol–gel-derived bioactive glass. Although the number of blind pores caused by processing of the glass ceramic was greater than that of the commercial one, the flexural strength was of the same order. The presence of the bioactive glass induced the crystallization of Ca-P phases, while after sintering the leucite content did not exceed the optimum (30 wt%) according to international standards. Furthermore, the *in vitro* bioactivity evaluation of the sintered specimens indicated the onset of apatite formation after 9 days, while a dense apatite layer developed on the surface of the specimens after 21 days of immersion in SBF.

7.5 Conclusions and future trends

Sol-gel-derived bioactive glasses and glass ceramics represent an extensive new field of bioactive materials with numerous applications in medicine and dentistry. The sol-gel technique is a versatile method used successfully in different applications including the fabrication of coatings and the preparation of new composite bioactive systems. In the field of dental restoration and regeneration, the sol-gel method is used extensively, while new compositions of sol-gel-derived bioactive glasses and glass-ceramic composites have started to emerge. The need to mimic and regenerate the complex biological structure of bone and teeth is contributing to the development of new composites with more desirable properties and controlled microstructural characteristics. The development of new systems of bactericidal behavior, able to form 3D porous structures and to incorporate growth factors, therapeutic drugs and seeded stem cells represents a challenge for future studies in which sol-gel-derived silicate systems discussed in this chapter will be required.

7.6 References

Ääritalo V, Areva S, Jokinen M, Lindén M and Peltola T (2007), 'Sol-gel-derived TiO_2–SiO_2 implant coatings for direct tissue attachment. Part I, design, preparation and characterization', *J Mater Sci Mater Med*, **18**, 1863–73.

Abiraman S, Kumari HK, Umashankar PR and John A (2002), 'Preliminary *in vitro* and *in vivo* characterizations of a sol-gel derived bioactive glass-ceramic system', *Bull Mater Sci*, **25**, 419–29.

Andersson J, Areva S, Spliethoff B and Linden M (2005), 'Sol-gel synthesis of a multifunctional, hierarchically porous silica/apatite composite', *Biomaterials*, **26**, 6827–35.

Aoba T, Moreno EC and Shimoda S (1992), 'Competitive adsorption of magnesium and calcium ions onto synthetic and biological apatites', *Calcif Tissue Int*, **51**, 143–50.

Arcos D, Greenspan DC and Vallet-Regí M (2002), 'Imfluence of the stabilization temperature on textural and structural features and ion release in SiO_2–CaO–P_2O_5 sol-gel glasses', *Chem Mater*, **14**, 1515–22.

Arcos D, Greenspan DC and Vallet-Regí M (2003), 'A new quantitative method to evaluate the *in vitro* bioactivity of melt and sol-gel-derived silicate glasses', *J Biomed Mater Res A*, **65**, 344–51.

Areva S, Ääritalo V, Tuusa S, Jokinen M, Lindén M and Peltola T (2007), 'Sol-gel-derived TiO_2–SiO_2 implant coatings for direct tissue attachment. Part II, Evaluation of cell response', *J Mater Sci Mater Med*, **18**, 1633–42.

Attia SM, Wang J, Ma J, Shen J and Ma J (2002), 'Review on sol-gel derived coatings, process, techniques and optical applications', *J Mater Sci Technol*, **18**, 211–18.

Balamurugan A, Balossier G, Kannan S, Michel J, Rebelo AH and Ferreira JM (2007a), 'Development and *in vitro* characterization of sol-gel derived CaO–P_2O_5–SiO_2–ZnO bioglass', *Acta Biomater*, **3**, 255–62.

Balamurugan A, Balossier G, Laurent-Maquin D, Pina S, Rebelo AHS, Faure J and Ferreira JMF (2008), 'An *in vitro* biological and anti-bacterial study on a sol-gel derived silver-incorporated bioglass system', *Dent Mater*, **24**, 1343–51.

Balamurugan A, Balossier G, Michel J, Kannan S, Benhayone H, Rebelo A and Fereira J (2007b), 'Sol-gel derived SiO_2–CaO–MgO–P_2O_5 bioglass system-preparation and *in vitro* characterization', *J Biomed Mater Res B Appl Biomater*, **83**, 546–53.

Balamurugan A, Kannan S and Rajeswari S (2002), 'Bioactive sol-gel hydroxy-apatite surface for biomedical application—*in vitro* study', *Trends Biomater Artif Organs*, **16**(1), 18–20.

Balas F, Arcos D, Perez-Pariente J and Vallet-Regí M (2001), 'Textural properties of SiO_2–CaO–P_2O_5 glasses obtained by the sol-gel method', *J Mater Res*, **16**, 1345–8.

Ballarre J, Manjubala I, Schreiner WH, Orellano JC, Fratzl P and Ceré S (2010), 'Improving the osteointegration and bone-implant interface by incorporation of bioactive particles in sol-gel coatings of stainless steel implants', *Acta Biomater*, **6**, 1601–9.

Bao Q, Zhao K and Liu J (2010), 'Characterization of wollastonite coatings prepared by sol-gel on Ti substrate', *J Coat Technol Res*, DOI 10.1007/s11998-009-9236-7.

Bauer TW, Geesink RC, Zimmerman R and McMahon JT (1991), 'Hydroxyapatite-coated femoral stems. Histological analysis of components retrieved at autopsy', *J Bone Joint Surg Am*, **73**, 1439–52.

Belantone M, Coleman NJ and Hench LL (2000), 'Bacteriostatic action of a novel four-component bioactive glass', *J Biomed Mater Res*, **51**, 484–90.

Bieniaś J, Surowska B, Stoch A, Matraszek H and Walczak M (2009), 'The influence of SiO_2 and SiO_2-TiO_2 intermediate coatings on bond strength of titanium and Ti6Al4V alloy to dental porcelain', *Dent Mater*, **25**, 1128–35.

Bigi A, Falini G, Foresti E, Gazzano M, Ripamonti A and Roveri N (1993), 'Magnesium influence on hydroxyapatite crystallization', *J Inorg Biochem*, **49**, 69–78.

Bini M, Grandi S, Capsoni D, Mustarelli P, Saino E and Visai L (2009), 'SiO_2–P_2O_5–CaO glasses and glass-ceramics with and without ZnO, relationships among composition, microstructure, and bioactivity', *J Phys Chem C*, **113**, 8821–8.

Bogdanoviciene I, Jankeviciute A, Pinkas J, Beganskiene A and Kareiva A (2008), 'Study of alumosilicate porcelains, Sol-gel preparation, characterization and erosion evaluated by gravimetric method', *Mater Res Bull*, **43**, 2998–3007.

Bonnelye E, Chabadel A, Saltel F and Jurdic P (2008), 'Dual effect of strontium ranelate, stimulation of osteoblast differentiation and inhibition of osteoclast formation and resorption *in vitro*', *Bone*, **42**, 129–38.

Brinker CJ and Scherer GW (1990), *The Physics and Chemistry of Sol-Gel Processing*, Academic Press, New York.

Catauro M and Laudisio G (1998), 'Sol-gel processing and crystallization of calcium silicate glasses', *J Mater Sci Lett*, **17**, 311–12.

Catauro M, Laudisio G, Costantini A, Fresa R and Branda F (1997), 'Low temperature synthesis, structure and bioactivity of $2CaO–3SiO_2$ glass', *J Sol-Gel Sci Technol*, **10**, 231–7.

Chang YL, Lew D, Park JB and Keller JC (1999) 'Biomechanical and morphometric analysis of hydroxyapatite-coated implants with varying crystallinity', *J Oral Maxillofac Surg*, **57**, 1096–108.

Chatzistavrou X, Esteve D, Hatzistavrou E, Kontonasaki E, Paraskevopoulos KM and Boccaccini AR (2010), 'Sol-gel based fabrication of novel glass-ceramics and composites for dental applications', *Mater Sci Eng, C*, **30**, 730–9.

Chatzistavrou X, Esteve D, Hatzistavrou E, Kontonasaki E, Paraskevopoulos KM and Boccaccini AR (2011), 'Sol-gel fabrication of glass-ceramic composite materials for dental application', *Bioceram Dev Appl*, **1**, Article ID D110156, doi,10.4303/bda/D110156.

Chen X, Meng Y, Li Y and Zhao N (2008), 'Investigation on bio-mineralization of melt and sol-gel derived bioactive', *Appl Surface Sci*, **255**, 562–4.

Chen X, Liao X, Huang Z, You P, Chen C, Kang Y and Yin G (2010), 'Synthesis and characterization of novel multiphase bioactive glass-ceramics in the CaO–MgO–SiO_2 system', *J Biomed Mater Res, Part B*, **93B**, 194–202.

Cho S, Miyaji F, Kokubo T, Nakanishi K, Soga N and Nakamura T (1998), 'Apatite formation on silica gel in simulated body fluid, effects of structural modification with solvent-exchange', *J Mater Sci, Mater Med*, **9**, 279–84.

Cholewa-Kowalska K, Kokoszka J, Laczka M, Niedzwiedzki L, Madej W and Osyczka AM (2009), 'Gel-derived bioglass as a compound of hydroxyapatite composites', *Biomed Mater*, **4**, 055007 (11pp).

Christodoulou I, Buttery LDK, Tai G, Hench LL and Polak JM (2006), 'Characterization of human fetal osteoblasts by microarray analysis following stimulation with 58S bioactive gel–glass ionic dissolution products', *J Biomed Mater Res, Part B*, **77B**, 431–46.

Chrysafi R, Perraki Th and Kakali G (2007), 'Sol-gel preparation of $2CaO \cdot SiO_2$', *J Eur Ceram Soc*, **27**, 1707–10.

Chu P and Liu X (2008), *Biomaterials Fabrication and Processing Handbook*, CRC Press/Taylor & Francis, Boca Raton.

Courthéoux L, Lao J, Nedelec J-M and Jallot E (2008), 'Controlled bioactivity in Zn-doped sol-gel derived SiO_2–CaO bioactive glasses', *J Phys Chem C*, **112**, 13663–7.

Creedon A, Flynn A and Cashman K (1999), 'The effect of moderately and severely restricted dietary magnesium intakes on bone composition and bone metabolism in the rat', *Br J Nutr*, **82**, 63–71.

Czarnobaj K and Sawicki W (2011), 'The sol-gel prepared SiO_2–CaO–P_2O_5 composites doped with Metronidazole for application in local delivery systems', *Pharm Deve Technol*, doi,10.3109/10837450.2011.572894.

De Aza PN, Guitian Fand De Aza S (1994), 'Bioactivity of wollastonite ceramics, *in vitro* evaluation', *Scripta Metall Mater*, **31**, 1001–5.

Di Giampaolo Conde AR, Puerta M, Ruiz H and Olivares J-L (1992), 'Thick aluminosilicate coatings on carbon steel via sol-gel', *J Non-Crystal Sol*, **147–8**, 467–73.

Dorozhkin SV and Epple M (2002), 'Biological and medical significance of calcium phosphates', *Angew Chem, Int Ed*, **41**, 3130–46.

Ebisawa Y, Kokubo T, Ohura K and Yamamuro T (1990), 'Bioactivity of CaO–SiO_2 based glasses *in vitro* evaluation', *J Mater Sci, Mater Med*, **1**, 239–44.

Erol M, Özyuguran A and Çelebican Ö (2010), 'Synthesis, characterization, and *in vitro* bioactivity of sol-gel-derived Zn, Mg, and Zn-Mg Co-doped bioactive glasses', *Chem Eng Technol*, **33**, 1066–74.

Federman SR, Costa VC, Vasconcelos DCL and Vasconcelos WL (2007), 'Sol-Gel SiO_2–CaO–P_2O_5 biofilm with surface engineered for medical application', *Mater Res*, **10**, 177–81.

Fredholm YC, Karpukhina N, Brauer DS, Jones JR, Law RV and Hill RG (2012), 'Influence of strontium for calcium substitution in bioactive glasses on degradation, ion release and apatite formation', *J R Soc Interface*, **9**(70), 880–9.

Gan L and Pilliar R (2004), 'Calcium phosphate sol-gel-derived thin films on porous-surfaced implants for enhanced osteoconductivity. Part I, Synthesis and characterization', *Biomaterials*, **25**, 5303–12.

Gerhardt L-C and Boccaccini A (2010), 'Bioactive glass and glass-ceramic scaffolds for bone tissue engineering', *Materials*, **3**, 3867–910.

Gil-Albarova J, Garrido-Lahiguera R, Salinas AJ, Román J, Bueno-Lozano AL, Gil-Albarova R and Vallet-Regí M (2004), 'The *in vivo* performance of a sol-gel glass and a glass-ceramic in the treatment of limited bone defects', *Biomaterials*, **25**, 4639–45.

Gil-Albarova J, Salinas AJ, Bueno-Lozano AL, Román J, Aldini-Nicolo N, García-Barea A, Giavaresi G, Fini M, Giardino R and Vallet-Regí M (2005), 'The *in vivo* behaviour of a sol-gel glass and a glass-ceramic during critical diaphyseal bone defects healing', *Biomaterials*, **26**,4374–82.

Goller G, Demirkiran H, Oktar F N and Demirkesen E (2003), 'Processing and characterization of bioglass reinforced hydroxyapatite composites', *Ceram Int*, **29**, 721–4.

Gorustovich A, Steimetz T, Cabrini RL and Porto-López JM (2007), 'Osteoconductivity of strontium-doped bioactive glass particles', *Bone*, **41**, S3–4.

Goudouri OM, Kontonasaki E, Kantiranis N, Chatzistavrou X, Papadopoulou L, Koidis P and Paraskevopoulos KM (2009), 'A bioactive glass/dental porcelain system by the sol gel route, fabrication and characterization', *Key Eng Mater*, **396–8**, 95–8.

Goudouri OM, Kontonasaki E, Theocharidou A, Kantiranis N, Chatzistavrou X, Koidis P and Paraskevopoulos KM (2011a). 'Dental ceramics/bioactive glass composites, characterization and mechanical properties investigation', *Bioceram Develop Appl*, **1**, Article ID D110257, doi,10.4303/bda/D110257.

Goudouri OM, Kontonasaki E, Theocharidou A, Papadopoulou L, Kantiranis N, Chatzistavrou X, Koidis P and Paraskevopoulos KM (2011b), 'Modifying a dental ceramic by bioactive glass via the sol-gel route, characterization and bioactivity investigation', *Mater Chem Phys*, **125**, 309–13.

Goudouri OM, Kontonasaki E, Papadopoulou L, Kantiranis N, Manda M, Lazaridis N, Chrissafis K, Chatzistavrou X, Koidis P and Paraskevopoulos KM (2011c), 'Towards the synthesis of an experimental bioactive dental ceramic. Part I. Crystal structure and bioactive behavior evaluation', submitted for publication.

Goudouri OM, Kontonasaki E, Papadopoulou L, Manda M, Triantafyllidis KS, Stefanidou M, Koidis P and Paraskevopoulos KM (2011d), 'An experimental bioactive dental ceramic for metal-ceramic restorations. Part II, Textural characterization and mechanical properties Investigation', submitted for publication.

Gough JE, Jones JR and Hench LL (2004), 'Nodule formation and mineralization of human primary osteoblasts cultured on a porous bioactive glass scaffold', *Biomaterials*, **25**, 2039–46.

Greenspan D and Hench LL (1976), 'Chemical and mechanical behavior of bioglass-coated alumina', *J Biomed Mater Res*, **10**, 503–9.

Haase H and Rink L (2009), 'The immune system and the impact of zinc during aging', *Immun Ageing*, **6**, 9.

Hamadouche M, Meunier A, Greenspan DC, Blanchat C, Zhong JP, La Torre GP and Sedel L (2000), 'Bioactivity of sol-gel bioactive glass coated alumina implants', *J Biomed Mater Res*, **52**, 422–9.

Hamadouche M, Meunier A, Greenspan DC, Blanchat C, Zhong JP, La Torre JP and Sedel L (2001), 'Long-term *in vivo* bioactivity and degradability of bulk sol-gel bioactive glasses', *J Biomed Mater Res*, **54**, 560–6.

Hattar S, Loty S, Gaisser D, Berdal A and Sautier J-M (2006), 'Effects of 58S sol-gel glasses on the temporal expression markers during mouse osteoblastic differentiation', *J Biomed Mater Res, Part A*, **76**, 811–19.

Hayashi T and Saito H (1980), 'Preparation of CaO-SiO glasses by the gel method', *J Mater Sci*, **15**, 1971–7.

Hench LL (1991), Bioceramics, 'From concept to clinic', *J Am Ceram Soc*, **74**, 1487–510.

Hench LL (1998), Biomaterials, 'A forecast for the future', *Biomaterials*, **19**, 1419–23.

Hench LL and West JK (1990), 'The sol-gel process', *Chem Rev*, **90**, 33–72.

Hesaraki S, Safari M and Shokrgozar MA (2009), 'Development of β-tricalcium phosphate/sol-gel derived bioactive glass composites, physical, mechanical, and *in vitro* biological evaluations', *J Biomed Mater Res, Part B*, **91B**, 459–69.

Hesaraki S, Alizadeh M, Nazarian H and Sharifi D (2010), 'Physico-chemical and *in vitro* biological evaluation of strontium/calcium silicophosphate glass', *J Mater Sci Mater Med*, **21**, 695–705.

Hoppe A, Güldal NS and Boccaccini AR (2011), 'A review of the biological response to ionic dissolution products from bioactive glasses and glass-ceramics', *Biomaterials*, **32**, 2757–74.

Hu S, Ning C, Zhou Y, Chen L, Lin K and Chang J (2011), 'Antibacterial activity of silicate bioceramics', *J Wuhan Univ Technol-Mater Sci Ed*, **26**, 226–30.

Huang Y, Jin X, Zhang X, Sun H, Tu J, Tang T, Chang J and Dai K (2009), '*In vitro* and *in vivo* evaluation of akermanite bioceramics for bone regeneration', *Biomaterials*, **30**, 5041–8.

Iimori Y, Kameshima Y, Yasumori A and Okada K (2004), 'Effect of solid/solution ratio on apatite formation from $CaSiO_3$ ceramics in simulated body fluid', *J Mater Sci Mater Med*, **15**, 1247–53.

Ilican S, Caglar Y and Caglar M (2008), 'Preparation and characterization of ZnO thin films deposited by sol-gel spin coating method', *J Optoelectron Adv Mater*, **10**, 2578–83.

Innocenzi PC, Guglielmi M, Gobbin M and Colombo P (1992), 'Coating of metals by the sol-gel dip-coating method', *J Eur Ceram Soc*, **10**, 431–6.

Isaac J, Nohra J, Lao J, Jallot E, Nedelec JM, Berdal A and Sautier JM (2011), 'Effects of strontium-doped bioactive glass on the differentiation of cultured osteogenic cells', *Eur Cell Mater*, **8–21**, 130–43.

Izquierdo-Barba I, Asenjo A, Esquivias L and Vallet-Regí M (2003a), 'SiO_2–CaO films deposited onto Ti6Al4V substrates', *Eur J Inorg Chem*, **2003**, 1608–13.

Izquierdo-Barba I, Rojo JM, Blanco E, Vallet-Regí M and Esquivias L (2003b), 'The role of precursor concentration on the characteristics of SiO_2–CaO films', *J Sol-Gel Sci Technol*, **26**, 1179–82.

Izquierdo-Barba I, Conde F, Olmo N, Lizarbe MA, García MA and Vallet-Regí M (2006), 'Vitreous SiO_2–CaO coatings on Ti6Al4V alloys, reactivity in simulated body fluid versus osteoblast cell culture', *Acta Biomater*, **2**, 445–55.

Jaroch DB and Clupper DC (2007), 'Modulation of zinc release from bioactive sol-gel derived SiO_2-CaO-ZnO glasses and ceramics', *J Biomed Mater Res, Part A*, **82A**, 575–88.

Jugdaohsingh R (2007), 'Silicon and bone health', *J Nutr Health Aging*, **11**, 99–110.

Kim HW, Kim HE and Knowles J (2003), 'Sol gel apatite films on titanium', *Key Eng Mater*, **254–6**, 423–6.

Kim HW, Knowles JC, Salih V and Kim HE (2004), 'Hydroxyapatite and fluor-hydroxyapatite layered film on titanium processed by a sol-gel route for hard-tissue implants', *J Biomed Mater Res, Part B*, **71**, 66–76.

Kokoti M, Sivropoulou A, Koidis P and Garefis P (2001), 'Comparison of cell proliferation on modified dental ceramics', *J Oral Rehabil*, **28**, 880–7.

Kokubo T, Kim H-M and Kawashita M (2003), 'Novel bioactive materials with different mechanical properties', *Biomaterials*, **24**, 2161–75.

Kondo N, Ogose A, Tokunaga K, Umezu H, Arai K, Kudo N, Hoshino M, Inoue H, Irie H, Kuroda K, Mera H and Endo N (2006), 'Osteoinduction with highly purified b-tricalcium phosphate in dog dorsal muscles and the proliferation of osteoclasts before heterotopic bone formation', *Biomaterials*, **27**, 4419–27.

Kontonasaki E, Papadopoulou L, Zorba T, Pavlidou E, Paraskevopoulos K and Koidis P (2003), 'Apatite formation on dental ceramics modified by a bioactive glass', *J Oral Rehabil*, **30**, 893–902.

Kweh SW, Khor KA and Cheang P (2002), 'An *in vitro* investigation of plasma sprayed hydroxyapatite (HA) coatings produced with flame-spheroidized feed-stock', *Biomaterials*, **23**, 775–85.

Laczka M, Cholewa K and Laczka-Osyczka A (1997), 'Gel-derived powders of CaO–P_2O_5–SiO_2 system as a starting material to production of bioactive ceramics', *J Alloy Compd*, **248**, 42–51.

Laczka M, Cholewa-Kowalska K, Laczka-Osyczka A, Tworzydlo M and Turyna B (2000), 'Gel-derived materials of a CaO–P_2O_5–SiO_2 system modified by boron, sodium, magnesium, aluminum, and fluorine compounds', *J Biomed Mater Res*, **52**, 601–12.

Lao J, Jallot E and Nedelec JM (2008), 'Strontium-delivering glasses with enhanced bioactivity, a new biomaterial for antiosteoporotic applications?', *Chem Mater*, **20**, 4969–73.

Lao J, Nedelec JM and Jallot E (2009), 'New strontium-based bioactive glasses, physicochemical reactivity and delivering capability of biologically active dissolution products', *J Mater Chem*, **19**, 2940–9.

Legeros RZ, Lin S, Rohanizadeh R, Mijares D and Legeros JPJ (2003), 'Biphasic calcium phosphate bioceramics, preparation, properties and applications', *Mater Sci Mater Med*, **14**, 201–9.

Leivo J, Meretoja V, Vippola M, Levänen E, Vallittu P and Mäntylä TA (2006), 'Sol-gel derived aluminosilicate coatings on alumina as substrate for osteoblasts', *Acta Biomater*, **2**, 659–68.

Li R, Clark AE and Hench LL (1991), 'An investigation of bioactive glass powders by sol-gel processing', *J Appl Biomater*, **2**, 231–9.

Li P, Zhang F and Kokubo T (1992), 'The effect of residual glassy phase in a bioactive glass-ceramic on the formation of its surface apatite layer *in vitro*', *J Mater Sci Med*, **3**, 452–6.

Li R, Clark AE, Hench LL (1992), 'Effect of structure and surface area on bioactive powders made by sol-gel process', In *Chemical Processing of Advanced Materials*, Hench LL and West JK (eds), Wiley, New York, 627–33.

Linati L, Lusvardi G, Malavasi G, Menabue L, Menziani MC, Mustarelli P and Segre U (2005), 'Qualitative and quantitative structure–property relationships analysis of multicomponent potential bioglasses', *J Phys Chem B*, **109**, 4989–98.

Liu X and Ding C (2002), 'Characterization of plasma sprayed wollastonite powder and coatings', *Surf Coat Technol*, **153**, 173–7.

Liu J and Miao X (2004), 'Sol-gel derived bioglass as a coating material for porous alumina scaffolds', *Ceram Int*, **30**, 1781–5.

Liu XY, Ding CX and Chu PK (2004), 'Mechanism of apatite formation on wollastonite coatings in simulated body fluids', *Biomaterials*, **25**, 1755–61.

Ma J, Chen CZ, Wang DG, Meng XG and Shi JZ (2010), '*In vitro* degradability and bioactivity of mesoporous $CaO–MgO–P_2O_5–SiO_2$ glasses synthesized by sol-gel method', *J Sol-Gel Sci Technol*, **54**, 69–76.

Maggini S, Wenzlaff S and Hornig D (2010), 'Essential role of vitamin C and zinc in child immunity and health', *J Int Med Res*, **38**, 386–414.

Maguire ME and Cowan JA (2002), 'Magnesium chemistry and biochemistry', *Biometals*, **15**, 203–10.

Marie PJ, Hott M, Modrowski D, Graulet AM and Gueris J (1993), 'An uncoupling agent containing strontium prevents bone loss by depressing bone resorption and maintaining bone formation in estrogen-deficient rats', *J Bone Miner Res*, **8**, 607–15.

Martínez A, Izquierdo-Barba I and Vallet-Regí M (2000), 'Bioactivity of a $CaO–SiO_2$ binary glasses,' *Syst Chem Mater*, **12**, 3080–8.

Meiszterics A, Rosta L, Peterlik H, Rohonczy J, Kubuki S, Henits P and Sinkó K (2010), 'Structural characterization of gel-derived calcium silicate systems', *J Phys Chem A*, **114**, 10403–11.

Meseguer-Olmo L, Ros-Nicolas MJ, Vicente-Ortega V, Alcaraz-Banos M, Clavel-Sainz M, Arcos D, Ragel CV, Vallet-Regi M and Meseguer-Oritz CI (2006), 'A bioactive sol-gel glass implant for *in vivo* gentamicin release'; experimental model in rabbit, *J Orthop Res*, **24**, 454–60.

Meunier PJ, Roux C, Seeman E, Ortolani S, Badurski JE, Spector TD, Cannata J, Balogh A, Lemmel EM, Pors- Nielsen S, Rizzoli R, Genant HK and Reginster JY (2004), 'The effects of strontium ranelate on the risk of vertebral fracture in women with postmenopausal osteoporosis', *N Engl J Med*, **350**, 459–68.

Muromachi T, Tsujino T, Kamitani K and Maeda K (2006), 'Application of functional coatings by sol-gel method', *J Sol-Gel Sci Technol*, **40**, 267–72.

Nakajima S, Harada Y, Kurihara Y, Wakatsuki T and Noma H (1989), 'Physicochemical characteristics of new reinforcement ceramic implant', [Article in Japanese], *Shikwa Gakuho*, **89**, 1709–17.

Nonami T and Tsutsumani S (1999), 'Study of diopside ceramics for biomaterials', *J Mater Sci Mater Med*, **10**, 475–9.

O'Donnell MD and Hill RG (2010), 'Influence of strontium and the importance of glass chemistry and structure when designing bioactive glasses for bone regeneration', *Acta Biomater*, **6**, 2382–5.

Ohura K, Nakamura T, Yamamuro T, Kokubo T, Ebisawa Y, Kotoura Y and Oka M (1991), 'Bone-bonding ability of P_2O_5-free $CaO{\cdot}SiO_2$ glasses', *J Biomed Mater Res*, **25**, 357–65.

Oki A, Parveen B, Hossain S, Adeniji S and Donahue H (2004). 'Preparation and *in vitro* bioactivity of zinc containing sol-gel-derived bioglass materials', *J Biomed Mater Res, Part A*, **69**, 216–21.

Otsuka M, Sawada M, Matsuda Y, Nakamura T and Kokubo T (1997), 'Antibiotic delivery system using bioactive bone cement consisting of Bis-GMA/TEGDMA resin and bioactive glass ceramics', *Biomaterials*, **18**, 1559–64.

Ou J, Kang Y, Huang Z, Chen X, Wu J, Xiao R and Yin G (2008), 'Preparation and *in vitro* bioactivity of novel merwinite ceramic', *Biomed Mater*, **3**, 015015.

Papadopoulou L, Kontonasaki E, Zorba T, Chatzistavrou X, Pavlidou E, Paraskevopoulos K, Sklavounos S and Koidis P (2003), 'Dental ceramics coated with bioactive glass, surface changes after exposure in a simulated body fluid under static and dynamic conditions', *Phys Status Solidi A*, **198**, 65–75.

Pasteris JD, Wopenka B, Freeman JJ, Rogers K, Valsami-Jones E, van der Houwen AM and Silva MJ (2004), 'Lack of OH in nanocrystalline apatite as a function of degree of atomic order, implications for bone and biomaterials', *Biomaterials*, **25**, 229–38.

Peitl O, LaTorre GP and Hench LL (1996), 'Effect of crystallization on apatite-layer formation of bioactive glass 45S5', *J Biomed Mater Res*, **30**, 509–14.

Pereira M and Hench LL (1996), 'Mechanisms of hydroxyapatite formation on porous gel-silica matrices', *J Sol-Gel Sci Technol*, **7**, 45–51.

Pereira MM, Clark AE and Hench LL (1994), 'Homogeneity of bioactive sol-gel-derived glasses in the system $CaO–P_2O_5–SiO_2$', *J Mater Synthesis Proc*, **2**, 189–96.

Pereira MM, Clark AE and Hench LL (1995), 'Effect of texture on the rate of hydroxyapatite formation on gel-silica surface', *J Am Ceram Soc*, **78**, 2463–8.

Pérez-Pariente J, Balas F, Roman J, Salinas AJ and Vallet-Reg M (1999), 'Influence of composition and surface characteristics on the *in vitro* bioactivity of SiO_2–$CaO–P_2O_5$–MgO sol-gel glasses', *J Biomed Mater Res*, **47**, 170–6.

Pérez-Pariente J, Balas F and Vallet-Regí M (2000), 'Surface and chemical study of $SiO_2–P_2O_5$–CaO-(MgO) bioactive glasses', *Chem Mater*, **12**, 750–55.

Porter AE, Best SM and Bonfield W (2004), 'Ultrastructural comparison of hydroxyapatite and silicon-substituted hydroxyapatite for biomedical applications', *J Biomed Mater Res*, **68**, 133–41.

Radev L, Hristov V, Michailova I and Samuneva B (2009), 'Sol-gel bioactive glass-ceramics Part II, Glass-ceramics in the $CaO–SiO_2–P_2O_5–MgO$ system', *Cent Eur J Chem*, **7**, 322–7.

Radin SR and Ducheyne P (1992), 'Plasma spraying induced changes of calcium phosphate ceramic characteristics and the effect on *in vitro* stability', *J Mater Sci Mater Med*, **3**, 33–42.

Radin S, Ducheyne P, Reicin KE and Lee MH (1997), 'The effect of composition and *in vitro* immersion on the formation of a bioactive surface on sol-gel derived glass', in *Transactions of the 23rd Annual Meeting of the Society for Biomaterials*, Society for Biomaterials, New Orleans.

Radin S, El-Bassyouni G, Vresilovic EJ, Schepers E and Ducheyne P (2005), '*In vivo* tissue response to resorbable silica xerogels as controlled-release materials', *Biomaterials*, **26**, 1043–52.

Reginster JY, Felsenberg D, Boonen S, Diez-Perez A, Rizzoli R, Brandi ML, Spector TD, Brixen K, Goemaere S, Cormier C, Balogh A, Delmas PD and Meunier PJ (2008), 'Effects of long-term strontium ranelate treatment on the risk of non-vertebral and vertebral fractures in postmenopausal osteoporosis. Results of a five-year, randomized, placebo-controlled trial', *Arthritis Rheum*, **58**, 1687–95.

Román J, Padilla S and Vallet-Regí M (2003), 'Sol-gel glasses as precursors of bioactive glass ceramics', *Chem Mater*, **15**, 798–806.

Roseberry HH, Baird Hastings A and Morse JK (1931), 'X-ray analysis of bone and teeth', *J Biol Chem*, **90**, 395–407.

Saboori A, Rabiee M, Moztarzadeh F, Sheikhi M, Tahriri M and Karimi M (2009), 'Synthesis, characterization and *in vitro* bioactivity of sol-gel-derived $SiO_2–CaO–P_2O_5–MgO$ bioglass', *Mater Sci Eng C*, **29**, 335–40.

Salinas AJ, Vallet-Regí M and Izquierdo-Barba I (2001), 'Biomimetic apatite deposition on calcium silicate gel glasses', *J Sol-Gel Sci Technol*, **21**, 13–25.

Saravanapavan P and Hench LL (2000), 'Low temperature synthesis, structure and bioactivity of gel derived glasses in the binary $CaO–SiO_2$ system', *J Biomed Mater Res*, **54**, 608–18.

Saravanapavan P and Hench LL (2003), 'Mesoporous calcium silicate glasses. II. Textural characterization', *J Non-Cryst Solids*, **318**, 14–26.

Sepulveda P, Jones JR and Hench LL (2002), 'Characterization of melt-derived 45S5 and sol-gel-derived 58S bioactive glasses', *J Biomed Mater Res*, **58**, 734–40.

Sepulveda P, Jones JR and Hench LL (2002), '*In vitro* dissolution of melt-derived 45S5 and sol-gel-derived 58S bioactive glasses', *J Biomed Mater Res*, **61**, 301–11.

Siriphannon P, Kameshima Y, Yasumori A, Okada K and Hayashi S (2002), 'Formation of hydroxyapatite on $CaSiO_3$ powders in simulated body fluid', *J Eur Ceram Soc*, **22**, 511–20.

Suciu RC, Indrea E, Silipas TD, Dreve S, Rosu MC, Popescu V, Popescu G and Nascu HI (2009), 'TiO_2 thin films prepared by sol-gel method', *J Phys: Conf Ser*, **182**, 012080.

Tanaka Y and Yamashita K (2008), 'Fabrication processes for bioceramics', in *Bioceramics and Their Clinical Applications*, Kokubo T (ed.), CRC Press, Boca Raton, 41–5.

Tinsley D, Watson CJ and Russell JL (2001), 'A comparison of hydroxylapatite coated implant retained fixed and removable mandibular prostheses over 4 to 6 years', *Clin Oral Implants Res*, **12**, 159–66.

Torricelli P, Verné E, Vitale Brovarone C, Appendino P, Rustichelli F, Krajewski A, Ravaglioli A, Pierini G, Fini M, Giavaresi G and Giardino R (2001), 'Biological glass coating on ceramic materials, *in vitro* evaluation using primary osteoblast cultures from healthy and osteopenic rat bone', *Biomaterials*, **22**, 2535–43.

Vallet-Regí M, Salinas AJ, Román J and Gil M (1999), 'Effect of magnesium content on the in vitro bioactivity of $CaO–MgO–SiO_2–P_2O_5$ sol-gel glasses', *J Mater Chem*, **9**, 515–18.

Vulpoi A, Baia L, Simon S and Simon V (2012), 'Silver effect on the structure of $SiO_2–CaO–P_2O_5$ ternary system', *Mater Sci Eng C*, **32**, 178–83.

Wheeler SL (1996), 'Eight-year clinical retrospective study of titanium plasma-sprayed and hydroxyapatite-coated cylinder implants', *Int J Oral Maxillofac Impl*, **11**, 340–50.

Wu CT and Chang J (2004), 'Synthesis and apatite-formation ability of akermanite', *Mater Lett*, **58**, 2415–17.

Wu CT and Chang J (2006), 'A novel akermanite bioceramic, preparation and characteristics', *J Biomater Appl*, **21**, 119–29.

Wu C, Chang J, Wang J, Ni S and Zhai W (2005), 'Preparation and characteristics of a calcium magnesium silicate (bredigite) bioactive ceramic', *Biomaterials*, **26**, 2925–31.

Wu C, Chang J, Ni S and Wang J (2006), '*In vitro* bioactivity of akermanite ceramics', *J Biomed Mater Res, Part A*, **76**, 73–80.

Wu C, Ramaswamy Y, Gale D, Yang W, Xiao K, Zhang L, Yin Y and Zreiqat H (2008), 'Novel sphene coatings on Ti-6Al-4V for orthopedic implants using sol-gel method', *Acta Biomater*, **4**, 569–76.

Wu C, Fan W, Gelinsky M, Xiao Y, Simon P, Schulze R, Doert T, Luo Y and Cuniberti G (2011), 'Bioactive $SrO–SiO_2$ glass with well-ordered mesopores, characterization, physiochemistry and biological properties', *Acta Biomater*, **7**, 1797–806.

Xie H, Wang X, Wang Y, Zhang F, Chen C and Xia Y (2009), 'Effects of sol-gel processed silica coating on bond strength of resin cements to glass-infiltrated alumina ceramic', *J Adhes Dent*, **11**, 49–55.

Yamaguchi M (2010), 'Role of nutritional zinc in the prevention of osteoporosis', *Mol Cell Biochem*, **338**, 241–54.

Yamane M and Kojima T (1981), 'Low temperature synthesis of non-crystalline solids of the system $SrO–SiO_2$', *J Non-Cryst Solids*, **44**, 181–90.

Yamashita K, Yagi T and Umegaki T (1996), 'Bonelike coatings onto ceramics by reactive magnetron sputtering', *J Am Ceram Soc*, **79**, 3313–16.

Yoshida K, Kamada K, Sato K, Hatada R, Baba K and Atsuta M (1999a), 'Thin sol-gel-derived silica coatings on dental pure titanium casting', *J Biomed Mater Res*, **48**, 778–85.

Yoshida K, Tanagawa M, Kamada K, Hatada R, Baba K, Inoi T and Atsuta M (1999b), 'Silica coatings formed on noble dental casting alloy by the sol-gel dipping process', *J Biomed Mater Res*, **46**, 221–7.

Yun HS, Park JW, Kim SH, Kim YJ and Jang JH (2011), 'Effect of the pore structure of bioactive glass balls on biocompatibility *in vitro* and *in vivo*', *Acta Biomater*, **7**, 2651–60.

Zhai W, Lu H, Chen L, Lin X, Huang Y, Dai K, Naoki K, Chen G and Chang J (2012), 'Silicate bioceramics induce angiogenesis during bone regeneration', *Acta Biomater*, **8**, 341–9.

Zhang K, Washburn NR and Simon CG Jr (2005), 'Cytotoxicity of three-dimensionally ordered macroporous sol-gel bioactive glass (3DOM-BG)', *Biomaterials*, **26**, 4532–9.

Zhang W, Chen X, Liao X, Huang Z, Dan X and Yin G (2011), 'Electrophoretic deposition of porous CaO–MgO–SiO_2 glass–ceramic coatings with B_2O_3 as additive on Ti–6Al–4V alloy', *J Mater Sci Mater Med*, **22**, 2261–71.

Zhong J and Greenspan DC (2000), 'Processing and properties of sol-gel bioactive glasses', *J Biomed Mater Res, Part B*, **53**, 694–701.

Zhong JP, Greenspan DC and Feng JW (2002), 'A microstructural examination of apatite induced by bioglass *in vitro*', *J Mater Sci Mater Med*, **13**, 321–6.

Part III

Dental composites for tooth repair and replacement

8

Composite adhesive restorative materials for dental applications

MICHAEL F. BURROW, The University of Hong Kong, PR China

DOI: 10.1533/9780857096432.3.235

Abstract: This chapter is a broad overview of adhesive or tooth-coloured restorative materials currently used in dental practice. The materials introduced are resin composites, polyacid-modified resin composites or compomers and glass ionomer cements (GIC). The different classifications of each of these materials are described. Brief outlines are provided of their physical properties, the effect of biofilm formation on each of the materials, as well as current research data on the clinical use of the materials. From current research evidence, it would appear that resin composite materials have steadily improved and when used as directed by manufacturers this group of materials is becoming a suitable substitute for amalgam in most instances. Polyacid-modified resin composites have limited use clinically. Although a useful material for small restorations in permanent teeth, their use is finding a place in paediatric dental treatment. The GIC have also found a place in the restoration of small non-loading bearing restorations as well as in those locations where resin-based materials may not adhere reliably to tooth structure, such as root surfaces.

Key words: glass ionomer cement, polyacid-modified resin composite, resin composite, tooth-coloured filling material.

8.1 Introduction

Adhesive restorative materials have now become a mainstay of direct restoration placement in all parts of the oral cavity. This has come about with the development of a wide variety of materials exhibiting improved physical properties, reduction of technique sensitivity and, importantly, the development of excellent, reliable adhesive resins for bond filling materials to enamel and dentine surfaces. In addition, demands from patients have meant practitioners have had to re-evaluate clinical procedures and material use to provide more aesthetic restorations.

Adhesive restorative materials cover not only resin composite restorative materials but also the polyacid-modified resin composites (compomers) and glass ionomer (polyalkenoate) cements. In all these tooth-coloured materials not only have the physical and mechanical properties continued to improve, but also the aesthetic qualities have shown great improvement over recent years.

The use of dental amalgam continues to decline and the influence of the United Nations environment programme in reduceing the use of mercury-containing products worldwide may eventually see the end of dental amalgam use (UNEP, 2008). In certain parts of the world, the use of amalgam has all but, or will soon, disappear from dentists' clinics. Therefore, it is important for researchers and manufacturers to provide clinicians with better clinical evidence and improved materials that allows appropriate selection of adhesive restorative materials to ensure long-lasting restorations for a wide variety of treatments.

This chapter provides an overview of commonly used tooth-coloured restorative materials, namely, resin composite, polyacid-modified resin composite and glass ionomer cements (GIC). The following sections outline the advantages and disadvantages of each material and finally the clinical evidence indicating where each of these materials may be used successfully.

8.2 Resin composite restorative materials

The first tooth-coloured filling materials were based on silicate cements that are no longer used in clinical practice. The problem with the silicate cements was their high solubility and pulpal toxicity. This led researchers to look for alternatives resulting in the development of resin-based materials. These resins were also not particularly successful in the beginning. The first resin-based materials were based on polymethymethacrylate (PMMA). PMMA-based materials were plagued with poor marginal sealing, since no 'true' adhesion was achieved and the polymerization shrinkage was high owing to the lack of filler particles (Söderholm, 2007). However, outcomes using PMMA-based filling materials were more successful than the silicate cements. At about the same time as the PMMA materials were being introduced, Hagger (1948) was also experimenting with new monomers and polymerization systems. He developed glycerophosphoric acid dimethacrylate (GPDM) which was used with polymethylmethacrylate and marketed as Sevriton Cavity Seal. The GPDM was believed to bond the PMMA-based filling material to the tooth surface. This was possibly the first 'adhesive' resin-based restorative material available to the dental profession.

Resin-based restorative materials underwent the greatest change during the 1960s when Bowen introduced new resin monomers consisting of bisphenol-A glycidylmethacrylate (bis-GMA) (Bowen, 1962). Bis-GMA still remains one of the major matrix resins used in filling materials. Shortly after, the urethane dimethacrylate (UDMA) resin monomer was also introduced as an alternative matrix resin and has become more popular in recent years. Although very successful, the polymerization of these monomers to polymeric structures leads to reduction in the overall volume and shrinkage of a restoration in the confined space of a cavity. This problem has been and continues to be a major concern for clinicians and researchers alike. Recently, more viable alternative resins have been introduced through the development of new monomers such as the 'ring-opening' monomers, for example, spiro-orthocarbonates, and epoxy-based resins used in the silorane-based composites (Weinmann *et al.*, 2005; Ilie and Hickel, 2006) and organically-modified ceramics (Ormocers) (Manhart *et al.*, 2000). The nature of these newer resins will be discussed in subsequent chapters.

The other major component of resin-composite materials, namely the filler particles and the linking agents that bind the fillers to the resin matrix are also extremely important to the success of these materials clinically as the mechanical properties together with the aesthetic qualities can be altered by modifying the fillers. A subsequent chapter will deal with the different filler systems available.

8.2.1 Classification

Resin-based composite filling materials have been classified in order to aid practitioners by providing information that assists material selection depending on its use, for example, restoration of a posterior tooth compared with a small anterior tooth restoration. Most classification systems have been centred on the filler particles/systems used, specifically the size of the fillers. Other classifications have been based on the consistency (viscosity) of the composite before it is cured.

The original resin-composite filling materials contained very large filler particles of between 10–50 μm in size. These glass fillers imparted great strength to the cured material but owing to the size of the fillers, the volume occupied by the resin was substantial, meaning that these materials tended to wear quickly when subjected to occlusal loading and could not be polished to a high lustre. These composite filling materials have now been relegated to history and have been commonly referred to as 'macrofil' materials. (Bayne *et al.*, 1994; Ferracane, 2011) (see Fig. 8.1).

Because the early materials showed high wear rates and poor aesthetics, manufacturers searched for new types of fillers to achieve restorations with highly polished surfaces that better mimic an enamel surface. In the late 1970s, the so-called 'microfill' composites were introduced (Williams, 1980). These composites used a new filler in the form of very small particles of silicon dioxide, approximately 0.04 μm in diameter. It could be said that these resin composites were the first 'nano-filled' composites, although such terminology had yet to be introduced into the scientific community. The use of the sub-micrometre particles was hailed a great success for dentistry as it allowed the composite to be polished to a high lustre, which fulfilled the desires of dentists for anterior restorations that required high aesthetic outcomes. 'Aesthetic' dentistry started at this time and could be realised for patients with unsightly restorations and/or teeth that were stained or misshapen. The downside though was that the volume percentage of filler particles in the bulk of the resin composite had to remain low, meaning these materials were quite brittle, could not be used for load-bearing restorations and still showed quite high wear (Brosh *et al.*, 1996). However, the introduction of the microfilled composites allowed practitioners to use these materials for various 'new' aesthetic procedures such as direct resin veneers and tooth build-ups. Another problem with the new microfilled materials was they also showed a large difference in coefficient of thermal expansion compared with tooth structure, meaning marginal staining around restorations tended to develop quite quickly and a retention form in some cavity shapes was needed to hold the restoration in place owing to expansion and shrinkage of the restorative material and the adhesive systems which at that time were not very good.

Therefore, because of the shortcomings of these materials, manufacturers continued to develop resin-composite restorative materials in order to fulfil the requirements of excellent aesthetics, high physical strength and low wear. The next version of resin composites that were introduced to the profession were termed 'hybrid' resin composites, as they combined the good points of the macrofill and microfill materials (Christensen, 1999).

With the development of so many variations of restorative materials, a variety of classification systems were developed based on mode of polymerization, average particle size of fillers, filler type, filler content, filler morphology, mechanical properties or type of restoration use. Some examples of classifications are outlined below.

An early classification based on filler type identified four major groups, namely, (i) traditional resin composite, (ii) hybrid resin composite, (iii) homogeneous microfilled and (iv) heterogeneous microfilled resin composites (Lutz *et al.*, 1983). With the changes in composition of fillers, this classification has been superseded.

Another classification, based on Young's modulus of elasticity, Vickers hardness and surface roughness (Willems *et al.*, 1992), concluded that five groups of composites were appropriate, these were so-called: (i) densified composite, (ii) microfine composite, (iii) miscellaneous composites, (iv) traditional composites and (v) fibre-reinforced composites. The 'densified' resin composites were further subdivided by volume per cent of filler. Those materials with less than 60 vol% were referred to as 'midway-filled' whilst those materials with greater than 60 vol% were called 'compact filled'. Each class was also subdivided according to filler size: ultrafine (<3 μm) and fine (>3 μm).

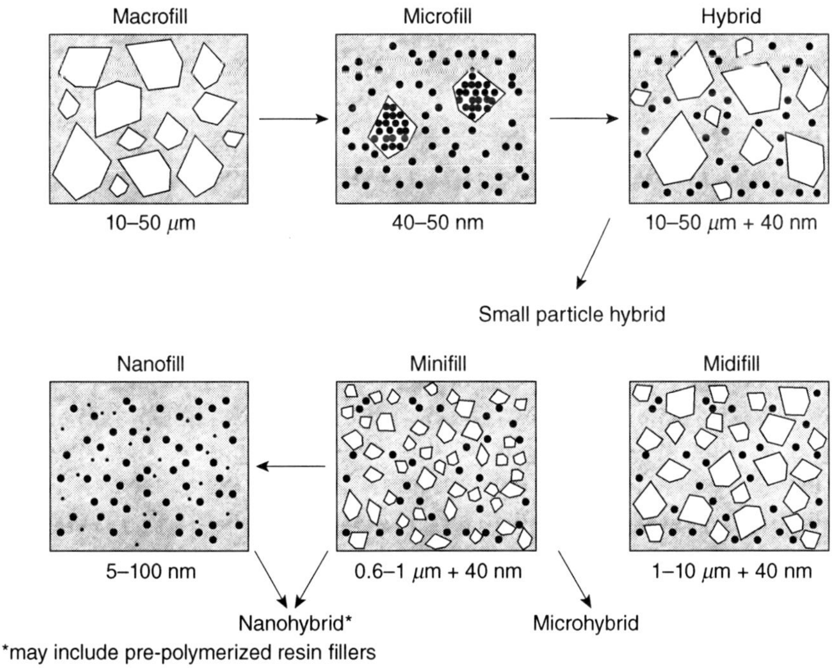

8.1 Outline of resin composite development and filler particle distribution (reproduced with permission from Ferracane, 2011.)

Possibly the most popular classification was developed and introduced by Bayne *et al.* (1994) who based their classification on filler particle size. They classified resin composites into six groups: megafill (0.5–2 mm), macrofill (10–100 μm), midifill (1–10 μm), minifill (01.1–1 μm), microfill (0.01–0.1 μm) and nanofill (0.005–0.01 μm). A recent review by Ferracane (2011) outlines the development of composite filling materials as well as providing an excellent diagram of the groupings of materials based on filler systems (Fig. 8.1).

The most recent classification of resin composites was based on the filler shape (Kim *et al.*, 2002). The authors developed three groups and found that the amount of filler loading was dependent on the morphology of the particles. The three groups in this classification are composites containing prepolymerized particles (which have the lowest filler content), composites with spherical filler particles (this group has the highest filler content) and finally those composites that have irregular-shaped particles (the filler content is intermediate) (Kim *et al.*, 2002).

From a clinical standpoint, a very simple classification can be centred on the viscosity of the resin composite before polymerization. This classification (Christensen, 1999) has three broad groups, namely: flowable, universal and so-called packable composites. The clinical application of each of these groups tends to vary. The flowable materials are more suited to non-load bearing locations such as cervical restorations or lining of cavities and the universal materials can be applied in any location in the oral cavity. The 'packable' composites are used in posterior restorations and have been developed for practitioners who prefer to have a composite with some resistance during placement that gives a feel similar to that of condensing dental amalgam into a cavity.

8.2.2 Physical properties

One of the common misconceptions related to use of resin composites for restoration of posterior teeth is that they lack a similar strength to dental amalgam. Current materials are now able to provide strengths that can withstand most occlusal loads and some composites have a higher compressive strength than some amalgams. Certainly, the early strengths of polymerized composite restorations are far better than the 1-hour strength of amalgam restorations, so the problem of early failure of a composite restoration is not a problem compared with an amalgam restoration (see Table 8.1).

The most recent work investigating the strength of resin-based materials has tended to centre on resin composites used for cores (Yüzügüllü *et al.*, 2008). This recent study compared diametral and compressive strengths of six materials which included four resin composites, a high copper amalgam and a silver-reinforced GIC. The outcomes showed the amalgam was at the lower scale for strength compared with the resin-based materials. However, the outcomes of this study would seem to vary from other published strength studies (Yüzügüllü *et al.*, 2008). The strengths recorded for the amalgam were somewhat lower than expected compared with the generally accepted strength of amalgam. In general the accepted 7-day compressive strength for high copper amalgams ranges between 340 and 500 MPa (Anusavice, 1996).

A recent comprehensive study investigated numerous aspects of resin composite material strength (Ilie and Hickel, 2009). This study provides data on physical properties of 72 resin composite materials of all types. Contrary to the paper by Yüzügüllü *et al.* (2008), outcomes indicate that the compressive strengths of resin-composite filling materials are less than dental amalgam, showing the lowest physical properties in the micro-filled hybrid materials, whereas all other groups (hybrid, nano-hybrid, packable and ormocer) were not significantly different. They concluded that most categories of resin composite, except the microfilled materials, can be regarded as being suitable for loading in posterior restorations, but care is needed for large restorations and for those patients that show

Table 8.1 Summary of various published physical properties of adhesive restorative materials

Material type	Flexural strength (MPa)	Flexural modulus (GPa)	Diametral tensile strength (MPa)	Compressive strength (MPa)
Composites				
Hybrid	116.6	7.3	32.5	211.5
				202.2
Packable	105.9	8.4	34.3	217.4
Ormocer	104.3	7.5	35.2	216.0
Nano-hybrid	103.1	5.0	40.5	210.8
Flowable composites	99.8	4.4	38.3	264.2
Microfilled composites	73.5	3.8	24.2	246.9
Core material	–	–	42.4	279
	84.2 9		34.8	
Compomer				
Compomer	94.7	9.2	33.9	230.9
				153.9
				243.5
Flowable compomer	89.1	4.2	33.5	237.8
Glass ionomer cement				
Conventional GIC	40.7		22.8	170.7
	24.4			226.5
Resin-modified GIC	75.9		43.3	156.7
				271.7
High viscosity GIC	46.5			176
				240
Metal-reinforced GIC	22.9		22.1	122
				211.8
Dental amalgam				
	85	15.7	35.6	432.2 (dispersed phase)
				539.2; 485 (unicompositional)
				424.6; 387(admix)
				486 (admix)

Information in the table is taken from various publications: Bryant (1979); Combe *et al.* (1999); el-Kalla and Garcia-Godoy (1999); Xie *et al.* (2000); Peez and Frank (2006); Craig (1997), Yüzügüllü *et al.* (2008); Ilie and Hickel (2009); Silva and Dias (2009).

occlusal functional habits such as bruxism. It is known that microfilled materials tend to chip more easily than 'conventional' composite materials (Lambrechts *et al.*, 1982) and therefore should not be used in load bearing restorations.

The predominant reason for failure of resin-composite restorations in large restorations has been shown to be fracture of the restoration (van Dijken, 2000; Van Nieuwenhuysen *et al.*, 2003). For restorations of moderate size, caries was the main reason for replacement for periods up to 17 years of clinical function, but for less than five years, it seems restoration fracture is the more common failure mode (Brunthaler *et al.*, 2003).

Wear

When composites were first used for the restoration of posterior teeth, wear was identified as perhaps the most significant problem, particularly when microfilled materials were used. Much of the early work on wear was undertaken by Leinfelder, whose scale was adopted for use in clinical studies (Leinfelder *et al.*, 1986). Braem *et al.* (1986) showed that posterior composite wear after one year was related to contact areas with opposing teeth. More recent long-term studies seem to indicate that wear rates are acceptable, with the exception of patients displaying occlusal functional habits such a bruxism or clenching (van Dijken, 2000; Pallesen and Qvist, 2003). The review paper by Ferracane (2006) concluded that concern still remains for wear of large resin composite restorations, however the evidence remains limited. Therefore, careful diagnosis and planning is necessary when considering a resin composite for large restorations in posterior teeth. A recent study compared the five-year volumetric wear performance of nanofilled and microhybrid resin composite materials (Palaniappan *et al.*, 2011). These authors determined that volumetric wear was related to such factors as operator, cavity type, a combination of these two factors as well as tooth location by quadrant. They also showed that the vertical wear rate and loss of volume were generally not constant during the life of the study (Palaniappan *et al.*, 2011).

Polymerization shrinkage

The conversion of long chain monomers to a polymer will always induce shrinkage in a resin-based material. The outcome of shrinkage in a resin-based restoration can be gap formation beneath a restoration that may lead to sensitivity, opening of the margin of the filling-tooth interface, which can allow the ingress of bacteria and therefore subsequent pulpal inflammation or even caries. A further consequence of polymerization shrinkage is that contraction forces can cause cuspal deflection (especially thin cusps), which can also lead to sensitivity of a restored tooth (Fleming *et al.*, 2007; Kim and Park, 2011). Polymerization contraction has been at the centre of a large amount of research and is perhaps one of the most difficult problems to overcome when using resin-based materials for the restoration of teeth.

Manufacturers have also spent a large amount of time creating new materials that can overcome the shrinkage problem. Changes have ranged from modifying and using new monomer formulations to increasing the volume of filler particles to the more recent introduction of 'ring opening' polymerization systems of resins that have been to shown to produce less shrinkage (Weinmann *et al.*, 2005). However, as these changes to materials are introduced, other characteristics of the composite may change.

A common problem associated with polymerization shrinkage in cavities is maintaining the bond of the composite to the walls during curing. This requires the composite to flow while it is in the gel state of polymerization. Davidson *et al.* (1984) first described this phenomenon. Further work showed the greater the number of cavity walls that are bonded, the greater the chance of the filling being pulled off the cavity wall during polymerization. This has been referred to as the configuration factor, or C-factor by Feilzer *et al.* (1987) (see Fig. 8.2).

The role of the C-factor, which is essentially the number of walls a restoration must adhere to compared with the number of surfaces that are not bonded, is an important consideration when placing resin-composite restorations. This has become a well-known and frequently quoted phenomenon. To reduce the effect of the C-factor, is it important to attempt to increase the area of the non-bonded surface area of the composite as much as possible, reduce the volume of resin by placing, for example, a GIC base, or slowing the initial rate of polymerization of the composite. This

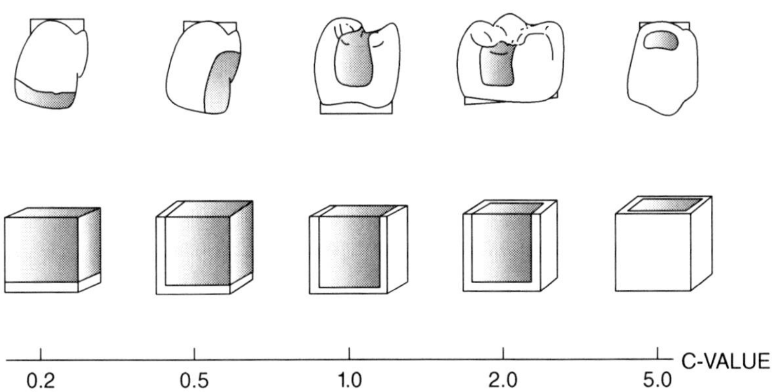

8.2 Effect of the C-factor on adhesion to cavity walls. The greater the number of cavity walls the increased chance of the composite debonding (reproduced with permission from Dr T Yoshikawa).

latter approach essentially allows the composite to release stresses during the polymerization phase by slowing the rate of polymerization and is often referred to as 'slow-start curing' (Yoshikawa *et al.*, 2003). Thus the type and intensity of curing light can influence the rate of cure and hence the rate of polymerization stress (Ilie *et al.*, 2005). A number of studies have shown that strong intensity lights cause greater shrinkage stress (Calheiros 2004; Sakaguchi and Berge, 1998).

Other studies have shown reduced marginal leakage/gap formation of the so-called 'soft-start' curing method. This technique can allow some viscoelastic movement within the composite as the polymer chains lengthen slowly allowing lower internal stress in the curing composite (Boaro *et al.*, 2010; Yoshikawa *et al.*, 2001, 2003). One of the common misconceptions of gap formation concerns the degree of shrinkage and bond strength of the composite. The shrinkage problem is related to the rate of stress and strain produced in the resin composite during polymerization (Logercio *et al.*, 2004). This is a factor related to the polymerization rate, composite formulation and geometry of the cavity (Ferracane, 2008). The size of the monomer molecule is another factor affecting shrinkage, namely, a larger monomer molecule and greater quantity of such monomers in the matrix means less shrinkage. Also, the greater the degree of conversion of monomer to polymer, the greater the amount of overall shrinkage. This rather complex topic is described well in the review by Stansbury *et al.* (2005).

Polishing

The surface finish of a tooth coloured restoration is an important feature when the restoration is located in the aesthetic zone. In addition, surface finish will determine the degree of roughness. If the restoration surface is microscopically rough, then it is more likely to become stained as well as to aid bacterial adherence. Part of the surface roughness will be related to the size and volume of filler particles of the filling material. The composites with the best surface finish are the microfill materials, but they are not strong enough for use in posterior teeth. Hence, to solve this issue, micro- and nano-hybrid resin composites that are able to withstand occlusal loads were introduced and these also achieve a relatively glossy surface after polishing. The surface finish has usually been measured as the surface roughness of the composite after proprietary polishing systems have been used. Most of these systems use various grits of aluminium oxide or even diamond suspensions. Some systems also use a polishing paste of either a suspension of aluminium oxide or diamond particles. A recent study compared three different polishing systems on three resin composites: a nanofill, microfill and minifill (Berger *et al.*, 2011). This study concluded that, '. . . surface roughness and staining are not solely influenced by filler size of the composite resin . . .' (Berger *et al.*, 2011). A further study found no interaction between tested resin composites (three minifills, a microfill and a nanofill) in six polishing systems (Da Costa *et al.*, 2007). They did find an interaction between surface gloss values of composites and the polishing systems used. The smaller the average filler particle size in the composite, the smoother the surfaces produced (Da Costa *et al.*, 2007). An investigation of polishing six nanocomposite materials also found little difference between the commercially available polishing systems evaluated (Korkmaz *et al.*, 2008). The authors found, however, that the smoothest surface that could be achieved was when the composite was polymerized against a Mylar strip. However, the 'strip-finished' surface was also the softest when subjected to a microhardness test, meaning it could be abraded more quickly than the 'polishing system finished' surfaces (Korkmaz *et al.*, 2008). Therefore, it is not recommended that a 'resin-rich' surface be left on the restoration as it will quickly wear off.

Biofilm formation

Biofilms are known to form on surfaces of any material placed in the oral cavity. The growth of the biofilm on the surface of a tooth or restoration can lead to dental caries or have an impact on the health of the gingival and periodontal tissues if the right conditions are present. It is known that biofilm forms on dental composites leading to changes in the surface of the composite material, in addition to possible progression of dental caries at the restoration margin. A recent study by Pereira *et al.* (2011) studied the adherence of *Streptococcus mutans* on three types of resin composite: a nanofilled, nanohybrid and microhybrid after using three surface finishing methods: Mylar strip, aluminium oxide discs or 30-bladed tungsten carbide bur and silicon carbide brush. Samples stored either in saliva for 1 hour or placed in a growth medium without saliva storage showed that saliva storage increased bacterial adhesion for all composites irrespective of the finishing method. The nanofilled composite showed the lowest bacterial adhesion to the surface. When samples were not stored in saliva, the mylar strip finished surface samples showed the least bacterial adhesion. Overall, it seemed the nanofilled composite showed the lowest degree of bacterial adhesion. This same phenomenon has been reported in other studies (Ikeda *et al.*, 2007; Montanaro *et al.*, 2004; Eick *et al.*, 2004). The adhesion of *S mutans*, which seems to be the most common bacteria studied, is influenced by the composition of the resin composite, the finishing and polishing undertaken as well as saliva. A review paper by Busscher *et al.* (2010) found that the presence of biofilm on the surface of resin composite can lead to a deterioration of the material surface. This leads to increased surface roughness and a decrease in the microhardness. Work by Beyth *et al.* (2008)

using atomic force microscopy, demonstrated increased roughness over one month in a microfilled resin composite. Roughness changes could be observed within one week of exposure to the bacteria (Beyth *et al.*, 2008). These changes may lead to change in wear patterns of the composite and possibly to increased surface staining.

8.2.3 Clinical performance

The clinical performance of resin composite restorations in posterior teeth has been a great source of debate amongst practitioners and researchers alike. The general belief has been that resin composite restorations do not last as long as dental amalgam restorations. This is definitely true for the older materials, but recent data now question this long held and somewhat anecdotal belief. A paper in 2001 by Hickel and Manhart (2001) reviewed longitudinal clinical trials of load-bearing restorations and reported failure rates for dental amalgam ranging from 0–7% and resin composite ranging from 0–9%. The longevity of the compared studies did vary somewhat, but the data of approximately 10 years ago was starting to demonstrate that there was not a lot of difference between these two materials. A later review by the same authors (Manhart *et al.*, 2004) reported mean annual failure rates for restorations in posterior teeth. Here the annual failure rates were 3% for amalgam and 2.2% for resin composite for the materials reviewed. They also reported that studies conducted after 1990 showed better outcomes, possibly owing to better materials and understanding of clinical techniques. Hence it would seem that the belief that composites are not an equivalent alternative to amalgam is perhaps misguided.

A recent paper by Opdam *et al.* (2011) reported that 'the median age of failed restorations may be considered as a deceptive measure of restoration longevity'. They went on to say, 'Kaplan–Meier statistics is still the preferred method of calculating longevity of a group of dental restorations'. Although prospective studies are the best alternative to evaluate material performance, retrospective clinical studies can also provide useful information and build up the evidence base of clinical performance of materials, which is still lacking.

A recent paper reported the 22-year clinical performance of a midifilled resin composite (Herculite XR, Kerr, USA) and a minifilled hybrid resin composite (P-50 APC, 3M-ESPE, USA) (Da Rosa Rodolpho *et al.*, 2011). This study was from one dental practice with one operator who placed 392 posterior composite restorations in 61 patients. The outcomes showed that of the failed restorations, 61 were repaired, while 49 were replaced. A further ten teeth/restorations had failed owing to loss of the tooth. Kaplan–Meier statistics showed that the annual failure rate changed over time. For

Herculite, the failure rate was 1.5% at ten years increasing to 2.2% at 20 years and for P-50 it was 1.6% at ten years and 1.5% at 20 years. Statistical analysis showed no difference in longevity between the two materials. However, if a P-50 restoration was present at ten-years, it was statistically more likely to be present at 20 years. This study also showed that premolars demonstrated a better survival rate compared with molars. Smaller restorations showed better survival compared with larger restorations and the more surfaces a restoration covered the greater the chance of failure. This is one of the few long-term studies that shows the performance of materials is not constant over time. Their earlier 17-year report showed both materials were equally successful but at 22 years the midifill material P-50 showed a better success rate with less marginal deterioration. It seems a material with a higher fracture toughness is likely to provide longer term survival.

Another recent retrospective long-term study compared amalgam and resin composite restoration survival over 12 years (Opdam *et al.*, 2010). This study also examined whether caries risk had any influence on longevity. The study evaluated 1949 restorations (1202 amalgam and 747 resin composite) placed in 273 patients between 1983 and 1990. The restorations ranged from three surface to larger 4/5 surface restorations for either material. It was noted that there was no difference in failure pattern for either material used for the high caries risk group, although the annual failure rate for composite was higher. For the low caries risk group, the composite restorations showed a better survival after 12 years for either the three or 4/5 surface restorations. No difference was found for premolar or molars in the high or low caries risk groups. They concluded in their study that, 'caries risk . . . plays a significant role in restoration survival. In the high risk group composite and amalgam showed comparable performance . . . with amalgam performing better in smaller restorations' (Opdam *et al.*, 2010). The outcomes question the widely held belief that composite restorations exhibit a higher failure rate than amalgam.

One of the issues, outlined earlier, is the problem associated with polymerization shrinkage of resin composites. One method promulgated to reduce this problem is the use of a low viscosity flowable resin composite to line the cavity before filling with a restorative composite. A prospective study examined the survival of 107 resin composite restorations over seven years in 48 patients who needed at least two resin composite restorations in posterior teeth with and without the use of a flowable composite lining material (van Dijken and Pallesen, 2011). The study concluded that the use of flowable composite as an intermediate afforded no benefit to the longevity of the restorations. However, the hybrid composite used showed 'good clinical performance'.

8.3 Polyacid-modified resin composite (compomer)

This group of materials has often been seen as an intermediate material between resin composite and GIC restorative materials. A polyacid-modified resin composite (PAMRC) was first proposed by McClean *et al.* in 1994. Commercially, these materials are termed 'compomers' from 'composite ionomer'. However, nowadays PAMRCs should be regarded as a distinct group of materials with specific applications. PAMRC comprise an ion-leachable glass within a polymeric matrix, making them a composite material (Meyer *et al.*, 1998). The glass is usually a calcium-aluminosilicate glass which is able to leach ions, usually fluoride, not unlike that in GIC (Meyer *et al.*, 1998). They are light activated and polymerize the resin to form a polymer matrix. The resin matrix is made up of either Bis-GMA or UDMA with sometimes the addition of triethyleneglycol dimethacrylate (TEG-DMA). In addition, bifunctional monomers, which have carboxylate groups and two double bond functional groups, for example, tetracarboxylic acid butane or citric acid dimethacrylate are also incorporated into the matrix structure (Meyer *et al.*, 1998; Young *et al.*, 2004). These bifunctional monomers are able to react with the methacrylate components of the PAMRC. In addition, an acid–base neutralization reaction occurs (Eliades *et al.*, 1998). However, a recent paper indicated there may be no acid–base reaction as they were unable to detect the COO^- group that indicated an acid–base reaction had occurred (Arrondo *et al.*, 2009). The PAMRC do not bond chemically to the tooth structure as it takes time for the acid–base reaction to occur (Mount and Hume, 2005), because it only occurs in association with the sorption of water into the polymeric matrix (Meyer *et al.*, 1998). PAMRCs have the ability to change the pH of storage solutions containing lactic acid by buffering and increasing the pH, thus showing that ion release from the glass occurs (Nicholson *et al.*, 1999).

8.3.1 Physical properties

Water sorption

One of the main differences of PAMRCs compared with resin composite filling materials is the amount of water absorbed and how this may affect the material. A second delayed cure occurs during the first few months as the PAMRC absorbs water (Small *et al.*, 1998). Hygroscopic expansion of PAMRCs has been shown to be significantly greater than in resin composites (Martin and Jedynakiewicz, 1998). This has potentially been a draw back for the older compomers, which showed significant marginal staining in clinical evaluations when they were not bonded with an intermediary adhesive (Tyas, 2000).

The water sorption of resin composite materials tends to be controlled and surface restricted (Mair, 1999), whereas the PAMRC contain acid-modified monomers that are hydrophilic and thus allow move water sorption (Nicholson and Alsarheed, 1998). In comparison with resin-modifed GIC, the uptake of water in PAMRC was shown to be statistically less after one week. (Meyer *et al.*, 1998). This water uptake may have some advantages, as it does in resin composites, as it can help compensate for the contraction occurring during polymerization and therefore provide a closer adaptation to cavity walls.

Abrasion

Studies investigating the wear resistance of PAMRCs have shown they wear at higher rates than resin composites, although the degree of wear varies depending on the PAMRC tested (Latta *et al.*, 2001). Another study demonstrated that the material Hytac (3M-ESPE) showed a wear rate equal to the resin composite materials evaluated (Frazier *et al.*, 1998). The higher wear rate of PAMRCs has been attributed to the reduced filler loading as well as different polymers in the matrix (Yap *et al.*, 2004).

With the development of Dyract AP (Dentsply), wear resistance was improved by adding a cross-linking monomer and reducing the glass filler particle size (Luo *et al.*, 2002). A toothbrush abrasion study showed the wear of Dyract AP was between microfilled and hybrid composites. This was a marked improvement in abrasion resistance compared with the early versions of PAMRC materials (Turssi *et al.*, 2003). There is no clear conclusion about the pH of the environment the PAMRC might be subjected to. One study has shown PAMRCs abrade more quickly in an acidic environment (Attin *et al.*, 1998), whereas another study using the earlier version of Dyract found no significant differences (Correr *et al.*, 2006).

Mechanical properties

In general, the microhardness, fracture toughness, modulus of elasticity, flexural and compressive strengths of PAMRCs fall between resin composites and glass ionomers. For this reason, these materials have not been recommended for load-bearing restorations in adult teeth, but seem to be a useful alternative tooth-coloured restorative material for primary teeth where long restoration life is not essential.

It would appear that the water absorption of PAMRCs leads to a reduction in flexural strength compared with resin composites (Yap *et al.*, 2000). However, another study showed the flexural strength of F2000 (3M-ESPE) increased after ageing in water (Yap *et al.*, 2002). A similar observation that water ageing increased strength was made for the shear punch strength of

Dyract Posterior (Yap *et al.*, 2003). The flexural strength and elastic flexural modulus of a range of PAMRCs was not affected by storage in either air or water (Meyer *et al.*, 1998).

When subjected to food simulating solutions (water, ethanol, heptane or citric acid) the resin composite materials were significantly stronger than either the PAMRCs and GIC tested, whilst the PAMRCs were stronger than the GIC (Yap *et al.*, 2005). The effect of accelerated ageing in various solutions on a resin composite, a PAMRC and a resin-modified glass ionomer cement demonstrated surface hardness was highest for the PAMRC F2000, whilst the shear punch test strength was lowest for the PAMRC and resin-modified GIC compared with the resin composites (Point 4, Kerr Sybron; Ceram-X, Dentsply) (Bagheri *et al.*, 2007). An investigation of fracture toughness of resin composite, PAMRC and GIC concluded that the fracture toughness of the resin composite and PAMRC significantly decreased as the time of immersion in water increased. The outcome for the GIC was more variable showing decreased fracture toughness at four weeks and then a slight increase after eight weeks (Bagheri *et al.*, 2010).

Polishing

The smoothest surface for PAMRCs, like most other tooth-coloured materials, can be obtained by applying a Mylar strip to the material's surface during polymerization (Rosen *et al.*, 2001). It has been shown that when subjected to polishing with silicon carbide discs and finished with diamond polishing pastes, the surface roughness of the PAMRC tested (F2000) was significantly greater than the two composites used (Z100 and A110, 3M-ESPE). It was concluded that this was due to the average size of the filler particles in the individual materials, that is, the larger the particle size the rougher the surface (Chung and Yap, 2005). This test may not replicate the clinical scenario so well. Other studies have used commercial dental polishing systems. When the 'Enhance system' (rubber polishing points impregnated with aluminium oxide average particle size 100 μm) was used followed by Prisma Gloss pastes it was found that the PAMRC (Dyract AP) was significantly rougher than the resin composite tested (Esthet-X) (Joniot *et al.*, 2006). One study has recommended that the polishing of PAMRC be delayed.

In a recent review paper on the polishing of GIC and PAMRCs in paediatric dentistry, the authors concluded there was still no ideal system available. It seems aluminium oxide coated discs provide the best outcome in laboratory-based studies (Koupis *et al.*, 2007), however, clinical outcomes tend to be more subjective and are influenced by numerous other factors such as size, shape and contour of the restoration evaluated.

8.3.2 Clinical performance

Most clinical evaluations have been carried out on paediatric patients, although there are a few trials on adult patients. A six-year study investigated the clinical performance and wear of two PAMRCs (Lund *et al.*, 2007). Seventy-two restorations in 33 patients were inserted using either F2000 (3M-ESPE) or Dyract AP (Dentsply). After six years, only 27 restorations were available for review. No difference existed between the two materials for colour match, caries, surface roughness and marginal staining. The only point where a slight, but insignificant, difference existed was anatomical form. It was noted that occlusal wear, using the Linefelder test, increased for both materials as the restorations aged. Another two-year study compared a microfilled resin composite (A110, 3M-ESPE) with a compomer (Dyract AP) for restoring anterior approximal cavities (Demirci *et al.*, 2008). A total of 96 restorations were placed in 32 patients. The restorations were evaluated by two persons using modified Ryge criteria. At two years, 90.6% of patients could attend recall with only one restoration of each material needing replacement due to poor colour match and marginal staining. Apart from this, all other restorations were deemed satisfactory at two years based on the criteria of colour match, caries, marginal staining, anatomical form and surface texture. It would seem PAMRC can be a suitable alternative material for restorations that are non-load bearing such as in anterior teeth in adult patients.

A two-year trial investigation of restoration of primary molars looked at four materials, even though the authors reported that only three tooth-coloured materials were used (Daou *et al.*, 2009). The materials used were amalgam (Permite C, SDI Ltd), a PAMRC (Dyract AP, Dentsply), resin-modified GIC (Fuji IILC, GC Corp) and a high viscosity GIC (Fuji IX, GC) (Daou *et al.*, 2009). The study initially included 149 occlusal and posterior approximal restorations (Class II) in 45 patients. At two years only 93 restorations in 31 patients were available for recall. The amalgam restorations survived better than the other three materials. All other materials showed degradation of the margins as well as loss of anatomic form between the one and two year recalls. The posterior approximal (Class II) cavities showed a higher failure rate. However, the authors concluded that the resin-modified GIC 'had the best scores for restoration of primary molars ... in a high caries risk population', thus indicating the PAMRC may not be the ideal material for this group of patients (Daou *et al.*, 2009). A seven-year trial in primary teeth comparing three resin-modified GICs and one PAMRC (Dyract) in the Danish Public Dental Service has been reported (Qvist *et al.*, 2004). This large study, that started with 1565 Class II restorations in 971 children, concluded that any of the materials tested were suitable for the restoration of primary teeth. The median longevity of the restorations was five years (Qvist *et al.*, 2004). The greatest factor related to restoration survival seemed to relate to the clinician rather than the material.

The use of PAMRC for paediatric patients seems a valid treatment option, unless they have a high caries risk. PAMRC can be placed relatively quickly in comparison to traditional bonding with an adhesive and resin composite. Long lasting restorations (e.g. greater than 10 years) is not a high priority for primary teeth. Hence PAMRC does have a place in clinical practice, even for small restorations in adult patients based on current evidence.

8.4 Glass ionomer (polyalkenoate) cements

Glass ionomer cements (GIC) were introduced to the profession in the 1970s after the initial work by Wilson and Kent (1972) and then McClean and Wilson (1977). Since the original cements appeared, a lot of work has been undertaken for improvement including modifications such as the inclusion of resins to form the resin-modified GICs (RM-GIC). Therefore, GICs, as a material, fall into two broad groups, namely conventional GICs and RM-GICs containing a resin monomer that polymerizes in addition to the acid–base setting reaction.

8.4.1 Conventional glass ionomer cement

The original development of GICs started from the idea of using silicate cements and looking at the chemistry of the setting of these materials (Wilson and Prosser, 1982). In addition, their development also arose from the knowledge of zinc polycarboxylate cements that were formed by mixing polyacrylic acid with zinc oxide powder instead of the phosphoric acid used in zinc phosphate cement (Smith, 1968). The subsequent development of GICs saw a modification of the glass powder by melting alumina (Al_2O_3), silicon dioxide (SiO_2), metal oxides, metal fluorides and phosphates to make a fluoroaluminosilicate glass that is mixed and then reacts with a polyacrylic acid (Saito *et al.*, 1999). The powders have been modified further to include calcium, strontium or even zinc. However, even though there may be variation in the glass powder, essentially the GICs remain very similar in terms of reaction and physical characteristics from that originally developed. The term GIC, which has become a commonly used term amongst dentists and researchers is not truly correct. These cements are better referred to as 'glass polyalkenoate cements' (McClean *et al.*, 1994).

Classification

GICs have various uses and because of this Wilson and McClean developed a classification of the cements which is still commonly used (Mount, 1994):

- Type I: luting and bonding materials;
- Type II: restorative, this group has two sub-categories;
  - II.1 restorative aesthetic where highly aesthetic restorations are required;
  - II.2 restorative material where aesthetic concerns are minimal;
- Type III: lining or base cements.

All of the above classifications can be applied to either conventional or resin-modified GICs.

In recent years, the classification has changed a little with the inclusion of the so-called 'packable' or 'high viscosity' materials. These materials usually have a high powder:liquid ratio and the glass powder particle size is smaller than for the other GICs (Guggenberger *et al.*, 1998). They are classed as Type II cements.

Setting reaction

The setting reaction is an acid–base reaction of the glass, which has a common structure of SiO_2-Al_2O_3-CaF_2, although the Ca can be varied to strontium or some other metal. The glass degrades in the presence of the polyalkenoic acid (Wilson and McClean, 1988). The setting reaction is quite complex, however, and in its simplest form it can be described as follows. The hydrogen ions from the acid attack the glass which in turn causes release of metal ions such as Al, Ca or St. These metal ions then combine with the carboxylate groups of the polyalkenoic acid to form a matrix of polyacid salts. In turn the surface of the glass changes, forming a silica hydrogel (Saito *et al.*, 1999). The core of the glass powder particles remains intact with the particle's surface being rich in Si. The initial setting reaction of the GIC takes about 24 hours with the final hardening taking up to seven days to complete (Wasson and Nicholson, 1993).

8.4.2 Physical properties

One of the main advantages of the GICs is their ability to release fluoride ions (Swartz *et al.*, 1984; Mickenautsch *et al.*, 2011; Neelakantan *et al.*, 2011) as well as their ability to interact chemically with tooth structure giving rise to a stable and reliable bond to all parts of the tooth (McClean *et al.*, 1994; Powis *et al.*, 1982; Smith, 1992). Whether or not the fluoride is enough to inhibit caries initiation or progression, the evidence remains less than convincing. One feature that has prevented this group of materials becoming a 'universal' restorative material is its brittle nature and poor wear resistance.

Strength

GICs are brittle materials, showing a lower diametral tensile strength compared with compressive strength. Xie *et al.* (2000) demonstrated that failure occurred more readily by crack propagation when specimens were subjected to tensile rather than compressive stresses.

It has been suggested that the best method for testing the strength of GICs is flexural strength. Peutzfeldt (1996) investigated the flexural strength of seven conventional GICs. It was shown that the powder:liquid ratio is a critical factor in determining the overall strength of set GICs. Therefore it is important to follow the manufacturer's recommended powder:liquid ratio carefully to ensure that the optimum strength of the cement can be achieved (Denisova *et al.*, 2004). It is also important to minimise the degree of porosity so the highest strength possible can be obtained (Kerby and Knobloch, 1992). Thus the method of mixing is important to ensure porosities can be minimised.

A further test method has been suggested as being suitable for testing the strength of GICs. This is the shear punch test where a metal punch is pushed through a disc of the set cement (Roydhouse, 1970). This test method has been used as an alternative to the compressive test, although limited research using this method has been published (Mount *et al.*, 1996; Nomoto *et al.*, 2001). Nevertheless, it would seem this assessment is a suitable technique for evaluating materials and is quite simple to undertake. This test showed that the conventional GICs have the lowest strength compared with other tooth-coloured restorative materials (Bagheri *et al.*, 2007).

Microhardness

Microhardness is another means of evaluating strength. It has been reported that the hardness of GICs is related to the ratio of glass cores (unreacted glass particles) to the surrounding softer matrix. Hardness has also been used to determine the effect of fluids on the surface of GICs, especially water. The greater the water uptake the softer the surface of conventional GICs (Okada *et al.*, 2001). The same study, however, showed that when stored in artificial saliva for up to seven days, the surface hardness increased for the high powder:liquid ratio material, Fuji IX (GC Corp). Although not clear, it was believed the interaction of the ions in the saliva, particularly calcium and phosphate contributed to the increase in surface hardness.

The addition of metal into the GIC has been investigated with the aim of making the GIC stronger (McClean and Gasser, 1985; Yap *et al.*, 2001). This was done by sintering a metal, in this case silver, with the GIC glass to form a 'Cermet'. The polyacid then reacts with the glass–metal powder to form the set GIC (McClean and Gasser 1985). Alternatively, amalgam alloy powder has been added to the GIC powder to make what has been referred to as an admix cement. Beyls *et al.* (1991) showed the compressive strength could be improved but this was dependent on the size and distribution of the particles. However, other studies have shown no difference from other GICs (Mitra and Kedrowski, 1994; Bapna *et al.*, 2002). A study by Williams *et al.* (1992) evaluated flexural strength and demonstrated a reduction in strength, however, others have shown opposing outcomes. Azillah *et al.* (1998) showed an improved flexural strength shortly after the initial set of the cement. Hence, it would seem with respect to strength of the cements, the addition of a metal has little influence.

Erosion

One of the important qualities that needs to be assessed for water-based cements is the possible deterioration of the surface when exposed to various fluids in the oral cavity. Test solutions like acetic, citric and lactic acid have been used to evaluate erosion (Crisp *et al.*, 1980; Fukazawa *et al.*, 1987; Matsuya *et al.*, 1984). GICs have been observed to undergo erosion continuously in the oral cavity (Norman *et al.*, 1969).

Because conventional GICs are moisture sensitive during the initial setting phase, exposure to water at this time can damage and cause erosion of the surface (Gemalmaz *et al.*, 1998; Oilo, 1984). The surrounding pH of a GIC can also effect its erosion, for example, the presence of a cariogenic biofilm may damage/erode a cement surface, especially over the long-term or where saliva may be limited in quantity. Interestingly though, it was shown that as the pH decreased when exposed to lactic acid; dissolution of the GIC resulted in a subsequent increase of the surrounding pH. Hence GICs exhibit the 'side-effect' of having a minor ability to neutralize the effects of acid attack (Nicholson *et al.*, 2000). This effect may also aid the reduction of initiation and progression of dental caries as erosion of the cement will also cause release of fluoride ions to the surrounding environment. When erosion does occur, most damage appears to occur to the matrix of the GIC rather than the glass particles (De Moor *et al.*, 1998; Patel *et al.*, 2000). A recent paper investigating change in surface hardness of a high viscosity GIC used in atraumatic restorative treatment (ART) restorations showed there was no change in Vickers microhardness at the surface compared with cement hardness 90 μm beneath the surface. The specimens were compared with a control of the same GIC stored in water for 720 days. There was no difference in hardness between the control and ten-year clinical specimens (Zanata *et al.*, 2011).

Abrasion

In association with erosion, abrasion of the GIC is also a potential problem compared with other tooth-coloured restorative materials. It has been reported that GICs have a lower abrasion resistance compared with resin composite materials (Shabanian and Richards, 2002). Resistance to abrasion of the GICs has been reported to change as the maturation process continues, that is, the cement is more abrasion resistant once it has fully matured (Mount and Hume, 2005). Metal reinforced GICs have shown much better resistance to abrasion (Forss *et al.*, 1991). Wear (abrasion) resistance can also be improved by modifying the powder:liquid ratio, thus for the high powder:liquid ratio materials such as, Fuji IX (GC Corp) or Ketac Molar (3M-ESPE) a reduction in abrasive wear has been reported (Kunzelmann *et al.*, 2003). There has been a small amount of research investigating the effects of coating GICs and the effect of abrasion resistance. One study showed that if the resin glazing agent, Bellfeel Brightener was applied to the surface of a GIC, the surface hardness increased siginificantly and became more resistant to abrasion (Hotta and Hirukawa, 1994). More recent work investigating a proprietary system of a GIC and resin coating (Equia, GC Corp) which is a combination of Fuji IX restorative material and a nanofilled resin coating (G-Coat Plus) showed that both the strength and wear resistance of the GIC were improved by application of the coating agent. It is believed the resin agent was able to fill porosities and cracks, which therefore reduced crack propagation and thus increased the cement strength (Lohbauer *et al.*, 2001). Similar findings have also been noted when G-Coat Plus was applied to a RM-GIC subjected to a fracture toughness test, the strength was fracture toughness improved, but no such change was observed for the conventional GIC tested (Bagheri *et al.*, 2010).

8.5 Resin-modified glass ionomer cement (RM-GIC)

Researchers searched for a solution to overcome some of the problems of GICs, such as poor early strength, poor aesthetics and early moisture sensitivity. This led to the incorporation of a water-soluble monomer into the cement (Sidhu and Watson, 1995). The resin component in RM-GICs is the hydrophilic monomer, 2-hydroxyethylmethacrylate (HEMA) (Wilson, 1990). The RM-GICs should maintain the acid–base reaction in order to be considered a 'true' RM-GIC, as recent years have seen the introduction of several 'so-called RM-GICs' that have a high resin content which requires polymerization in some form (self or light activation) for the cement mix to set hard (Mount *et al.*, 2009). Current evidence indicates that RM-GICs are the best material for the restoration of non-carious cervical lesions over the long-term in comparison with other resin-based adhesive materials (Peumans *et al.*, 2005; van Dijken and Pallesen, 2008).

8.5.1 Physical properties

Strength

One of the major advantages of RM-GICs over GIC is the early 'command' set and initial high strength that can be achieved. Compressive, flexural and tensile strengths are reported to be higher than GIC (Burgess *et al.*, 1993; Iazetti *et al.*, 2001; Li *et al.*, 1995; Peutzfeldt, 1996; Resistancia, 2003; Sidhu and Watson, 1995; Xie *et al.*, 2000). The improved strength is due to the presence of the HEMA (Mitra, 1991). Xie *et al.* (2000) showed a marked improvement in the diametral tensile and compressive strengths of RM-GICs. To achieve this strength it is essential that the light-polymerization of the cement component is completed in addition to concurrently setting acid–base powder-liquid 'GIC' part of the cement (Li *et al.*, 1995). The acid–base reaction continues to mature in the same manner as conventional GICs. This has been demonstrated in studies investigating changes in strength over time. Shear-punch strength studies showed the RM-GIC strength steadily increased over nine days in one study (Mount *et al.*, 2002) or five days in another (Mount *et al.*, 1996). The strength of the RM-GICs is still not regarded as being great enough to withstand occlusal loads in restorations that replace anatomical features such as marginal ridges or incisal corners of teeth (Mount, 1994).

Hardness

The microhardness of RM-GICs has been reported in most studies to be less than that of resin composite materials (Attin *et al.*, 1996; Bayindir and Yildiz, 2004). When comparing the microhardness of GIC and RM-GIC, conclusions have been quite variable. Most studies seem to indicate, however, that the RM-GICs are not as hard as the conventional GICs (Momoi *et al.*, 1997; Peutzfeldt *et al.*, 1997; Yli-Urpo *et al.*, 2005). Only one study has reported higher microhardness values (McKinney *et al.*, 1987). The reasons for the lower hardness are not clear. It has been suggested that the differences are related to differences in the setting reaction and nature of the matrix (Ellakuria *et al.*, 2003). Others believe the presence of the HEMA in the polymer matrix of the RM-GIC absorbs a greater amount of water leading to an ionomer salt hydrogel that is not as hard as that of conventional GIC matrix (Momoi *et al.*, 1997). A long-term storage study showed the surface hardness of RM-GIC deteriorated over 360 days in an artificial saliva solution (Kanchanavasita *et al.*, 1998). It was speculated that the calcium polyacrylates produced during the set may be vulnerable owing to their solubility. The authors also reported that the plasticization effects of water by continuing the hardening process of the RM-GICs had an effect on the hardness (Kanchanavasita *et al.*, 1998).

Erosion

RM-GICs, like conventional GICs, are susceptible to erosion by various solutions including water. It has been shown that hydrolytic action of water on the surface of RM-GICs occurs leading to erosive loss of material (Cattani-Lorente *et al.*, 1999; Fano *et al.*, 2004). A study by Fano *et al.* (2004) indicated that the length of time of light irradiation influenced the rate of erosion. An irradiation time of less that 15 s caused worse erosion, leading to the opening of cracks. This study also showed that the pH of the solution influenced the rate of erosion. Similar outcomes were noted in the study by Czarnecka and Nicholson (2006). As mentioned for the conventional GICs, one potentially positive effect of increased erosion in an acidic environment is that it has also been demonstrated that the quantity of fluoride ions released increases. (Carey *et al.*, 2003) This may have some effect in helping to reduce demineralization of surrounding tooth tissue, although more research is needed on this point.

Abrasion

The addition of the resin into the RM-GIC has not been shown to improve abrasion resistance. Many studies have reported that the RM-GICs abrade more quickly than GIC (Cho and Cheng, 1999; Xie *et al.*, 2000; Pelka *et al.*, 1996; Momoi *et al.*, 1997; Sunnegardh-Gronberg *et al.*, 2002; Peutzfeldt *et al.*, 1997). This is believed, in part, to be caused by the glass particles being loosely bonded to the matrix as well as their distribution not being uniform throughout the set cement (Xie *et al.*, 2000). This phenomenon was also observed clinically when the wear of a RM-GIC was compared with that of a PAMRC (Chinelatti *et al.*, 2004). A recent study of a 35-day exposure of various restorative materials to pH cycling in a cola drink and artificial saliva showed both the GIC and RM-GIC exibited a greater degree of erosion compared with either the amalgam and resin composite (Honório *et al.*, 2008).

Biofilm formation

A study investigating a 30-day old *Streptococcus mutans* biofilm growth on various aesthetic restorative materials showed increased roughness and decreased hardness for the GIC (Ketac Molar easymix, 3M-ESPE) and RM-GIC (Vitremer, 3M-ESPE) in the biofilm group (Fúcio *et al.*, 2008). No measure was made of whether there was any variation in bioflim growth over the 30 days of the test. The surface degradation was believed to be caused by the production of lactic acid from the *S. mutans*.

Another investigation using *Streptococcus sobrinus* evaluated biofilm formation on various materials, including a GIC (Fuji II, GC Corp) and RM-GIC (Fuji IILC, GC Corp) (Steinberg and Eyal, 2002). They observed the GIC had the lowest affinity of salivary protein adsorption, while the RM-GIC had a greater affinity. It was noted though that the GIC demonstrated the greatest adhesion capability and viability of *S. sobrinus*. The RM-GIC showed an intermediate viability and adhesion level of the bacterial species. However, the authors reported that both GIC 'accumulated most bacteria ... but did not exhibit the highest protein affinity' (Steinberg and Eyal, 2002). It is thought that the increased bacterial numbers were associated with the increased roughness of the GICs. Poggio *et al.* (2009), also investigating *S. mutans* growth on various restorative materials, showed a GIC (Fuji IX, GC Corp) was in the group exhibiting the greatest bacterial adhesion, whereas a GIC with a resin coating (Equia, GC Corp) was in the group showing lower levels of bacterial adhesion. The latter GIC showed a lower surface roughness than the uncoated GIC. They also observed there was no reduced bacterial adhesion even though the GIC released fluoride, which has, in the past, been thought to influence bacterial adhesion. The coated GIC was smoother, so it was concluded that part of the reason why the difference in bacterial adhesion observed was most likely related to the roughness of the material (Poggio *et al.*, 2009).

8.5.2 Clinical performance

This section will discuss clinical evaluation of all GICs, that is, conventional and resin-modified materials. ART (atraumatic restorative treatment) has become a popular method for restoration of teeth in countries where dental facilities may be limited in non-urban regions. GIC is the usual and recommended material of choice for this clinical technique. A recent paper reported the ten-year outcomes of restoration of permanent teeth (Zanata *et al.*, 2011). This study was centred in public health centres in Bauru, Brazil where 167 single surfaced and 107 multi-surface restorations were placed. After ten years only 129 restorations were available for evaluation. Of these, 86.5% of the single surface and 57.6% of the multi-surface restorations were deemed satisfactory using United States Public Health Services (USPHS) criteria. The authors concluded that this method shows the 'potential of the ART approach for restoring and saving posterior permanent teeth' (Zanata *et al.*, 2011).

A similar study using ART on primary teeth over 31 months (range of 6–48 months), but using a RM-GIC, showed using survival analysis that the

25–48 month recall group had a restoration survival rate of 72%. This study also concluded that ART was 'an appropriate treatment option for primary teeth . . .' (Faccin *et al.*, 2009).

A further investigation using RM-GIC in primary molars for indirect pulp capping and restoration over a mean clinical observation time of up to 32 months, showed that 96.5% of the teeth remained asymptomatic and that 76 of the 83 class II restorations were acceptable but exhibited 'varying levels of occlusal wear' (Kotsanos and Arizos, 2011).

The most common clinical evaluation of RM-GICs has been the restoration of non-carious cervical lesions. Much of this work was completed some years ago. A recent two-year study compared a single-bottle etch and rinse resin adhesive system with a RM-GIC. One-hundred percent of RM-GIC restorations were intact for those that could be evaluated at two years (59 of 70 for both materials compared with 78.8% intact resin-based restorations) (Santiago *et al.*, 2010). An extensive review by Peumans *et al.* (2005) also concluded that GICs were the 'best' material for restoration of NCCL when retention was the criterion for success.

Evidence of the inhibition of caries remains unclear. The original analysis by Randall and Wilson (1999) showed 50% of papers they reviewed showed a positive effect whilst the other 50% did not. Another more recent review also has similar conclusions (Weigand *et al.*, 2007). A very recent trial studied a split mouth approach to investigate the use of GIC to prevent early (incipient) caries from occurring (Trairatvorakul *et al.*, 2011). This 12-month study of 7- to 19-year-olds placed a coating on the proximal surfaces of teeth using a high-fluoride content GIC (Fuji VII, GC Corp). Forty-one teeth were coated and a further 41 were control teeth. Radiographs were obtained, digitized and changes were evaluated. A significant reduction in early caries lesion depth was observed for the GIC coated teeth. However, the authors did report that a long-term follow-up was still needed to confirm the overall benefits of such a technique (Trairatvorakul *et al.*, 2011). This study does lend support to the anecdotal evidence that proximal surfaces adjacent to GIC restorations seem to have less caries formation.

8.6 Conclusion

This chapter has covered an overview of adhesive restorative materials currently available for clinical use. Manufacturers are continuing to develop new materials with the aim of simplifying clinical procedures and at the same time creating restorations with greater clinical longevity. One area that is seeing an increase in new materials is the self-adhesive resin composites. These composite restoratives combine the adhesion of the enamel-dentine bonding agents with the qualities of a restorative material. Few data exist with regard to the success or otherwise of this new group of self-adhesive restorative materials. However, should they show successful clinical performance, it will make restorative procedures somewhat simpler, but not necessarily overcome some of the current common problems present in the resin-based materials.

Each of the broad groups of materials introduced have yet to fulfil all of the criteria needed for placing an 'ideal' restoration that is long lasting and can inhibit further caries occurrence. However, each of the materials has its strong and weak points. Until we have created the 'ideal' material, the important point is to select an adhesive restorative material that is most likely to be able to achieve the best clinical outcome for a particular clinical scenario. Hence it is important to know and understand the various aspects of material durability such as strength, shrinkage, hardness and so on when placing restorations with the aim to achieve the greatest longevity.

8.7 References

Anusavice KJ (1996) *Phillips' Science of Dental Materials*, 10th edn, WB Saunders, Philadelphia, USA.

Arrondo JL, Collado MI, I S, Triana R and Ellacuria J (2009) 'Setting reaction of polyacid modified composite resins or compomers'. *Open Dent J*, **16**, 197–201.

Attin T, Vatschki M and Hellwig F (1996) 'Properties of reisn-modified glass-ionomer restorative materials and two polyacid-modified resin composite materials'. *Quintessence Int*, **27**, 203–9.

Attin T, Buchalla W, Trett A and Hellwig E (1998) 'Toothbrushing abrasion of polyacid-modified composites in neutral and acidic buffer solutions'. *J Prosthet Dent*, **80**, 148–50.

Azillah MA, Anstice HM and Pearson GJ (1998) 'Long-term flexural strength of three direct aesthetic restorative materials'. *J Dent*, **26**, 177–82.

Bagheri R, Tyas MJ and Burrow MF (2007) 'Comparison of the effect of storage media on hardness and shear punch strength of tooth-colored restorative materials'. *Am J Dent*, **20**, 329–34.

Bagheri R, Azar MR, Tyas MJ and Burrow MF (2010) 'The effect of aging on the fracture toughness of esthetic restorative materials'. *Am J Dent* **23**, 142–6.

Bapna MS, Gadia CM and Drummond JL (2002) 'Effects of aging and cyclic loading on the mechanical properties of glass ionomer cements'. *Eur J Oral Sci*, 330–4.

Bayindir YZ and Yildiz M (2004) 'Surface hardness properties of resin-modified glass ionomer cements and polyacid modified composite resins'. *J Contemp Dent Pract*, **5**, 42–9.

Bayne SC, Heymann HO and Swift EJ Jr (1994) 'Update on dental composite restorations'. *J Am Dent Assoc* **125**, 687–701.

Berger SB, Palialol ARM, Cavalli V and Giannini M (2011) 'Surface roughness and staining susceptibility of composite resins after finishing and polishing'. *J Esthet Restor Dent*, **23**, 34–45.

Beyls HM, Verbeeck RM, Martens LC and Lemaitre L (1991) 'Compressive strength of some polyalkenoates with or without dental alloy incorporation'. *Dent Mater* **7**, 151–4.

Beyth N, Bahir R, Matalon S, Domb AJ and Weiss EI (2008) '*Streptococcus mutans* biofilm changes surface-topography of resin composites'. *Dent Mater*, **24**, 732–6.
Boaro LC, Goncalves F. Guimarães TC, Ferracane JL, Versluis A and Braga RR (2010) 'Polymerization stress, shrinkage and elastic modulus of current low-shrinkage restorative composites'. *Dent Mater*, **26**, 1144–50.
Bowen RL (1962) *Dental Filling Material Comprising Vinyl Silane Treated Fused Silica and a Binder Consisting of the Reaction Product of Bis Phenol and Glycidyl Acrylate*, US Patent No. 3,066,112.
Braem M, Lambrechts P, Van Doren V and Vanherle G (1986) '*In vivo* evaluation of four posterior composites: quantitative wear measurements and clinical behavior'. *Dent Mater*, **2**, 106–13.
Brosh T, Pilo R and Arcan M (1996) 'Shear modulus – measurement methodology with application of light-cured resin composites'. *Dent Mater*, **12**, 52–7.
Brunthaler A, König F, Lucas T, Sperr W and Schedle A (2003) 'Longevity of direct resin composite restorations in posterior teeth'. *Clin Oral Investig*, **7**, 63–70.
Bryant RW (1979) 'The strength of fifteen amalgam alloys'. *Aus Dent J*, **24**, 244–52.
Burgess JO, Barghi N, Chan DC and Hummert T (1993) 'A comparative study of three glass ionomer base materials'. *Am J Dent*, **6**, 137–41.
Busscher HJ, Rinastiti M, Siswomihardjo W and van der Mei HC (2010) 'Biofilm formation on dental restorative and implant materials'. *J Dent Res*, **89**, 657–65.
Calheiros FC, Braga RR, Kawano Y and Ballester RY (2004) 'Relationship between contraction stress and degree of conversion in restorative composites'. *Dent Mater*, **20**, 939–46.
Carey CM, Spencer M, Give RJ and Eichmiller FC (2003) 'Fluoride release from a resin-modified glass-ionomer cement in a continuous-flow system. Effect of pH'. *J Dent Res*, **82**, 829–32.
Cattani-Lorente MA, Dupuis V, Payan J, Moya F and Meyer JM (1999) 'Effect of water on the physical properties of resin-modified glass ionomer cements'. *Dent Mater*, **15**, 132–7.
Chinelatti MA, Ramos RP, Chimello DT and Palma-Dibb RG (2004) 'Clinical performance of a resin-modified glass ionomer and two polyacid modified resin composites in cervical lesion restorations; 1-year follow-up'. *J Oral Rehabil*, **31**, 251–7.
Cho SY and Cheng AC (1999) 'A review of glass ionomer restorations in the primary dentition'. *J Can Dent Assoc*, **65**, 491–5.
Christensen GJ (1999) 'Sorting out the confusing array of resin-based composites in dentistry'. *J Am Dent Assoc*, **130**, 275–7.
Chung SM and Yap AU (2005) 'Effects of surface finish on indentation modulus and hardness of dental composite restoratives'. *Dent Mater*, **21**, 1008–16.
Combe EC, Shaglouf A-MS, Watts DC and Wilson NHF (1999) 'Mechanical properties of direct core build-up materials'. *Dent Mater*, **15**, 158–65.
Correr GM, Bruschi Alonso RC, Correr Sobrinho L, Puppin-Rontani RM and Ferracane JL (2006) '*In vitro* wear of resin-based materials–simultaneous corrosive and abrasive wear'. *J Biomed Mater Res, Part B*, **78**, 105–14.
Craig RG (1997) *Restorative Dental Materials*, 10th edn, Mosby-Year Book Inc, St Louis, Missouri.
Crisp S, Lewis BG and Wilson AD (1980) 'Characterization of glass-ionomer cements. 6 A study of erosion and water absorption in both neutral and acidic media'. *J Dent*, **8**, 68–72.

Czarnecka B and Nicholson JW (2006) 'Ion release by resin-modified glass ionomer cements into water and lactic acid solutions'. *J Dent*, **34**, 539–43.

Da Costa J, Ferracane J, Paravina RD, Mazur RF and Roeder L (2007) 'The effect of different polishing systems on surface roughness and gloss of various resin composites'. *J Esthet Restor Dent*, **19**, 214–26.

Daou MH, Tavernier B and Meyer JM (2009) 'Two-year clinical evaluation of three restorative materials in primary molars'. *J Clin Pediatr Dent*, **34**, 53–8.

Da Rosa Rodolpho PA, Donassollo TA, Cenci MS, Loguércio AD, Moraes RR, Bronkhorst EM, Opdam NJ and Demarco FF (2011) '22-year clinical evaluation of the performance of two posterior composites with different filler characteristics'. *Dent Mater*, **27**, 955–63.

Davidson CL, de Gee AJ and Feilzer A (1984) 'The competition between the composite-dentin bond strength and the polymerization contraction stress'. *J Dent Res*, **63**, 1396–9.

De Moor RJ and Verveeck RM (1998) 'Effect of acetic acid on the fluoride release profiles of restorative glass ionomer cements'. *Dent Mater*, **14**, 261–8.

Demirci M, Yildiz E and Uysal O (2008) 'Comparative clinical evaluation of different treatment approaches using a microfilled resin composite and a compomer in Class III cavities: two-year results'. *Oper Dent*, **33**, 7–14.

Denisova LA, Maev RG, Poyurovskaya IY, Grineva TV, Denisov AF, Maeva EY and Bakulin EY (2004) 'The use of acoustic microscopy to study the mechanical properties of glass-ionomer cement'. *Dent Mater*, **20**, 358–63.

Eick S, Glockmann E, Brandl B and Pfister W (2004) 'Adherence of Streptococcus mutans to various restorative materials in a continuous flow system'. *J Oral Rehabil*, **31**, 278–85.

Eliades G, Kakaboura A and Palaghias G (1998) 'Acid-base reaction and fluoride release profiles in visible light-cured polyacid-modified composite restoratives (compomers)'. *Dent Mater*, **14**, 57–63.

el-Kalla IH and Garcia-Godoy F (1999) 'Mechanical properties of compomer restorative materials'. *Oper Dent*, **24**, 2–8.

Ellakuria J, Triana R, Minguez N, Soler I, Ibaseta G, Maza J and Garcia-Godoy F (2003) 'Effect of one-year water storage on the surface microhardness of resin-modified versus conventional glass-ionomer cements'. *Dent Mater*, **19**, 286–90.

Faccin ES, Ferreira SH, Kramer PF, Ardenghi TM and Feldens CA (2009) 'Clinical performance of ART restorations in primary teeth: a survival analysis'. *J Clin Pediatr Dent*, **33**, 295–8.

Fano L, Fano V, Ma W, Wang X and Zhu F (2004) 'Hydrolytic degradation and cracks in resin-modified glass-ionomer cements'. *J Biomed Mater Res, Part B*, **69**, 87–93.

Feilzer AJ, de Gee AJ and Davidson CL (1987) 'Setting stress in composite resin in relation to configuration of the restoration'. *J Dent Res*, **66**, 1636–9.

Ferracane JL (2006) 'Is the wear of dental composites still a clinical concern? Is there still a need for *in vitro* wear simulating devices?' *Dent Mater*, **22**, 689–92.

Ferracane JL (2008) 'Buonocore Lecture. Placing dental composites – a stressful experience'. *Oper Dent*, **33**, 247–57.

Ferracane JL (2011) 'Resin composite – state of the art'. *Dent Mater*, **27**(1), 29–38.

Fleming GJ, Cara RR, Palin WM and Burke FJ (2007) 'Cuspal movement and microleakage in premolar teeth restored with resin-based filling materials cured using a 'soft-start' polymerisation protocol'. *Dent Mater*, **23**, 637–43.

Forss H, Seppa I and Lappalainen R (1991) '*In vitro* abrasion resistance and hardness of glass ionomer cements'. *Dent Mater*, **7**, 36–9.

Frazier KB, Reuggeberg FA and Mettenburg DJ (1998) 'Comparison of wear-resistance of Class V restorative materials'. *J Esthet Dent*, **10**, 309–14.

Fúcio SB, Carvalho FG, Sobrinho LC, Sinhoreti MA and Puppin-Rontani RM (2008) 'The influence of 30-day-old *Streptococcus mutans* biofilm on the surface of esthetic restorative materials–an *in vitro* study'. *J Dent*, **36**, 833–9.

Fukuzawa M, Matsuya S and Yamane M (1987) 'Mechanism for erosion of glass-ionomer cements in acidic buffer solution'. *J Dent Res*, **66**, 1770–4.

Gemalmaz D, Yoruc B, Ozcan M and Alkumru HN (1998) 'Effect of early water contact on solubility of glass ionomer luting cements'. *J Prosthet Dent*, **80**, 474–8.

Guggenberger R, May R and Stefan KP (1998) 'New trends in glass-ionomer chemistry'. *Biomaterials*, **19**, 479–83.

Hagger O (1948) 'New catalyst for polymerization of ethylene at room temperature'. *Helv Chim Acta*, **31**, 1624–30.

Hickel R and Manhart J (2001) 'Longevity of restorations in posterior teeth and reasons for failure'. *J Adhes Dent*, **3**, 45–64.

Honório HM, Rios D, Francisconi LF, Magalhães AC, Machado MA and Buzalaf MA (2008) 'Effect of prolonged erosive pH cycling on different restorative materials'. *J Oral Rehabil*, **35**, 947–53

Hotta M and Hirukawa H (1994) 'Abrasion resistance of restorative glass-ionomer cements and a light-cured surface coating'. *Oper Dent*, **19**, 42–6.

Iazetti G, Burgess JO and Gardiner D (2001) 'Selected mechanical properties of fluoride releasing restorative materials'. *Oper Dent*, **26**, 21–6.

Ilie N and Hickel R (2006) 'Silorane-based dental composite: behavior and abilities'. *Dent Mater J*, **25**, 445–54.

Ilie N and Hickel R (2009) 'Investigations on mechanical behaviour of dental composites'. *Clin Oral Invest*, **13**, 427–38.

Ilie N, Felten K, Trixner K, Hickel R and Kunzelmann KH (2005) 'Shrinkage behavior of a resin-based composite irradiated with modern curing units'. *Dent Mater*, **21**, 483–9.

Ikeda M, Matin K, Nikaido T, Foxton RM and Tagami J (2007) 'Effect of surface characteristics on adherence of S. mutans biofilms to indirect resin composites'. *Dent Mater*, **26**, 915–23.

Joniot S, Salomon JP, Dejou J and Grégoire G (2006) 'Use of two surface analyzers to evaluate the surface roughness of four esthetic restorative materials after polishing'. *Oper Dent*, **31**, 39–46.

Kanchanavasita W, Anstice HM and Pearson GJ (1998) 'Long-term surface micro-hardness of resin-modified glass ionomers'. *J Dent*, **26**, 707–12.

Kerby RE and Knobloch L (1992) 'Strength characteristics of glass-ionomer cements'. *Oper Dent*, **17**, 170–4.

Kim KH, Ong JL and Okuno O (2002) 'The effect of filler loading and morphology on the mechanical properties of contemporary composites'. *J Prosthet Dent*. **87**, 642–9.

Kim ME and Park SH (2011) 'Comparison of premolar cuspal deflection in bulk or in incremental composite restoration methods'. *Oper Dent*, **36**, 326–34.

Korkmaz Y, Ozel E, Attar N and Aksoy G (2008) 'The influence of one-step polishing systems on the surface roughness and microhardness of nanocomposites'. *Oper Dent*, **33**, 44–50

Kotsanos N and Arizos S (2011) 'Evaluation of a resin modified glass ionomer serving both as indirect pulp therapy and as restorative material for primary molars'. *Eur Arch Paediatr Dent*, **12**, 170–5.

Koupis NS, Marks LAM, Verbeeck RMH and Martens LC (2007) 'Review: finishing and polishing procedures of (resin-modified) glass ionomers and compomers in paediatric dentistry'. *Eur Arch Paediatr Dent*, **8**, 22–8.

Kunzelmann KH, Burkle V and Bauer C (2003) 'Two-body and three-body wear of glass ionomer cements'. *Int J Paediatr Dent*, **13**, 434–40.

Lambrechts P, Ameye C and Vanherle G (1982) 'Conventional and microfilled composite resins. Part II. Chip fractures'. *J Prosthet Dent*, **48**, 527–38.

Latta MA, Barkmeier WW, Wilwerding TM and Blake SM (2001) 'Localized wear of compomer restorative materials'. *Am J Dent*, **14**, 238–40.

Leinfelder KF, Wilder AD Jr and Teixeira LA (1986) 'Wear rates of posterior composite resins'. *J Am Dent Assoc*, **112**, 829–33.

Li J, von Beetzen M and Sundstrom F (1995) 'Strength and setting behavior of resin-modified glass ionomer cements'. *Acta Odont Scand*, **53**, 311–17.

Loguercio AD, Reis A and Ballester RY (2004) 'Polymerization shrinkage: effects of constraint and filling technique in composite restorations'. *Dent Mater*, **20**, 236–43.

Lohbauer U, Krämer N, Siedschlag G, Schubert EW, Lauerer B, Müller FA, Petschelt A and Ebert J (2011) 'Strength and wear resistance of a dental glass-ionomer cement with a novel nanofilled resin coating'. *Am J Dent*, **24**, 124–8.

Lund RG, Sehn FP, Piva E, Detoni D, Moura FR, Cardoso PE and Demarco FF (2007) 'Clinical performance and wear resistance of two compomers in posterior occlusal restorations of permanent teeth: six-year follow-up'. *Oper Dent*, **32**, 118–23.

Luo Y, Lo EC, Fang DT, Smales RJ and Wei SH (2002) 'Clinical evaluation of Dyract AP restorative in permanent molars: 2-year results'. *Am J Dent*, **15**, 403–6.

Lutz F, Phillips RW, Rouilet JF and Imfeld T (1983) 'Composites – classification and assessment'. *SSO: Schweitz Monatsschr Zahnheilkd*, **93**, 914–29.

Mair LH (1999) 'The silver sorption layer in dental composites: three year results'. *Dent Mater*, **15**, 408–12.

Manhart J, Kunzelmann KH, Chen HY and Hickel R (2000) 'Mechanical properties of new composite restorative materials'. *J Biomed Mater Res*, **53**, 353–61.

Manhart J, Chen H, Hamm G and Hickel R (2004) 'Buonocore Memorial Lecture. Review of the clinical survival of direct and indirect restorations in posterior teeth of the permanent dentition'. *Oper Dent*, **29**, 481–508.

Martin N and Jedynakiewicz N (1998) 'Measurement of water sorption in dental composites'. *Biomaterials*, **19**, 77–83.

Matsuya S, Matsuya Y, Yamamoto Y and Yamane M (1984) 'Erosion process of a glass ionomer cement in organic acids'. *Dent Mater J*, **3**, 210–19.

McClean JW and Gasser O (1985) 'Glass–cermet cements'. *Quintessence Int*, **16**, 333–43.

McClean JW and Wilson AD (1977) 'The clinical development of the glass-ionomer cement III. The erosion lesion'. *Aust Dent J*, **22**, 190–5.

McClean JW, Nicholson JW and Wilson AD (1994) 'Proposed nomenclature for glass ionomer dental cements and related materials'. *Quintessence Int*, **25**, 587–9.

McKinney JE, Antonucci JM and Rupp NW (1987) 'Wear and microhardness of glass ionomer cements'. *J Dent Res*, **66**, 1134–9.

Meyer JM, Cattani-Lorente MA and Dupuis V (1998) 'Compomers: between glass-ionomer cements and composites'. *Biomaterials*, **19**, 529–39.

Mickenautsch S, Mount G and Yengopal V (2011) 'Therapeutic effect of glass-ionomers: an overview of evidence'. *Aust Dent J*, **56**, 10–15.

Mitra SB (1991) 'Adhesion to dentin and physical properties of a light-cured glass-ionomer liner/base'. *J Dent Res*, **70**, 72–4.

Mitra SB and Kedrowski BL (1994) 'Long-term mechanical properties of glass ionomers'. *Dent Mater*, **10**, 78–82.

Momoi Y, Hirosaki K, Kohno A and McCabe JF (1997) '*In vitro* toothbrush-dentifrice abrasion of resin-modified glass ionomers'. *Dent Mater*, **13**, 82–8.

Montanaro L, Campoccia D, Rizzi S, Donati ME, Breschi L, Prati C and Arciola CR (2004) 'Evaluation of bacterial adhesion of Streptococcus mutans on dental restorative materials'. *Biomaterials*, **25**, 4457–63.

Mount GJ (1994) *An Atlas of Glass Ionomer Cements. A Clinician's Guide*. 2nd edn, Martin Dunitz, London.

Mount GJ and Hume WR (2005) *Preservation and Restoration of Tooth Structure*. 2nd edn, Knowledge Boos and Software, Queensland.

Mount GJ and Makinson OF and Peters MC (1996) 'The strength of auto-cured and light-cured materials. The shear punch test'. *Aust Dent J*, **41**, 118–23.

Mount GJ, Patel C and Makinson OF (2002) 'Resin-modified glass-ionomers: strength, cure depth and tarnsluncency'. *Aust Dent J*, **47**, 339–43.

Mount GJ, Tyas MJ, Ferracane JL, Nicholson JW, Berg JH, Simonsen RJ and Ngo HC (2009) 'A revised classification for direct tooth-colored restorative materials'. *Quintessence Int*, **40**, 691–7.

Neelakantan P, John S, Anand S, Sureshbabu N and Subbarao C (2011) 'Fluoride release from a new glass-ionomer cement'. *Oper Dent*, **36**, 80–5.

Nicholson JW and Alsarheed M (1998) 'Changes on storage of polyacid-modified composite resins'. *J Oral Rehabil*, **25**, 616–20.

Nicholson JW, Millar BJ, Czarnecka B and Limanowska-Shaw H (1999) 'Storage of polyacid-modified resin composites ("compomers") in lactic acid solution'. *Dent Mater*, **15**, 413–16.

Nicholson JW, Aggarwal A, Czarnecka B and Limanowska-Shaw H (2000) 'The rate of change of pH of lactic acid exposed to glass-ionomer dental cements'. *Biomaterials*, **21**, 1989–93.

Nomoto R, Carrick TE and McCabe JF (2001) 'Suitability of a shear punch test for dental restorative materials'. *Dent Mater*, **17**, 415–21.

Norman RD, Swartz ML, Phillips RW and Virmani R (1969) 'A comparison of the intraoral disintegration of three dental cements'. *J Am Dent Assoc*, **78**, 777–82.

Oilo G (1984) 'Early erosion of dental cements'. *Scand J Dent Res*, **92**, 539–43.

Okada K, Tosaki S, Hirota K and Hume WR (2001) 'Surface hardness change of restorative materials stored in saliva'. *Dent Mater*, **17**, 34–9.

Opdam NJM, Bronkhurst EM, Loomans BAC and Huysmans M-CDNJM (2010) '12-year survival of composite *vs* amalgam restorations'. *J Dent Res*, **89**, 1063–7.

Opdam NJ, Bronkhorst EM, Cenci MS, Huysmans MC and Wilson NH (2011) 'Age of failed restorations: A deceptive longevity parameter'. *J Dent*, **39**, 225–30.

Palaniappan S, Bharadwaj D, Mattar DL, Peumans M, Van Meerbeek B and Lambrechts P (2011) 'Nanofilled and microhybrid composite restorations: Five-year clinical wear performances'. *Dent Mater*, **27**, 692–700.

Pallesen U and Qvist V (2003) 'Composite resin fillings and inlays. An 11-year evaluation'. *Clin Oral Investig*, **7**, 71–9.
Patel M, Tawfik H, Myint Y, Brocklehurst D and Nicholson JW (2000) 'Factors affecting the ability of dental cements to alter pH of lactic acid solutions'. *J Oral Rehabil*, **27**, 1030–3.
Peez R and Frank S (2006) 'The physical-mechanical performance of the new Ketac Molar easymix compared to commercially available glass ionomer restoratives'. *J Dent*, **34**, 582–7.
Pelka M, Ebert J, Schneider H, Kramer N and Petschelt A (1996) 'A comparison of two- and three-body wear of glass ionomers and composites'. *Eur J Oral Sci*, **104**, 132–7.
Periera CA, Eskelson E, Cavalli V, Liporoni PCS, Jorge AOC and do Rego MA (2011) 'Streptococcus mutans biofilm adhesion on composite resin surfaces after different finishing and polishing techniques'. *Oper Dent*, **36**, 311–17.
Peumans M, Kanumilli P, De Munck J, Van Landuyt K, Lambrechts P and Van Meerbeek B (2005) 'Clinical effectiveness of contemporary adhesives: a systematic review of current clinical trials'. *Dent Mater*, **21**, 864–81.
Peutzfeldt A (1996) 'Compomers and glass ionomers bond strength to dentin and mechanical properties'. *Am J Dent*, **9**, 259–63.
Peutzfeldt A, Garcia-Godoy F and Asmussen E (1997) 'Surface hardness and wear of glass ionomers and compomers'. *Am J Dent*, **10**, 15–17.
Poggio C, Arciola CR, Rosti F, Scribante A, Saino E and Visai L (2009) 'Adhesion of Streptococcus mutans to different restorative materials'. *Int J Artif Organs*, **32**, 671–7.
Powis DR, Folleras T, Merson SA and Wilson AD (1982) 'Improved adhesion of a glass ionomer cement to dentin and enamel'. *J Dent Res*, **61**, 1416–22.
Qvist V, Laurberg L, Poulsen A and Teglers PT (2004) 'Class II restorations in primary teeth: 7-year study on three resin-modified glass ionomer cements and a compomer'. *Eur J Oral Sci*, **112**, 188–96.
Randall RC and Wilson NH (1999) 'Glass-ionomer restoratives: a systematic review of a secondary caries treatment effect'. *J Dent Res*, **78**, 628–37.
Resistencia A (2003) 'Diametral tensile strength and water sorption of glass ionomer cements used in atraumatic restorative treatment'. *J Appl Oral Sci*, **11**, 96–101.
Rosen M, Grossman ES, Cleaton-Jones PE and Volchansky A (2001) 'Surface roughness of aesthetic restorative materials: an *in vitro* comparison'. *SADJ*, **56**, 316–20.
Roydhouse RH (1970) 'Punch-shear test for dental purposes'. *J Dent Res*, **49**, 131–6.
Saito S, Tosaki T and Hirota K (1999) 'Characteristic of glass-ionomer cements'. In: *Advances in Glass-ioinomer Cements*. Davidson CL and Mjor I (eds), Quintessence Publishing Carol Stream IL, USA.
Sakaguchi RL and Berge HX (1998) 'Reduced light energy density decreases post-gel contraction while maintaining degree of conversion in composites'. *J Dent*, **26**, 695–700.
Santiago SL, Passos VF, Vieira AH, Navarro MF, Lauris JR and Franco EB (2010) 'Two-year clinical evaluation of resinous restorative systems in non-carious cervical lesions'. *Braz Dent J*, **21**, 229–34.
Shabanian M and Richards LC (2002) '*In vitro* wear rates of materials under different loads and varying pH'. *J Prosthet Dent*, **87**, 650–6.

Sidhu SK and Watson TF (1995) 'Resin-modified glass ionomer materials. A status report for the American Journal of Dentistry'. *Am J Dent*, **8**, 59–67.

Silva CM and Dias KRHC (2009) 'Compressive strength of esthetic restorative materials polymerized with quartz-tungsten-halogen light and blue LED'. *Braz Dent J*, **20**, 54–7.

Small IC, Watson TF, Chadwick AV and Sidhu SK (1998) 'Water sorption in resin-modified glass-ionomer cements: an *in vitro* comparison with other materials'. *Biomaterials*, 19, 545–50.

Smith DC (1968) 'A new dental cement'. *Br Dent J*, **124**, 381–4.

Smith DC (1992) 'Polyacrylic acid-based cements: adhesion to enamel and dentin'. *Oper Dent*, **5**, 177–183.

Söderholm KJ (2007) 'Dental adhesives ... how it all started and later evolved'. *J Adhes Dent Suppl*, **2**, 227–30.

Stansbury JW, Trujillo-Lemon M, Lu H, Ding X, Lin Y and Ge J (2005) 'Conversion-dependent shrinkage stress and strain in dental resins and composites'. *Dent Mater*, **21**, 57–67.

Steinberg D and Eyal S (2002) 'Early formation of *Streptococcus sobrinus* biofilm on various dental restorative materials'. *J Dent*, **30**, 47–51.

Sunnegardh-Gronberg K, Peutzfeldt A and van Dijken JW (2002) 'Hardness and *in vitro* wear of a novel ceramic restorative cement'. *Eur J Oral Sci*, **110**, 175–8.

Swartz ML, Phillips RW and Clark HE (1984) 'Long-term F release from glass ionomer cements'. *J Dent Res*, **63**, 158–60.

Trairatvorakul C, Itsaraviriyakul S and Wiboonchan W (2011) 'Effect of glass-ionomer cement on the progression of proximal caries'. *J Dent Res*, **90**, 99–103.

Turssi CP, Hara AT, de Magalhães CS, Serra MC and Rodrigues AL Jr (2003) 'Influence of storage regime prior to abrasion on surface topography of restorative materials'. *J Biomed Mater Res, Part B*, **65**, 227–32.

Tyas MJ (2000) 'Three-year clinical evaluation of a poly-acid modified resin composite (Dyract)'. *Oper Dent*, **25**, 152–4.

UNEP (2008). *United Nations Environmental Program: Awareness Package Module 4: Mercury Use in Healthcare Settings and Dentistry*. www.unep.org

van Dijken JW (2000) 'Direct resin composite inlays/onlays: an 11-year follow-up'. *J Dent*, **28**, 299–306.

van Dijken JW and Pallesen U (2008) 'Long-term retention of etch-and-rinse adhesives and a resin-modified glass ionomer cement in non-carious cervical lesions.' *Dent Mater*, **24**, 915–22.

van Dijken JW and Pallesen U (2011) 'Clinical performance of a hybrid resin composite with and without an intermediate layer of flowable resin composite: a 7-year evaluation'. *Dent Mater*, **27**, 150–6.

Van Nieuwenhuysen JP, D'Hoore W, Carvalho J and Qvist V (2003) 'Long-term evaluation of extensive restorations in permanent teeth'. *J Dent*, **31**, 395–405.

Wasson EA and Nicholson JD (1993) 'New aspects of the setting of glass-ionomer cements'. *J Dent Res*, **72**, 481–3.

Weinmann W, Thalacker C and Guggenbergeer R (2005) 'Siloranes in dental composites'. *Dent Mater*, **21**, 68–74.

Wiegand A, Buchalla W and Attin T (2007) 'Review on fluoride-releasing restorative materials–fluoride release and uptake characteristics, antibacterial activity and influence on caries formation'. *Dent Mater*, **23**, 343–62.

Willems G, Lambrechts P, Braem M, Celis JP and Vanherle G (1992) 'A classification of dental composites according to their morphological and mechanical characteristics'. *Dent Mater*, **8**, 310–19.

Williams PT (1980) 'Microfill resins'. *J Can Dent Assoc*, **46**, 665–7.

Williams JA, Billington RW and Pearson GJ (1992) 'The comparative strengths of commercial glass-ionomer cements with and without metal additions'. *Br Dent J*, **172**, 279–82.

Wilson AD (1990) 'Resin-modified glass ionomer cements'. *Int J Prosthodont*, **3**, 425–9.

Wilson AD and Kent BE (1972) 'A new translucent cement for dentistry. The glass ionomer cement'. *Br Dent J*, **132**, 133–5.

Wilson AD and McClean JW (1988) *Glass Ionomer Cement*. Chicago Quintessence Publishing, Chicago.

Wilson AD and Prosser HJ (1982) 'Biocompatability of the glass ionomer cement'. *J Dent Assoc S Afr*, **37**, 872–9.

Xie D, Brantley WA, Culbertson BM and Wang G (2000) 'Mechanical properties and microstructures of glass ionomer cements'. *Dent Mater*, **16**, 129–38.

Yap AU, Tan DT, Goh BK, Kuah HG and Goh M (2000) 'Effect of food-simulating liquids on the flexural strength of composite and polyacid-modified composite restoratives'. *Oper Dent*, **25**, 202–8.

Yap AU, Teo JC and Teoh SH (2001) 'Comparative wear resistance of reinforced glass ionomer restorative materials'. *Oper Dent*, **26**, 343–8.

Yap AU, Chandra SP, Chung SM and Lim CT (2002) 'Changes in flexural properties of composite restoratives after aging in water'. *Oper Dent*, **27**, 468–74.

Yap AU, Lee MK, Chung SM, Tsai KT and Lim CT (2003) 'Effect of food-simulating liquids on the shear punch strength of composite and polyacid-modified composite restoratives'. *Oper Dent*, **28**, 529–34.

Yap AU, Tan CH and Chung SM (2004) 'Wear behavior of new composite restoratives'. *Oper Dent*, **29**, 269–74.

Yap AU, Lim LY, Yang TY, Ali A and Chung SM (2005) 'Influence of dietary solvents on nanofill and ormocer composites'.*Oper Dent*, **30**, 129–33.

Yli-Urpo H, Lassila LV, Narhi T and Vallitu PK (2005) 'Compressive strength and surface characterization of glass ionomer cements modified by particles of bioactive glass'. *Dent Mater*, **21**, 201–9.

Yoshikawa T, Burrow MF and Tagami J (2001) 'The effects of bonding system and light curing method on reducing stress of different C-factor cavities'. *J Adhes Dent*, **3**, 177–83.

Yoshikawa T, Nakaoki Y, Takada T, Burrow MF and Tagami J (2003) 'Effect of light-curing method and irradiation time on marginal sealing and cavity wall adaptation of resin composite restorations'. *Am J Dent*, Spec No 63A-67A.

Young AM, Rafeeka SA and Howlett JA (2004) 'FTIR investigation of monomer polymerisation and polyacid neutralisation kinetics and mechanics in various aesthetic dental restorative materials'. *Biomaterials*, **25**, 823–33.

Yüzügüllü B, Ciftci Y, Saygili G and Canay S (2008) 'Diametral tensile compressive strengths of several types of core materials'. *J Prosthodont*, **17**, 102–7.

Zanata RL, Fagundes TC, Freitas MC, Lauris JR and Navarro MF (2011) 'Ten-year survival of ART restorations in permanent posterior teeth'. *Clin Oral Investig*, **15**, 265–71.

9

Antibacterial composite restorative materials for dental applications

IDRIS MOHAMED MEHDAWI, Benghazi University, Libya and ANNE YOUNG, UCL Eastman Dental Institute, UK

DOI: 10.1533/9780857096432.3.270

Abstract: This chapter begins with a brief discussion of the factors involved in dental caries and the general limitations of current aesthetic restorative materials. It reviews the antibacterial activity of current commercial aesthetic dental materials and the methods employed for their evaluation. Thereafter, various different approaches used to develop an aesthetic dental material that might reduce the risk of bacterial microleakage and secondary caries are described. Furthermore, the chapter discusses calcium phosphate-based dental composites, their limitations and potential carious dentine remineralisation activity. Finally, recently formulated dental composites containing reactive calcium phosphate fillers and chlorhexidine (which is both antimicrobial and a matrix metalloproteinase inhibitor) are discussed.

Key words: antibacterial adhesive materials, reactive calcium phosphates, remineralizing composites.

9.1 Introduction

With improvements in aesthetic restorative materials and increasing patient demand for 'white fillings', resin-based composites and glass ionomer cements (GIC) have now largely replaced the use of dental amalgam. A major weakness, however, of these aesthetic materials is the restoration tooth interface (hybrid bonding region). After damage, bacterial microleakage and secondary caries beneath the restoration can occur. This is the main cause of dental restoration replacement.

It has been stated that 'the treatment of carious teeth by insertion of simple direct restorations costs the NHS in England and Wales about £173 million per year'.[1] The replacement of fillings accounts for 60% of all restorative work.[2] Furthermore, it has been reported that restoration replacement consumes 60–75% of dentists' operating time.[3] The replacement of restorations tends to involve additional reduction of remaining tooth structures with potential effects on the longevity of the restoration and health of pulpal tissues. Subsequently, the tooth may require endodontic management with further substantial increase in treatment costs.

Restorative materials with antibacterial and remineralizing properties could help overcome these issues.

In this chapter, a brief introduction to factors affecting caries and current aesthetic dental material limitations is first described. Thereafter, mechanisms for producing antibacterial materials followed by remineralizing restorative materials are reviewed. Finally, new composites, with potential antibacterial, enzyme inhibiting and remineralizing capacity are discussed.

9.2 Current direct aesthetic restorative materials

9.2.1 Etiological factors involved in dental caries

The main aetiological factors involved in dental caries are the dental biofilm (dental plaque), dietary and salivary factors. A dental biofilm is a community of microorganisms, embedded in extracellular matrix that adheres to the surface of the tooth.[4] It can be classified as either supra- or sub-gingival. The development of the dental biofilm occurs by a sequence of events including the formation of salivary pellicle, bacterial adhesion to the pellicle and co-adhesion and co-aggregation of secondary colonizers.[5,6]

Although the dental biofilm is known to be essential for caries formation, most of the bacteria present are not an etiologic factor. Only specific cariogenic microorganisms are involved in the carious process. Among the various biofilm communities, several microorganisms, including *Streptococcus mutans*, *Lactobacilli* and *Actinomyces* species, have been correlated with the cariogenicity of the dental biofilm.[7–9]

Dietary carbohydrate is essential for bacteria to produce acids that initiate demineralization of tooth structure. Sucrose, being readily fermentable by oral bacteria, is the most important carbohydrate to consider.[10] In addition, sucrose is required by bacteria for production of an intracellular and extracellular polysaccharide matrix.[11] The latter is a contributing factor to bacterial adhesion to the tooth surface and in establishing the biofilm microstructure.[12] There are well-known correlations between sucrose exposure and prevalence of dental caries.[13]

Caries initiation and progression is affected by salivary flow rate and composition. Saliva has a buffering capacity that contributes to neutralization of acids generated by bacteria.[14] In addition, the calcium, phosphate and fluoride content of saliva can help in remineralization activity. Once salivary secretion function is impaired (xerostomia), the risk of dental caries is enhanced.[15]

9.2.2 Dental biofilm adhesion to direct restorative materials

A dental biofilm can develop on the surface of various restorative materials, in a similar sequence to that on tooth surfaces. This biofilm can initiate the process of secondary caries either at the tooth surface or at the tooth restoration interface. Higher levels of more cariogenic biofilms have been observed on the surfaces of composite resin compared to other restorative materials, such as amalgam and glass ionomers.[16–19] This is mainly due to the limited antibacterial action of composite resin.[20] In addition, use of composite restorations in sub-gingival spaces (instead of perhaps with GIC) may enhance the incidence of periodontal diseases.[21] Furthermore, it has been reported that the resin component of composite may increase the growth of some cariogenic species.[22] Therefore, the composite resins develop secondary caries at higher rates than any other restorative materials.[23]

9.2.3 Current direct aesthetic restorative material limitations

Composites are essentially composed of an organic resin matrix, inorganic filler and silane agent which bonds the two parts together. They are bonded to the tooth using various procedures usually involving acid-containing resin-based adhesives. Dental composite polymerization shrinkage, however, affects bonding integrity and can lead to gaps at the adhesive/tooth interface. These gaps increase the possibility of bacterial microleakage[24] leading to discoloration of the restoration, hypersensitivity of restored teeth, secondary caries and pulpal inflammation.

Conventional glass ionomer cements (GICs) consist of fluoroaluminosilicate glass fillers and an aqueous solution of polyalkenoic acid. They set via an acid–base reaction mechanism.[25] These materials exhibit early moisture sensitivity,[26] delays in final strength development and low mechanical properties.[27,28] Therefore, their use is limited to non-stress bearing areas.[29]

Resin-modified glass ionomer cements (RMGICs) are chemically similar to conventional GICs, but with additional photopolymerizable monomers, frequently 2-hydroxyethylmethacrylate (HEMA).[30] The RMGICs are vulnerable to some of the limitations of resin-based materials, including polymerization shrinkage and heat generation. The mechanical properties of RMGICs are, however, still generally below those of the composite.[31]

Compomers or polyacid-modified composite resins were introduced to overcome the low mechanical properties and moisture sensitivity of GICs. The compomers however, exhibit lower mechanical properties compared to dental composites.[32] They are therefore mostly indicated for restoration of primary teeth or non-stress bearing areas.

9.3 Antibacterial properties of aesthetic restorative materials

9.3.1 Assessment of restorative material antibacterial activity

Several methods have been used to assess the antibacterial activity of dental restorative materials, mostly through measurement of the minimum inhibitory concentration (MIC),[33] direct contact and agar diffusion tests.[18,34–36] The later test is readily available, inexpensive and widely accepted as a simple screening method. It has been used to evaluate the antibacterial activity of materials that release water-soluble components in surrounding medium. The direct contact test is largely used to quantify the ability of materials to inhibit bacterial growth upon surface contact. Unfortunately, these assays may poorly reflect the actual status in an oral cavity. Here the bacteria exist as a biofilm with increased resistance to antibacterial agents. The constant depth film fermentor (CDFF), however, was developed to grow microbial biofilms in the laboratory, under controlled conditions. This model is particularly suitable for studying antibacterial properties of restorative materials as it enables biofilms similar to those in the oral cavity to be grown on their surfaces.[37]

9.3.2 Dental composites

Studies carried out on conventional, cured dental composites have revealed little or no antibacterial activity.[18,35,38] This is to be expected as the ingredients of dental composites have no[22,39–41] or very low antibacterial action.[40,42]

9.3.3 Dental adhesives

Several ingredients of dental adhesives may exhibit antibacterial activity. Examples include glutaraldehyde and acidic comonomers. Glutaraldehyde was primarily incorporated into dental adhesives to enhance the bond strength and reduce the risk of postoperative hypersensitivity.[43,44] *In vivo* studies have shown, however, that dental adhesives containing glutaraldehyde could eliminate a variety of cariogenic bacteria.[45,46] This antibacterial activity was attributed to glutaraldehyde release. Unfortunately, glutaraldehyde, is known to induce toxic effects,[47] which has given major concern regarding its use in clinical applications.

Methacrylate monomers containing phosphoric and carboxylic acid groups are incorporated into many composite adhesives. The acidity enables partial dentine demineralization generating a rough surface into which the adhesive can penetrate and bond via micromechanical interlocking.[48] Studies have shown that some uncured adhesive components have antibacterial activity against cariogenic bacteria.[49,50] This antibacterial activity was attributed to low pH. It is, however, significantly reduced after light curing or buffering by dentinal fluid.[41,51] It may therefore contribute to eradication of residual bacteria in the cavity but is unlikely to affect longer term bacterial microleakage. In addition, the bactericidal effect was not observed with *Lactobacillus casei*[49] which are known to be acid tolerant and cariogenic bacteria.

9.3.4 Glass ionomer cements

Several *in vitro* studies have provided evidence that glass ionomers can inhibit the growth of known cariogenic species.[52–54] Various other studies, however, have given conflicting results about the antibacterial benefits of GICs.[55–57] This was attributed to the decline of fluoride release with time and increase in material surface roughness. The GICs potentially reduce bacterial microleakage through a combination of an initial lower pH of freshly mixed cement, fluoride and other element release, direct adhesion to enamel and dentine[52–54] and minimal dimensional change during set.[54] Although these materials release fluoride, their anticariogenic effects have been attributed to formation of less soluble fluoroapatite more than to direct antibacterial action.[58] Recurrent caries, however, still remains the main cause for GIC restoration replacement.[58]

9.3.5 Compomers

Several studies have been carried out to evaluate the antibacterial properties of compomers *in vitro*.[59–64] Many studies, however, revealed that compomers have no or limited antibacterial effect against cariogenic bacteria *in vitro*[60,62] *in situ*[63] and *in vivo*.[64] The compomers mainly behave as composites rather than GICs.[65] They exhibit comparable polymerization shrinkage behaviour to composites[66] but low fluoride release.[59] The compomers are therefore not an ideal material solution to the problem of bacterial microleakage and secondary caries at the tooth restoration interface.

9.3.6 Clinical implications for antibacterial restorative materials

Mechanical and thermal stresses over time further enhance composite restoration microgaps, bacterial microleakage and the need for replacement.[67–69] Infiltration of the composite adhesives into the demineralized collagen network can also be incomplete.[70] This enables nanoleakage[71] and penetration of fluids and bacterial byproducts with subsequent degradation of the resin adhesive[72] and collagen fibrils.[73] This ultimately leads to deterioration of the dentine bond.[74,75]

An increasingly used approach in modern management of carious lesions relies on removal of only outer infected dentine, whilst inner remineralizable dentine is conserved.[76] The presence of residual caries within this dentine further increases the risk of reinfection and secondary caries. Whilst this is less of a risk with GIC use, these can only be used in small cavities owing to their low strength. Antibacterial inclusion in dental adhesives or composites might provide a solution.

9.3.7 Antibacterial composite resin

To obtain dental composites with antibacterial activity, various modifications have been attempted.

Direct addition of antibacterial agents

Various antibacterial agents, such as chlorhexidine, triclosan and benzalkonium chloride (BAC), have been incorporated into both commercial and experimental dental composites.

- Triclosan (2,4,4-trichloro-2-hydroxidiphenilethere): triclosan is a wide spectrum antibacterial agent that inhibits bacterial growth by interfering with their enzymatic activities.[77] Composites containing 1 wt% triclosan have been found to inhibit growth of *S. mutans*.[78]
- Benzalkonium chloride (BAC): BAC is a wide spectrum quaternary ammonium antibacterial agent that has been used in various dental composites.[79,80] It is cationically charged and induces antibacterial action through attraction to the negatively charged bacterial membrane.[81] Dental composite containing 0.25–2.5 wt% BAC exhibited antibacterial activity on *S. mutans* and *S. sorbinus*.[80] In addition, the mechanical properties, which are commonly reduced by component addition to and/or release from composites, were not affected.
- Chlorhexidine (CHX): Incorporation of either chlorhexidine gluconate or dihydrochloride into dental composites inhibited the growth of tested bacterial strains.[82] These authors, however, reported a decline in the mechanical properties with use of chlorhexidine gluconate. Other composites containing chlorhexidine diacetate had reduced oral biofilm growth on their surfaces after up to one week in a CDFF when compared with controls without chlorhexidine or commercial fluoride-releasing materials.[83] This study, however, relied upon addition of hydrophilic monomers to encourage water sorption to promote antibacterial

release. This strategy, however, usually leads to mechanical property deterioration. New approaches are therefore critical for the production of an effective antibacterial restorative material.

Immobilized antibacterial monomer

The antibacterial monomer 12-methacryloyloxydodecylpyridinium bromide (MDPB) is a quaternary amine derivative with a positive charge, which is attracted to and disrupts the negatively charged bacterial cell wall.[84] On curing, MDPB monomer copolymerizes with other methacrylate-based monomers in any resin phase. Dental composites containing 0.2–0.5 wt% MDPB monomer showed effective antibacterial effect with no adverse changes on mechanical, chemical and biological properties.[85–87] These antibacterial composites, however, unlike released antibacterial agents, can only act upon surface contact and are therefore unlikely to inhibit recurrent caries.

Silver-containing dental composites

The bactericidal effect of silver ions has been attributed to their interference with bacterial enzymatic activity.[88] Dental composites containing either silver–glass fillers, silver–apatite, silver–zeolite, silver–zirconium phosphate or silver–silica gel exhibited effective antibacterial properties.[89–96] In order to achieve this antibacterial property, the silver–apatite and silver–zeolite fillers had to be minimally loaded at 10 and 20 wt%, respectively. At these concentrations, however, the mechanical properties and colour stability are affected. Incorporation of silver–zirconium phosphate or silver–silica gel into composites had no adverse effect on mechanical properties. These composites, however, exhibited their antibacterial activity only upon direct contact with bacteria.

Antibacterial prepolymerized resin fillers

A filler system consisting of prepolymerized resin fillers (PPRF) with immobilized MDPB was investigated. This filler system contained milled prepolymerized methacrylate and antibacterial MDPB monomers (at 15.8 wt%) with glass silica particles.[97] A dental composite with 17.9 wt% PPRF suppressed accumulation of *S. mutans in vitro*.[98] This was attributed to interference with bacterial adhesion, glucan synthesis and bacterial growth. In addition, the authors reported no elution of unpolymerized MDPB. Furthermore, incorporation of this filler had no effect on either surface roughness or hydrophobicity, which are known contributing factors affecting adhesion of bacterial biofilms to surfaces.[99,100]

Polyethylenimine nanoparticles

Polyethylenimine (PEI) has quaternary ammonium groups that can exhibit antibacterial action through disruption of the bacterial cell membrane.[101] Dental composites containing 1 or 2 wt% PEI nanoparticles could strongly inhibit surface bacterial growth but gave no inhibition zones in an agar diffusion assay.[102,103] Therefore, these antibacterial composites have similar limitations to the other composites that act purely by direct surface contact.

Fluoride-releasing dental composites

Fluoride is well known to induce tooth remineralization and enhance their resistance to cariogenic bacteria.[104] It can also interfere with bacterial metabolic activities and adhesion to dental plaque.[105]

Various approaches have been described to develop fluoride-releasing composites. These include fluoride incorporation as inorganic water-soluble salts, addition to glass fillers, bonding to a resin component and as an organic fluoride salt.[106–112] Despite some success in the development of dental composites with sustained fluoride release, the levels achieved are generally very much lower compared to those gained with GICs and compomers.[104,113]

9.3.8 Antibacterial dental adhesives and glass ionomer cements

To achieve a dentine-bonding agent with antibacterial activity, several chemicals and antimicrobial agents have been blended into commercial or experimental adhesive systems, for example sodium fluoride, dodecylamine silver compound (protargin),[114] iron binding agent, 2,2-bipyridine[115] and antibiotics.[116] Although release of antibiotics was found to be effective, lower release of antibiotics may promote the development of resistant bacterial strains. Therefore, antibiotic incorporation is not an ideal strategy for developing dental adhesives with antibacterial activity.

In other studies, unpolymerized dental adhesive containing MDPB monomer exhibited strong antibacterial properties with no effect on either degree of conversion or bond strength.[117,118] Unpolymerized bonding systems, with MDPB antibacterial monomer, are clearly able to eliminate residual bacteria, following cavity preparation. After curing, however, the immobilized MDPB may have limited antibacterial benefit.

Several fluoride-releasing dentine adhesives are available for clinical application.[119] These adhesives release fluoride at restoration margins and in the hybrid layer.[120] Some reports, however, have indicated that fluoride-releasing adhesives have limited ability to inhibit secondary caries or maintain bond strength to dentine.[121] Incorporation of antimicrobial agents such as chlorhexidine to fluoride-releasing GICs has also been attempted.[122] Although the antibacterial activity of GICs improved upon addition of chlorhexidine, mechanical properties and bond strength can be reduced.[123] Furthermore, chlorhexidine release can be severely restricted by interaction with polyacrylic acid.[124]

9.4 Remineralizing dental composites

9.4.1 Introduction

The mineral composition of enamel and dentine [hydroxyapatite, $Ca_{10}(PO_4)_6(OH)_2$] is in dynamic equilibrium at neutral pH (6–7). Hydroxyapatite, however, will start to dissolve when the pH of the local environment declines below a critical level (~ pH 5.5).[125] This demineralization normally occurs every time sugary food is ingested.[126] It can, however, be reversed by the buffering effect of hydroxyapatite dissolution products[127] and the presence of sufficient Ca^{2+} and PO_4^{3-} in the surrounding environment. Environmental pH neutralization above the critical level enhances precipitation of Ca^{2+} and PO_4^{3-} within demineralized tooth structures. This phenomenon is known as remineralization. Providing additional calcium and phosphate to the oral environment may help increase this process and thereby reduce caries.

9.4.2 Calcium phosphates

Calcium phosphates include various salts of tribasic phosphoric acid (H_3PO_4). $H_2PO_4^-$, HPO_4^{2-} or PO_4^{3-} ions can all be formed through progressive removal of H^+ ions from this acid.[128] Their natural occurrence in skeletal tissues and teeth makes them of particular interest to both clinicians and biomedical scientists. These compounds are highly biocompatible and osteoconductive materials[129] and widely used as bone substitutes and as carriers in controlled drug delivery.[130]

Several calcium phosphate species are known to dissolve in neutral or basic solution and reprecipitate as hydroxyapatite, $Ca_{10}(PO_4)_6(OH)_2$, with a similar structure to apatite found in bone and teeth. The solubility of calcium phosphate phases in aqueous solution is an important property and mainly correlated with the calcium (Ca)/phosphorous (P) ratio.[131] Generally the higher the Ca/P ratio, the lower is the solubility. At physiological pH, the solubility of calcium phosphate species for example decreases in the order MCPM > DCPD = DCPA > OCP > β-TCP > HA (see Table 9.1).[132]

Table 9.1 Main calcium phosphates arranged according to calcium (Ca) and phosphorus (P) ratio (modified from Bohner[132])

Name	Abbreviation	Formula	Ca/P ratio
Monocalcium phosphate monohydrate	MCPM	$Ca(H_2PO_4)_2 \cdot H_2O$	0.5
Dicalcium phosphate anhydrate (monetite)	DCPA	$CaHPO_4$	1.0
Dicalcium phosphate dihydrate (brushite)	DCPD	$CaHPO_4 \cdot 2H_2O$	1.0
Octacalcium phosphate	OCP	$Ca_8H_2(PO_4)_6 \cdot 5H_2O$	1.3
β-Tricalcium phosphate	β-TCP	$Ca_3(PO_4)_2$	1.5
Amorphous calcium phosphate	ACP	$Ca_3(PO_4)_2 \cdot nH_2O$	1.5
α-Tricalcium phosphate	α-TCP	α-$Ca_3(PO_4)_2$	1.5
Hydroxyapatite	HA	$Ca_{10}(PO_4)_6(OH)_2$	1.7
Tetracalcium phosphate	TetCP	$Ca_4(PO_4)_2O$	2.0

9.4.3 Calcium phosphate dental composites

In order to formulate restorative materials with remineralizing activity, many studies have incorporated calcium phosphate species within dental monomers. If these phosphate fillers are more soluble than hydroxyapatite they may be released from the set resin and reprecipitate within a tooth lesion. Amorphous calcium phosphate (ACP) in particular, has been extensively studied.[133–135] Additionally, composites containing dicalcium phosphate anhydrate (DCPA), tetracalcium phosphate (TetCP)[136] and monocalcium phosphate monohydrate (MCPM) [137] have been investigated. The difficulty is to gain sufficient calcium and phosphate release without decline in composite strength.

Amorphous calcium phosphate (ACP) has been incorporated up to 40% in various methacrylate dental monomers. Upon immersion in water, the set ACP composites release calcium and phosphate which increase upon raising filler mass fraction[133] and filler particle size.[134] Furthermore, this release can advantageously be enhanced by lowering the pH of the storage media.[135] The levels of calcium and phosphate release from ACP composites were sufficient to promote tooth remineralization *in vitro*.[138] These composites however, exhibited lower biaxial flexure strength than the base polymer or conventional glass filled composites. This was attributed mainly to the tendency of the ACP filler particles to agglomerate within the composite and increase water sorption.[139]

Several studies, therefore, have been carried out to improve the mechanical properties, for example through enhancing interaction between the filler and resin matrix, ACP hybridization with glass fillers,[140] reduction in water sorption,[141] or lowering of filler particle size.[134] The maximum biaxial flexure strengths of these wet ACP composites, however, achieved to date is only ~50 MPa, which is in the range of GICs. Therefore, the current ACP composites are not suitable for use as restorative material in stress-bearing areas.

ACP composites however, have sufficient strength to be considered as dental adhesives or liner/base materials. In one study, the shear bond strength of an experimental ACP composite to dentine was 18 MPa.[142] Upon water storage, some decline in this strength was observed but the failure mechanism also changed from adhesive to adhesive/cohesive. Recently, ACP composites have been commercialized as an adhesive cement and pit and fissure sealant. With commercial ACP orthodontic adhesive (Aegis Ortho), the shear bond strength was 7 MPa. This was comparable with that of a commercial RMGIC-type orthodontic adhesive but approximately half that of a conventional resin adhesive.[143]

Dicalcium phosphate anhydrate (DCPA) and tetracalcium phosphate included in a dental resin also provided sustained release of calcium and phosphate.[136] This composite was capable of remineralizing tooth structure *in vitro*. A similar composite also showed less microleakage and higher shear bond strength compared to a commercial light cured calcium hydroxide liner material.[144]

Recently, DCPA nanoparticles have been combined with nano-silica-fused to silicon carbide[145] or silicon nitride[146] whiskers and added to dental resins. Chemical curing formulations were developed and proved to have wet flexural strengths that could exceed 100 MPa, in addition to calcium and phosphate release comparable with that of ACP composites. When DCPA in the earlier study was replaced by more soluble MCPM nanoparticles, higher levels of calcium and phosphate were observed while the flexure strength was comparable.[146]

9.5 Antibacterial, remineralizing and proteinase-inhibiting materials

9.5.1 Inhibition of matrix metalloproteinases (MMPs)

In addition to the problems mentioned above, deterioration of bond strength between adhesives and dentine has been partially attributed to enzymatic degradation of demineralized collagen fibrils, which are unprotected by adhesive resin. This collagenolytic activity is mediated through endogenous enzymes known as matrix metalloproteinases (MMPs).[147] In addition to its antibacterial properties, chlorhexidine has been reported to act as an inhibitor of MMPs.[148] It therefore has two mechanisms that help maintain the integrity of the dentine bond.[149]

One *in vivo* study showed that surface treatment of dentine with 2% chlorhexidine solution could help preserve the bond strength of dental adhesives.[150] In a further *in vitro* study, similar chlorhexidine pretreatment was found to decrease the deterioration in composite bond strength after six months' storage in artificial saliva.[151] Furthermore, a dental adhesive system used in association with either 0.2 or 2 wt% chlorhexidine digluconate showed less decline in bond strength following six months storage using *in vivo* like conditions.[152]

Chlorhexidine diacetate was previously added to various tetraethyleneglycol dimethacrylate (TEGDMA)/urethane dimethacrylate (UDMA)/HEMA/fluoralumino silicate composites.[83] Unfortunately CHX release was very low unless HEMA content was greater than 70 wt% of the monomer. Upon raising the HEMA content, water sorption increased. This process causes material swelling that may, if controlled, enable compensation for polymerization shrinkage. Water sorption enhances drug release via polymer plasticization but this also reduces mechanical properties.

In recent work it was also found that ACP slowly converted to hydroxyapatite directly within methacrylate composites.[135] Using a combination of tricalcium phosphate (TCP), $Ca_3(PO_4)_2$, and monocalcium phosphate monohydrate (MCPM), $Ca(H_2PO_4)_2$, however, a water sorption-catalysed, much faster, transition to dicalcium phosphate occurs.[153] The following demonstrates how these reactive fillers affect CHX release from and mechanical properties of systematically varying composites. In order to help interpret the observed results chemical changes and water sorption properties have also been described.

9.5.2 Antibacterial reactive calcium phosphate filler composites

The antibacterial reactive filler composites studied[153] used a liquid phase with UDMA:TEGDMA:HEMA in the weight ratio 1:1:2. Eight different formulations were prepared with a powder to liquid ratio (PLR) of 3:1 or 1:1 by weight. The powder consisted of MCPM and β-TCP of equal weight and 0 or 5 wt% chlorhexidine diacetate (CHX). The average MCPM particle diameter was 29 or 90 μm.

Upon light exposure, monomer conversion of 93 and 87% was observed with and without CHX, respectively. These high conversions will give large shrinkage. Upon placement in water, however, the sample mass increased in the first 24 h by up to 12 wt% due to water sorption. The associated volume change could help compensate for the polymerization shrinkage. Diffusion controlled release of over 70wt% of the encapsulated drug could

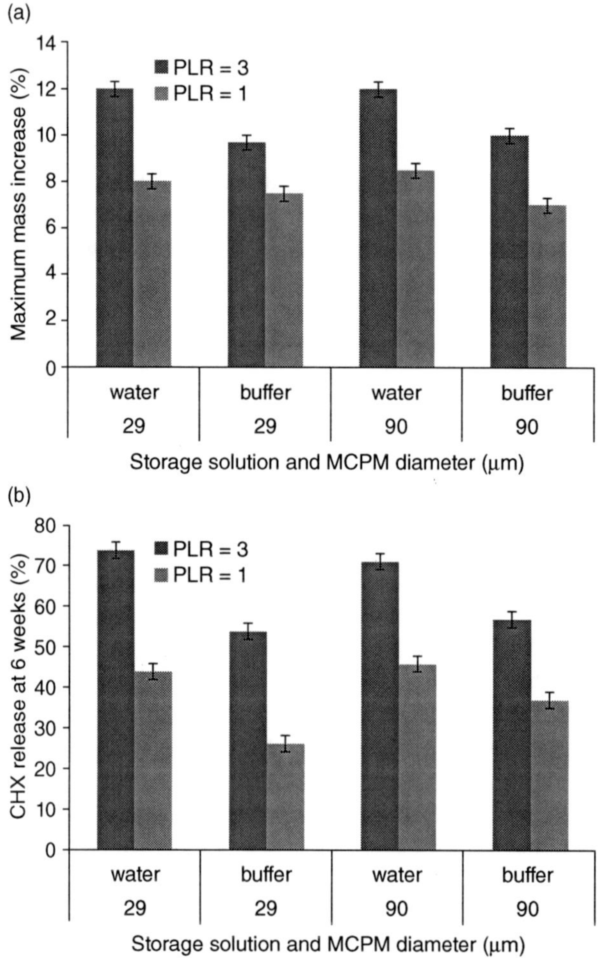

9.1 Effect of powder liquid ratio (PLR), monocalcium phosphate (MCPM) particle size and sample storage solution on (a) maximum mass increase and (b) chlorhexidine release after 6 weeks in reactive filler composites. (Figures generated from data in Mehdawi *et al.*[153]).

be observed over six weeks. Reducing the PLR ratio and adding buffer to the storage solution, however, decreased both water sorption and chlorhexidine release rate (see Fig. 9.1).

The initial composite compressive and biaxial flexural strengths were 87 and 61 MPa, respectively. These declined after 24 h water immersion to below 40 MPa (see Fig. 9.2). No variable in this study affected initial strength but a reduction in MCPM particle diameter reduced its early decline. After 24 hours, Raman studies showed that water was bound by bulk reactive

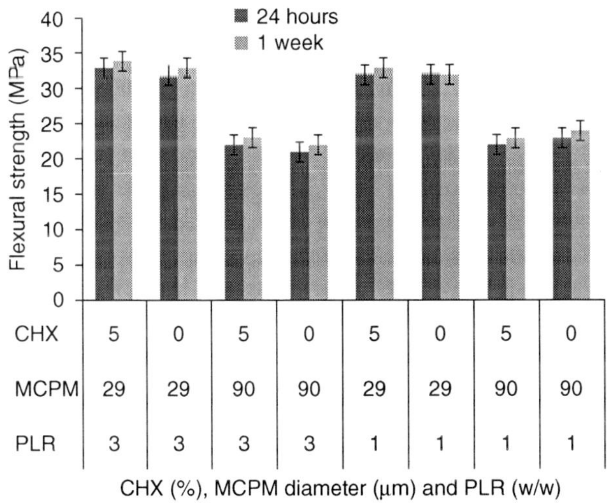

9.2 Effect of powder liquid ratio (PLR), chlorhexidine diacetate (CHX) content in the powder phase and monocalcium phosphate particle size on the flexural strength of reactive filler composites. (Figures generated from data in Mehdawi *et al.*[153]).

filler conversion to brushite. This corresponded to reduction in water sorption. After this period, on average a slight but consistent increase in strength was noted despite continuing release of drug (see Fig. 9.2). This suggests that brushite formation provides a novel means of reducing the effects of high water sorption and enabling material 'self-healing' during prolonged CHX release.

9.6 Conclusion and future trends

Given the increasing use of dental composites and their high failure rate caused by bacterial microleakage, new antibacterial composites that additionally provide remineralizing action could be of significant benefit. For effective action, the antibacterial agent needs to be released in sufficient quantities to affect bacteria within biofilms. Release rate as a function of time should also be carefully controlled. It has been suggested that positively charged antibacterial agents such as chlorhexidine, released underneath a restoration, can remain trapped to provide long term action.[83] If entrapment does occur, early high release could potentially provide long-term benefits.

As high water sorption is often required for high drug release from composites, novel mechanisms to 'self-heal' the bulk material and tooth restoration interface could be of benefit. Reactive calcium phosphate containing composites show promise in this respect but further work is required to increase their mechanical properties. The above results indicate that this may be achieved by reducing particle size. Other unpublished work suggests that altering both the monomer type and partial replacement of reactive fillers with more conventional fillers may further improve strength. Mechanical properties over a prolonged time, however, require evaluation, as do long-term antibacterial effectiveness *in vivo* and biocompatibility.

The ability of calcium phosphate-containing composites to remineralize carious enamel and dentine still needs greater investigation. The bond strength of various formulations to sound and carious enamel and dentine should also be evaluated. In addition, the polymerization shrinkage and stresses need to be assessed and water sorption induced swelling better controlled.

9.7 References

1 University of York NHS Centre for Reviews and Dissemination. 'Dental restoration: what type of filling?' *Effective Health Care*, 1999, **5**, 1–12.

2 Todd JE and Lader D. *Adult Dental Health in the United Kingdom 1988*. Office of Population Censuses and Surveys, Social Survey Division. HMSO, London, 1991.

3 Kidd EAM, Joyston-Bechal S and Beighton D. 'Diagnosis of secondary caries: a laboratory study'. *British Dental Journal*, 1994, **176**, 135–9.

4 Marsh PD. 'Dental plaque as a microbial biofilm'. *Caries Research*, 2004, **38**, 204–11.

5 Rosan B and Lamont RJ. 'Dental plaque formation'. *Microbes and Infection*, 2000, **2**, 1599–607.

6 Kolenbrander PE. 'Oral microbial communities: biofilms, interactions, and genetic systems'. *Annual Review of Microbiology*, 2000, **54**, 413–37.

7 Carlsson, P, Gandour IA, Olsson B, Rickardsson B and Abbas K. 'High prevalence of *Streptococci mutans* in a population with extremely low prevalence of dental caries'. *Oral Microbiology and Immunology*, 1987, **2**, 121–4.

8 Badet C and Thebaud NB. 'Ecology of lactobacilli in the oral cavity: a review of literature'. *The Open Microbiology Journal*, 2008, **2**, 38–8.

9 Nyvad B and Kilian M. 'Microbiology of the early colonization of human enamel and root surfaces *in vivo*'. *Scandinavian Journal of Dental Research*, 1987, **95**, 369–80.

10 Leme AFP, Koo H, Bellato CM, Bedi G and Cury JA. 'The role of sucrose in cariogenic dental biofilm formation – new insight'. *Journal of Dental Research*, 2006, **85**, 878–87.

11 Bowen WH. 'Do we need to be concerned about dental caries in the coming millennium?' *Critical Reviews in Oral Biology& Medicine*, 2002, **13**, 126–31.

12 Schilling KM and Bowen WH. 'Glucans synthesized *in situ* in experimental salivary pellicle function as specific binding sites for Streptococcus mutans'. *Infection and Immunity*, 1992, **60**, 284–95.

13 Aires CP, Tabchoury CPM, Del Bel Cury AA, Koo H and Cury JA. 'Effect of sucrose concentration on dental biofilm formed in situ and on enamel demineralization'. *Caries Research*, 2006, **40**, 28–32.
14 Humphrey SP and Williamson RT. 'A review of saliva: normal composition, flow and function'. *Journal of Prosthetic Dentistry*, 2001, **85,** 162–9.
15 Saini TS, Edwards PC, Kimmes NS, Carroll LR, Shaner JW and Dowd FJ. 'Etiology of xerostomia and dental caries among methamphetamine abusers'. *Oral Health and Preventive Dentistry*, 2005, **3**, 189–95.
16 Svanberg M, Mjör IA and Ørstavik D. '*Mutans streptococci* in plaque from margins of amalgam, composite, and glass-ionomer restorations'. *Journal of Dental Research*, 1990, **69**, 861–4.
17 Moura JS, Lima EM, Paes Leme AF, Del Bel Cury AA, Tabchoury CP and Cury JA. 'Effect of luting cement on dental biofilm composition and secondary caries around metallic restorations in situ'. *Operative Dentistry*, 2004, **29**, 509–14.
18 Beyth N, Domb AJ and Weiss EI. 'An *in vitro* quantitative antibacterial analysis of amalgam and composite resins'. *Journal of Dentistry*, 2007, **35**, 201–6.
19 Vermeersch G, Leloup G, Delmée M and Vreven J. 'Antibacterial activity of glass–ionomer cements, compomers and resin composites: relationship between acidity and material setting phase'. *Journal of Oral Rehabilitation*, 2005, **32**, 368–74.
20 Forss H, Jokinen J, Spets-Happonen S, Seppä L and Luoma H. 'Fluoride and *mutans streptococci* in plaque grown on glass ionomer and composite'. *Caries Research*, 1991, **25**, 454–8.
21 Paolantonio M, D'ercole S, Perinetti G, Tripodi D, Catamo G, Serra E, Brue C and Piccolomini R. 'Clinical and microbiological effects of different restorative materials on the periodontal tissues adjacent to subgingival class V restorations: 1-year results'. *Journal of Clinical Periodontology*, 2004, **31**, 200–7.
22 Hansel C, Leyhausen G, Mai UEH and Geurtsen W. 'Effects of various resin composite (co)monomers and extracts on two caries-associated micro-organisms *in vitro*'. *Journal of Dental Research*, 1998, **77**, 60–7.
23 Gama-Teixeira A, Simionato MR, Elian SN, Sobral MA and Luz MA. '*Streptococcus mutans*-induced secondary caries adjacent to glass ionomer cement, composite resin and amalgam restorations *in vitro*'. *Brazilian Oral Research*, 2007, **21**, 368–74.
24 Kidd EAM. 'Microleakage in relation to amalgam and composite restorations: a laboratory study'. *British Dental Journal*, 1976, **141**, 305–10.
25 Wasson EA and Nicholson JW. 'New aspects of the setting of glass-ionomer cements'. *Journal of Dental Research*, 1993, **72**, 481–3.
26 Phillips S and Bishop BM. 'An *in vitro* study of the effect of moisture on glass-ionomer cement'. *Quintessence International* 1985, **16**, 175–7.
27 Cattani-Lorente MA, Godin C and Meyer JM. 'Mechanical behavior of glass-ionomer cements affected by long-term storage in water'. *Dental Materials*, 1994, **10**, 37–44.
28 Cattani-Lorente MA, Godin C and Meyer JM. 'Early strength of glass ionomer cements'. *Dental Materials*, 1993, **9**, 57–62.
29 Wilson AD and McLean JW. *Glass Ionomer Cement*, Quintessence Publishing, Chicago, 1988.
30 Culbertson BM. 'Glass-ionomer dental restoratives'. *Progress in Polymer Science*, 2001, **26**, 577–604.

31 Musanje L, Shu M and Darvell BW. 'Water sorption and mechanical behaviour of cosmetic direct restorative materials in artificial saliva'. *Dental Materials*, 2001, **17**, 394–401.
32 Piwowarczyk A, Ottl P, Lauer HC and Büchler A. 'Laboratory strength of glass ionomer cement, compomers, and resin composites'. *Journal of Prosthodontics*, 2002, **11**, 86–91.
33 Imazato S, Kuramoto A, Kaneko T, Ebisu S and Russell RR. 'Comparison of antibacterial activity of simplified adhesive systems'. *American Journal of Dentistry*, 2002, **15**, 356–60.
34 Tobias RS. 'Antibacterial properties of dental restorative materials: a review'. *International Endodontic Journal*, 1988, **21**, 155–60.
35 Matalon S, Slutzky H and Weiss EI. 'Surface antibacterial properties of packable resin composites: part I'. *Quintessence International*, 2004, **35**, 189–93.
36 Slutzky H, Slutzky-Goldberg I, Weiss EI and Matalon S. 'Antibacterial properties of temporary filling material'. *Journal of Endodontics*, 2006, **32**, 214–17.
37 Wilson M. 'Susceptibility of oral bacterial biofilms to antimicrobial agents'. *Journal of Medical Microbiology*, 1996, **44**, 79–87.
38 Yap AUJ, Khor E and Foo SH. 'Fluoride release and antibacterial properties of new generation tooth colored restoratives'. *Operative Dentistry*, 1999, **24**, 297–305.
39 Bundy KJ, Butler MF and Hochman RF. 'An investigation of the bacteriostatic properties of pure metals'. *Journal of Biomedical Materials Research*, 1980, **14**, 653–63.
40 Orstavik D and Hensten-Pettersen A. 'Antibacterial activity of tooth-colored dental restorative materials'. *Journal of Dental Research*, 1978, **57**, 171–4.
41 Schmalz G, Ergücü Z and Hiller KA. 'Effect of dentin on the antibacterial activity of dentin bonding agents'. *Journal of Endodontics*, 2004, **30**, 352–8.
42 Imazato S. 'Antibacterial properties of resin composites and dentin bonding systems'. *Dental Materials*, 2003, **19**, 449–57.
43 Hansen EK and Asmussen E. 'Improved efficacy of dentin-bonding agents'. *European Journal of Oral Sciences*, 1997, **105**, 434–9.
44 Camps J, Pizant S, Dejou J and Franquin JC. 'Effects of desensitizing agents on human dentin permeability'. *American Journal of Dentistry*, 1998, **11**, 286–90.
45 Fraga RC, Siqueira JF Jr and de Uzeda M. '*In vitro* evaluation of antibacterial effects of photo-cured glass ionomer liners and dentin bonding agents during setting'. *Journal of Prosthetic Dentistry*, 1996, **76**, 483–6.
46 Meiers JC and Miller GA. 'Antibacterial activity of dentin bonding systems, resin-modified glass ionomers, and polyacid-modified composite resins'. *Operative Dentistry*, 1996, **21**, 257–64.
47 Schweikl H and Schmalz G. 'Glutaraldehyde-containing dentin bonding agents are mutagens in mammalian cells *in vitro*'. *Journal of Biomedical Materials Research*, 1997, **36**, 284–8.
48 Watanabe I, Nakabayashi N and Pashley DH. 'Bonding to ground dentin by a phenyl-P self-etching primer'. *Journal of Dental Research*, 1994, **73**, 1212–20.
49 Imazato S, Imai T and Ebisu S. 'Antibacterial activity of proprietary self-etching primers'. *American Journal of Dentistry*, 1998, **11**, 106–8.
50 Ohmori K, Maeda N and Kohno A. 'Evaluation of antibacterial activity of three dentin primers using an in vitro tooth model'. *Operative Dentistry*, 1999, **24**, 279–85.

51 Gondim JO, Duque C, Hebling J and Giro EM. 'Influence of human dentine on the antibacterial activity of self-etching adhesive systems against cariogenic bacteria'. *Journal of Dentistry*, 2008, **36**, 241–8.
52 Herrera M, Castillo A, Bravo M, Liébana J and Carrión P. 'Antibacterial activity of resin adhesives, glass ionomer and resin-modified glass ionomer cements and a compomer in contact with dentin caries samples'. *Operative Dentistry*, 2000, **25**, 265–9.
53 da Silva RC, Zuanon ACC, Spolidorio DMP and Campos JAD. 'Antibacterial activity of four glass ionomer cements used in a traumatic restorative treatment'. *Journal of Materials Science: Materials in Medicine*, 2007, **18**, 1859–62.
54 Davidovich E, Weiss E, Fuks AB and Beyth N. 'Surface antibacterial properties of glass ionomer cements used in a traumatic restorative treatment'. *Journal of the American Dental Association*, 2007, **138**, 1347–52.
55 Carlén A, Nikdel K, Wennerberg A, Holmberg K and Olsson J. 'Surface characteristics and *in vitro* biofilm formation on glass ionomer and composite resin'. *Biomaterials*, 2001, **22**, 481–7.
56 Al-Naimi OT, Itota T, Hobson RS and McCabe JF. 'Fluoride release for restorative materials and its effect on biofilm formation in natural saliva'. *Journal of Materials Science: Materials in Medicine*, 2008, **19**, 1243–8.
57 van Dijken JW, Kalfas S, Litra V and Oliveby A. 'Fluoride and *mutans streptococci* levels in plaque on aged restorations of resin-modified glass ionomer cement, compomer and resin composite'. *Caries Research*, 1997, **31**, 379–83.
58 Craig RG. *Restorative Dental Materials*, 10th edn, Mosby-Year Book, St Louis, 1997.
59 Wiegand A, Buchalla W and Attin T. 'Review on fluoride-releasing restorative materials–fluoride release and uptake characteristics, antibacterial activity and influence on caries formation'. *Dental Materials*, 2007, **23**, 343–62.
60 Karanika-Kouma A, Dionysopoulos P, Koliniotou-Koubia E and Kolokotronis A. 'Antibacterial properties of dentin bonding systems, polyacid-modified composite resins and composite resins'. *Journal of Oral Rehabilitation*, 2001, **28**, 157–60.
61 Vermeersch G, Leloup G, Delmee M and Vreven J. 'Antibacterial activity of glass–ionomer cements, compomers and resin composites: relationship between acidity and material setting phase'. *Journal of Oral Rehabilitation*, 2005, **32**, 368–74.
62 Matalon S, Weiss EI, Gozaly N and Slutzky H. 'Surface antibacterial properties of compomers'. *European Archives of Paediatric Dentistry*, 2006, **7**, 136–41.
63 Kielbassa AM, Schulte-Mönting J, Garcia-Godoy F and Meyer-Lueckel H. 'Initial in situ secondary caries formation: effect of various fluoride-containing restorative materials'. *Operative Dentistry*, 2003, **28**, 765–72.
64 Millar BJ, Abiden F and Nicholson JW. '*In vitro* caries inhibition by polyacid modified composite resins ('compomers')'. *Journal of Dentistry*, 1998, **26**, 133–6.
65 Trachtenberg F, Maserejian NN, Soncini JA, Hayes C and Tavares M. 'Does fluoride in compomers prevent future caries in children?' *Journal of Dental Research*, 2009, **88**, 276–9.
66 Meyer JM, Cattani-Lorente MA and Dupuis V. 'Compomers: between glass-ionomer cements and composites'. *Biomaterials*, 1998, **19**, 529–39.

67 Chen HY, Manhart J, Kunzelmann KH and Hickel R. 'Polymerization contraction stress in light-cured compomer restorative materials'. *Dental Materials*, 2003, **19**, 597–602.

68 Brunthaler A, König F, Lucas T, Sperr W and Schedle A. 'Longevity of direct composite restorations in posterior teeth'. *Clinical Oral Investigations*, 2003, **7**, 63–70.

69 Manhart J, Chen HY, Hamm G and Hickel R. 'Review of the clinical survival of direct and indirect restorations in posterior teeth of the permanent dentition'. *Operative Dentistry*, 2004, **29**, 481–508.

70 Burke FJT, Cheung SW, Mjör IA and Wilson NHF. 'Restoration longevity and analysis of reasons for the placement and replacement of restorations provided by vocational dental practitioners and their trainers in the United Kingdom'. *Quintessence International*, 1999, **30**, 234–42.

71 Yuan Y, Shimada Y, Ichinose S and Tagami J. 'Effect of dentin depth on hybridization quality using different bonding tactics *in vivo*'. *Journal of Dentistry*, 2007, **35**, 664–72.

72 Sano H, Takatsu T, Ciucchi B, Horner JA, Matthews WG and Pashley DH. 'Nanoleakage: leakage within the hybrid layer'. *Operative Dentistry*, 1995, **20**, 18–25.

73 Wang Y and Spencer P. 'Hybridization efficiency of the adhesive/dentin interface with wet bonding'. *Journal of Dental Research*, 2003, **82**, 141–5.

74 Pashley DH, Tay FR, Yiu C, Hashimoto M, Breschi L, Carvalho RM and Ito S. 'Collagen degradation by host-derived enzymes during aging'. *Journal of Dental Research*, 2004, **83**, 216–21.

75 Koshiro K, Inoue S, Tanaka T, Koase K, Fujita M, Hashimoto M and Sano H. '*In vivo* degradation of resin-dentin bonds produced by a self-etch vs. a total-etch adhesive system'. *European Journal of Oral Sciences*, 2004, **112**, 368–75.

76 Banerjee A, Watson TF and Kidd EA. 'Dentine caries: take it or leave it?' *Dental Update*, 2000, **27**, 272–6.

77 Yazdankhah SP, Scheie AA, Høiby EA, Lunestad B, Heir E, Fotland T, Naterstad K and Kruse H. 'Triclosan and antimicrobial resistance in bacteria: an overview'. *Microbial Drug Resistance*, 2006, **12**, 83–90.

78 Imazato S, Torii M and Tsuchitani Y. 'Antibacterial effect of composite incorporating Triclosan against *Streptococcus mutans*'. *Journal of Osaka University Dental School*, 1995, **35**, 5–11.

79 Sehgal V, Shetty VS, Mogra S, Bhat G, Eipe M, Jacob S and Prabu L. 'Evaluation of antimicrobial and physical properties of orthodontic composite resin modified by addition of antimicrobial agents – an *in-vitro* study'. *American Journal of Orthodontics and Dentofacial Orthopedics*, 2007, **131**, 525–9.

80 Othman HF, Wu CD, Evans CA, Drummond JL and Matasa CG. 'Evaluation of antimicrobial properties of orthodontic composite resins combined with benzalkonium chloride'. *American Journal of Orthodontics and Dentofacial Orthopedics*, 2002, **122**, 288–94.

81 McDonnell G and Russell AD. 'Antiseptics and disinfectants: activity, action, and resistance'. *Clinical Microbiology Reviews*, 1999, **12**, 147–79.

82 Jedrychowski JR, Caputo AA and Kerper S. 'Antibacterial and mechanical properties of restorative materials combined with chlorhexidines'. *Journal of Oral Rehabilitation*, 1983, **10**, 373–81.

83 Leung D, Spratt DA, Pratten J, Gulabivala K, Mordan NJ and Young AM. 'Chlorhexidine-releasing methacrylate dental composite materials'. *Biomaterials*, 2005, **26**, 7145–53.
84 Scheie AA. 'Modes of action of currently known chemical anti-plaque agents other than chlorhexidine'. *Journal of Dental Research*, 1989, **68**, 1609–16.
85 Imazato S, Torii M, Tsuchitani Y, McCabe JF and Russell RRB. 'Incorporation of bacterial inhibitor into resin composite'. *Journal of Dental Research*, 1994, **73**, 1437–43.
86 Imazato S and McCabe JF. 'Influence of incorporation of antibacterial monomer on curing behavior of a dental composite'. *Journal of Dental Research*, 1994, **73**, 1641–5.
87 Imazato S, Tarumi H, Kato S and Ebisu S. 'Water sorption and colour stability of composites containing the antibacterial monomer MDPB'. *Journal of Dentistry*, 1999, **27**, 279–83.
88 Lansdown ABG. 'Silver I: its antibacterial properties and mechanism of action'. *Journal of Wound Care*, 2002, **11**, 125–30.
89 Yamamoto K, Ohashi S, Aono M, Kokubo T, Yamada I and Yamauchi J. 'Antibacterial activity of silver ions implanted in SiO_2 filler on oral streptococci'. *Dental Materials*, 1996, **12**, 227–9.
90 Kawashita M, Tsuneyama S, Miyaji F, Kokubo T, Kozuka H and Yamamoto K. 'Antibacterial-silver containing silica glass prepared by sol–gel method'. *Biomaterials*, 2000, **21**, 393–8.
91 Syafiuddin T, Igarashi T, Shimomura H, Hisamitsu H and Goto N. 'Bacteriological and mechanical evaluation of antibacterial filler-containing composite resins'. *Journal of Showa University Dental Society*, 1993, **13**, 443–9.
92 Syafiuddin T, Igarashi T, Toko T, Hisamitsu H and Goto N. 'Bacteriological and mechanical evaluation of resin composites containing antibacterial filler (Apacider)'. *Journal of Showa University Dental Society*, 1995, **15**, 119–25.
93 Syafiuddin T, Hisamitsu H, Toko T, Igarashi T, Goto N, Fujishima A and Miyazaki T. '*In vitro* inhibition of caries around a resin composite restoration containing antibacterial filler'. *Biomaterials*, 1997, **18**, 1051–7.
94 Hotta M, Nakajima H, Yamamoto K and Aono M. 'Antibacterial temporary filling materials: the effect of adding various ratios of Ag-Zn zeolite'. *Journal of Oral Rehabilitation*, 1998, **25**, 485–9.
95 Yoshida K, Tanagawa M, Matsumoto S, Yamada T and Atsuta M. 'Antibacterial activity of resin composites with silver-containing materials'. *European Journal of Oral Sciences*, 1999, **107**, 290–6.
96 Yoshida K, Tanagawa M and Atsuta M. 'Characterization and inhibitory effect of antibacterial dental resin composites incorporating silver-supported materials'. *Journal of Biomedical Materials Research*, 1999, **47**, 516–22.
97 Imazato S, Ebi N, Takahashi Y, Kaneko T, Ebisu S and Russell RRB. 'Antibacterial activity of bactericide-immobilized filler for resin-based restoratives'. *Biomaterials*, 2003, **24**, 3605–9.
98 Ebi N, Imazato S, Noiri Y and Ebisu S. 'Inhibitory effects of resin composite containing bactericide-immobilized filler on plaque accumulation'. *Dental Materials*, 2001, **17**, 485–91.
99 Tanner J, Carlén A, Söderling E and Vallittu PK. 'Adsorption of parotid saliva proteins and adhesion of Streptococcus mutans ATCC 21752 to dental

fiber-reinforced composites'. *Journal of Biomedical Materials Research*, 2003, **66**, 391–8.

100 Buergers R, Schneider-Brachert W, Hahnel S, Rosentritt M and Handel G. 'Streptococcal adhesion to novel low-shrink silorane-based restorative'. *Dental Materials*, 2009, **25**, 269–75.

101 Lin J, Qiu S, Lewis K and Klibanov AM. 'Mechanism of bactericidal and fungicidal activities of textiles covalently modified with alkylated polyethylenimine'. *Biotechnology and Bioengineering*, 2003, **83**, 168–72.

102 Beyth N, Yudovin-Farber I, Bahir R, Domb AJ and Weiss EI. 'Antibacterial activity of dental composites containing quaternary ammonium polyethylenimine nanoparticles against *Streptococcus mutans*'. *Biomaterials*, 2006, **27**, 3995–4002.

103 Beyth N, Houri-Haddad Y, Baraness-Hadar L, Yudovin-Farber I, Domb AJ and Weiss EI. 'Surface antimicrobial activity and biocompatibility of incorporated polyethylenimine nanoparticles'. *Biomaterials*, 2008, **29**, 4157–63.

104 Itota T, Nakabo S, Iwai Y, Konishi N, Nagamine M and Torii Y. 'Inhibition of artificial secondary caries by fluoride-releasing adhesives on root dentin'. *Journal of Oral Rehabilitation*, 2002, **29**, 523–7.

105 Bowden GH. 'Effects of fluoride on the microbial ecology of dental plaque'. *Journal of Dental Research*, 1990, **69**, 653–9.

106 Cook PA and Youngson CC. 'A fluoride-containing composite resin-an in vitro study of a new material for orthodontic bonding'. *British Journal of Orthodontics*, 1989, **16**, 207–12.

107 Arends J and Ruben J. 'Fluoride-releasing from a composite resin'. *Quintessence International*, 1988, **19**, 513–14.

108 Arends J and van der Zee Y. 'Fluoride uptake in bovine enamel and dentin from a fluoride-releasing composite resin'. *Quintessence International*, 1990, **21**, 541–4.

109 Xu X and Burgess JO. 'Compressive strength, fluoride release and recharge of fluoride-releasing materials'. *Biomaterials*, 2003, **24**, 2451–61.

110 Rawls HR. 'Fluoride-releasing acrylics'. *Journal of Biomaterials Applications*, 1987, **1**, 382–405.

111 Glasspoole EA, Erickson RL and Davidson CL. 'A fluoride-releasing composite for dental applications'. *Dental Materials*, 2001, **17**, 127–33.

112 Ling L, Xu X, Choi GY, Billodeaux D, Guo G and Diwan RM. 'Novel F-releasing composite with improved mechanical properties'. *Journal of Dental Research*, 2009, **88**, 83–8.

113 Boeckh C, Schumacher E, Podbielski A and Haller B. 'Antibacterial activity of restorative dental biomaterials *in vitro*'. *Caries Research*, 2002, **36**, 101–7.

114 Bapna MS, Murphy R and Mukherjee S. 'Inhibition of bacterial colonization by antimicrobial agents incorporated into dental resins'. *Journal of Oral Rehabilitation*, 1988, **15**, 405–11.

115 Bapna M, Mukherjee S and Murphy R. 'The antimicrobial effect of an iron-binding agent on *Streptococcus mutans*'. *Journal of Oral Rehabilitation*, 1992, **19**, 111–13.

116 Kudou Y, Obara K, Kawashima T, Kubota M, Abe S, Endo T, Komatsu M and Okuda R. 'Addition of antibacterial agents to MMA-TBB dentin bonding systems-influences on tensile bond strength and antibacterial effect'. *Dental Materials Journal*, 2000, **19**, 65–74.

117 Imazato S, Kinomoto Y, Tarumi H, Torii M, Russell RRB and McCabe JF. 'Incorporation of antibacterial monomer MDPB into dentin primer'. *Journal of Dental Research*, 1997, **76**, 768–72.
118 Imazato S, Kinomoto Y, Tarumi H, Ebisu S and Tay FR. 'Antibacterial activity and bonding characteristics of an adhesive resin containing antibacterial monomer MDPB'. *Dental Materials*, 2003, **19**, 313–19.
119 Han L, Cruz E, Okamoto A and Iwaku M. 'A comparative study of fluoride-releasing adhesive resin materials'. *Dental Materials Journal*, 2002, **21**, 9–19.
120 Ferracane JL, Mitchem JC and Adey JD. 'Fluoride penetration into the hybrid layer from a dentin adhesive'. *American Journal of Dentistry*, 1998, **11**, 23–8.
121 Peris AR, Mitsui FHO, Lobo MM, Bedran-russo AKB and Marchi GM. 'Adhesive systems and secondary caries formation: Assessment of dentin bond strength, caries lesions depth and fluoride release'. *Dental Materials*, 2007, **23**, 308–16.
122 Frencken JA, Imazato S, Toi C, Mulder J, Mickenautsch S, Takahashi Y and Ebisu S. 'Antibacterial effect of chlorhexidine-containing glass ionomer cement *in vivo*: a pilot study'. *Caries Research*, 2007, **41**, 102–7.
123 Takahashi Y, Imazato S, Kaneshiro AV, Ebisu S, Frencken JE and Tay FR. 'Antibacterial effects and physical properties of glass-ionomer cements containing chlorhexidine for the ATR approach'. *Dental Materials*, 2006, **22**, 647–52.
124 Palmer G, Jones FH, Billington RW and Pearson GJ. 'Chlorhexidine release from an experimental glass ionomer cement'. *Biomaterials*, 2004, **25**, 5423–31.
125 Dawes C. 'What is the critical pH and why does a tooth dissolve in acid?' *Journal of the Canadian Dental Association*, 2003, **69**, 722–4.
126 Pecharki GD, Cury JA, Paes Leme AF, Tabchoury CPM, Del Bel Cury AA, Rosalen PL and Bowen WH. 'Effect of sucrose containing iron (II) on dental biofilm and enamel demineralization *in situ*'. *Caries Research*, 2005, **39**, 123–9.
127 Aiuchi H, Kitasako Y, Fukuda Y, Nakashima S, Burrow MF and Tagami J. 'Relationship between quantitative assessments of salivary buffering capacity and ion activity product for hydroxyapatite in relation to cariogenic potential'. *Australian Dental Journal*, 2008, **53**, 167–71.
128 Elliot JC. 'General chemistry of the calcium orthophosphate. Structure and Chemistry of apatites and other calcium orthophosphates'. *Studies in Inorganic Chemistry*, Elsevier, Amsterdam, 1994, volume 18, 1–61.
129 Goto K, Shinzato S, Fujibayashi S, Tamura J, Kawanabe K, Hasegawa S, Kowalski R and Nakamura T. 'The biocompatibility and osteoconductivity of a cement containing β-TCP for use in vertebroplasty'. *Journal of Biomedical Materials Research*, 2006, **78**, 629–37.
130 Ginebra MP, Traykova T and Planell JA. 'Calcium phosphate cements as bone drug delivery systems: A review'. *Journal of Controlled Release*, 2006, **113**, 102–10.
131 Vallet-Regi M. 'Ceramics for medical applications'. *Journal of the Chemical Society Dalton Transactions*, 2001, **2**, 97–108.
132 Bohner M. 'Calcium orthophosphates in medicine: from ceramics to calcium phosphate cements'. *Injury*, 2000, **31**, D37–D47.
133 Skrtic D, Antonucci JM and Eanes ED. 'Improved properties of amorphous calcium phosphate fillers in remineralizing resin composites'. *Dental Materials*, 1996, **12**, 295–301.

134 Lee SY, Regnault WF, Antonucci JM and Skrtic D. 'Effect of particle size of an amorphous calcium phosphate filler on the mechanical strength and ion release of polymeric composites'. *Journal of Biomedical Materials Research*, 2007, **80**, 11–17.
135 Regnault WF, Icenogle TB, Antonucci JM and Skrtic D. 'Amorphous calcium phosphate/urethane methacrylate resin composites. I. Physicochemical characterization'. *Journal of Materials Science: Materials in Medicine*, 2008, **19**, 507–15.
136 Dickens SH, Flaim GM and Takagi S. 'Mechanical properties and biochemical activity of remineralizing resin-based Ca–PO_4 cements'. *Dental Materials*, 2003, **19**, 558–66.
137 Xu HHK, Sun L, Weir MD, Takagi S, Chow LC and Hockey B. 'Effects of incorporating nanosized calcium phosphate particles on properties of whisker-reinforced dental composites'. *Journal of Biomedical Materials Research*, 2007, **81**, 116–25.
138 Skrtic D, Hailer AW, Takagi S, Antonucci JM and Eanes ED. 'Quantitative assessment of the efficacy of amorphous calcium phosphate/methacrylate composites in remineralizing caries-like lesions artificially produced in bovine enamel'. *Journal of Dental Research*, 1996, **75**, 1679–86.
139 O'Donnell JNR, Langhorst SE, Fow MD, Skrtic D and Antonucci JM. 'Light-cured dimethacrylate-based resins and their composites: Comparative study of mechanical strength, water sorption, and ion release'. *Journal of Bioactive and Compatible Polymers*, 2008, **23**, 207–26.
140 Skrtic D, Antonucci JM and Eanes ED. 'Amorphous calcium phosphate-based bioactive polymeric composites for mineralized tissue regeneration'. *Journal of Research of the National Institute of Standards and Technology*, 2003, **108**, 167–82.
141 Antonucci JM, Fowler BO, Weir MD, Skrtic D and Stansbury JW. 'Effect of ethyl-α-hydroxymethylacrylate on selected properties of copolymers and ACP resin composites'. *Journal of Materials Science: Materials in Medicine*, 2008, **19**, 3263–71.
142 Schumacher GE, Antonucci JM, O'Donnell JNR and Skrtic D. 'The use of amorphous calcium phosphate composites as bioactive basing materials. Their effect on the strength of the composite/adhesive/dentin bond'. *Journal of the American Dental Association*, 2007, **138**, 1476–84.
143 Foster JA, Berzins DW and Bradley TG. 'Bond strength of an amorphous calcium phosphate-containing orthodontic adhesive'. *The Angle Orthodontist*, 2008, **78**, 339–44.
144 Dickens SH, Kelly SR, Flaim GM and Giuseppetti AA. 'Dentin adhesion and microleakage of a resin-based calcium phosphate pulp capping and basing cement'. *European Journal of Oral Sciences*, 2004, **112**, 452–7.
145 Xu HHK, Sun L, Weir MD, Antonucci JM, Takagi S, Chow LC and Peltz M. 'Nano DCPA-whisker composites with high strength and Ca and PO_4 release'. *Journal of Dental Research*, 2006, **85**, 722–7.
146 Xu HHK, Weir MD, Sun L, Takagi S and Chow LC. 'Effects of calcium phosphate nanoparticles on Ca-PO_4 composite'. *Journal of Dental Research*, 2007, **86**, 378–83.
147 van Strijp AJ, Jansen DC, DeGroot J, ten Cate JM and Everts V. 'Host-derived proteinases and degradation of dentine collagen *in situ*'. *Caries Research*, 2003, **37**, 58–65.

148 Gendron R, Grenier D, Sorsa T and Mayrand D. 'Inhibition of the activities of matrix metalloproteinases 2, 8, and 9 by chlorhexidine'. *Clinical and Diagnostic Laboratory Immunology*, 1999, **6**, 437–9.
149 Hebling J, Pashley DH, Tjäderhane L and Tay FR. 'Chlorhexidine arrests subclinical degradation of dentin hybrid layers *in vivo*'. *Journal of Dental Research*, 2005, **84**, 741–6.
150 Carrilho MR, Geraldeli S, Tay F, de Goes MF, Carvalho RM, Tjäderhane L, Reis AF, Hebling J, Mazzoni A, Breschi L and Pashley D. '*In vivo* preservation of the hybrid layer by chlorhexidine'. *Journal of Dental Research*, 2007, **86**, 529–33.
151 Carrilho MR, Carvalho RM, de Goes MF, di Hipólito V, Geraldeli S, Tay FR. Pashley DH and Tjäderhane L. 'Chlorhexidine preserves dentin bond *in vitro*'. *Journal of Dental Research*, 2007, **86**, 90–4.
152 Campos EA, Correr GM, Leonardi DP, Barato-Filho F, Gonzaga CC and Zielak JC. 'Chlorhexidine diminishes the loss of bond strength over time under simulated pulpal pressure and thermo-mechanical stressing'. *Journal of Dentistry*, 2009, **37**, 108–14.
153 Mehdawi I, Abou Neel EA, Valappil, SP, Palmer G, Salih V, Pratten J, Spratt DA and Young AM. 'Development of remineralizing, antibacterial dental materials'. *Acta Biomaterialia*, 2009, **5**, 2525–39.

10
Effects of particulate filler systems on the properties and performance of dental polymer composites

JACK L. FERRACANE, Oregon Health & Science University, USA and WILLIAM M. PALIN, University of Birmingham, UK

DOI: 10.1533/9780857096432.3.294

Abstract: The filler component is the main determinant of the mechanical and wear properties of a dental composite. The filler also significantly influences curing shrinkage, thermal properties, optical properties, water uptake, handling and other physical properties. In general, maximizing filler reinforcement, specifically by using a high concentration of relatively small particulate fillers that have been coated with a silane agent to enhance the interfacial adhesion between the filler and resin matrix, is desirable to maximize the mechanical properties. It is generally believed that the result of this filler optimization will be superior clinical performance. But the specific manner in which the filler characteristics affect clinical outcomes of composites is not well understood or well described in the literature. However, there have been numerous studies and investigations into the role of the filler formulation on the properties and performance of dental composites, many of which will be reviewed in this chapter.

Key words: composition, dental composites, fillers, properties, size.

10.1 Introduction

The filler system plays a major role in determining the physical properties and ultimately the performance of a dental composite restoration. This chapter will provide information about the current state of dental composites in terms of their filler types, sizes and properties. The theoretical considerations of composite materials will be reviewed to provide a context for the specific information that follows. The specific types of filler used in today's dental composites will be described, as will the manner in which the fillers affect important mechanical properties, such as strength, stiffness, toughness, hardness, fatigue and wear, and other physical properties such as aesthetics, radiopacity, viscosity, thermal expansion and diffusivity, polymerization shrinkage, degree of conversion, and water sorption and solubility. The manner in which the fillers affect the stability of dental composites in various environments will then be addressed, followed by a presentation of current and future trends in filler technology for dental composites. While the properties of a composite are strongly dependent upon each of its components, the theme of this chapter will be to concentrate on a review of the literature that pertains directly to the filler and the interfacial coupling, and purposefully de-emphasizes the role of the resin matrix, as this has been covered in a previous chapter.

10.2 Current dental composite materials

10.2.1 Diversity of composite filler types and sizes

Perhaps the greatest advances in dental resin composites through the years have come from modifications of the reinforcing filler component. Early materials were filled with rather coarse, irregular-shaped particles, with a widely varied distribution of sizes but with many particles approaching or exceeding the dimension of a human hair (approximately 50–100 μm). These materials were strong, but also were difficult to polish and maintain smooth surfaces in the mouth. Further, they were prone to excessive wear due to the forces of mastication and abrasion from food and tooth brushing. Manufacturers' attempts to produce more wear resistant, polishable and aesthetically pleasing materials led to the development of fillers that were 100 to 1000 times smaller than those used in the original formulations, reaching the nanoscale size (1–100 nm). Today's commercial dental composites generally have particles with average sizes that remain in the nanoscale, or in the sub-micrometre range. These fillers are typically finely ground into irregular-shaped particulates, but more spherical-like particles formed by a pyrogenic process (fumed silica) or by the chemical sol–gel process also are common in many composites (Fig. 10.1). Short, chopped glass fibres have been used to reinforce some commercial formulations, but with minimal success owing to the inherently rougher surface produced.

The types of fillers employed in commercial dental composites also have changed significantly from those used in early formulations. Many early materials contained quartz because of its excellent refractive index match with the dimethacrylate resins used in the matrix phase and its high strength and hardness. However, as it is based entirely on silica, quartz is a non-radiopaque material and thus provides a significant diagnostic challenge to the clinician as the resultant composite appeared as a radiolucent area on a dental X-ray film. To address this deficiency, dental composites began to be formulated with radiopaque fillers comprising aluminium, strontium, zinc and other metallic oxide modified silica glasses. These fillers are produced by standard glass making processes by which oxide powders are melted to produce a homogeneous mixture and then cooled to a solid and prepared for wet grinding into finer particles. Other common fillers include zirconia silica particles, which are not produced by a melting of oxides, but

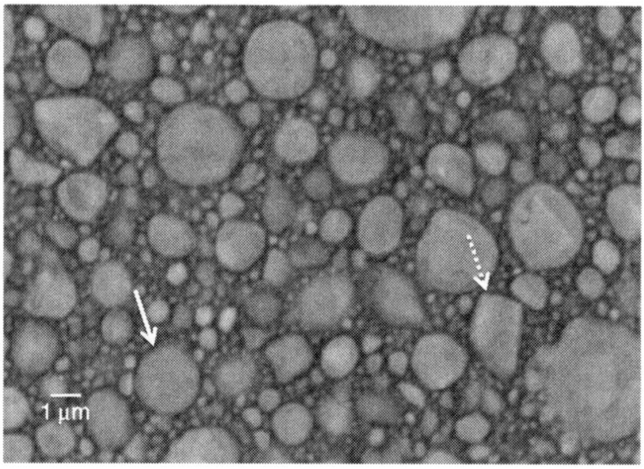

10.1 Backscatter scanning electron micrograph of a dental composite showing predominantly spherical-shaped fillers (solid arrow) and some irregular-shaped fillers (dotted arrow).

by the wet chemical sol–gel process. In this process, metallic precursor molecules, typically alkoxides, are chemically linked through condensation reactions in the solution phase into networks, ultimately forming a gel that is densified by the removal of water to produce a solid that can then be finely ground.

10.2.2 Range of properties produced

Based on the amount of reinforcing filler added, that is the proportion of filler and matrix, the properties of a dental composite can vary tremendously. In a general sense however, dental composites tend to have strength (tensile, flexure, compressive) and fracture resistance that is similar to that of other dental materials, such as amalgam and porcelain. But dental composites tend to have much lower stiffness (elastic modulus) owing to the relatively high content of the less stiff polymer matrix needed to bind the fillers. As the amount of filler increases, so do the properties; but filler level is limited by the ability to wet the high surface area particles with monomers during the blending process.

Dental composites do have excellent thermal insulating capabilities, as polymers are generally not good conductors of heat. Thermal conductivity does not vary greatly for different filler levels. The thermal expansion coefficient of dental composites varies between about twice as great as the tooth for the very highly filled materials, to several times as high for the very lightly filled materials. In this regard, composites are more similar to dental amalgam and other metallic dental materials than to porcelains or other ceramics, the latter having thermal expansion coefficients that are nearly the same as enamel.

Aesthetic properties can be finely tuned based on the types of fillers added. As the refractive index of the filler more closely matches that of the resin matrix, the composite can become nearly transparent. In contrast, the opposite effect (opacity) can be produced by using fillers with a large mismatch in the refractive index compared with the resin matrix. Thus, a wide range of translucencies is possible by altering the filler type. Water sorption and solubility can vary tremendously based on the formulation of the composite, but this is mainly due to the presence of more hydrophobic or hydrophilic monomers in the resin matrix component. Polymerization shrinkage is reduced as filler content is increased, but perhaps the greater concern about the dimensional change in dental composites is related to the stresses produced by the shrinkage, as opposed to the actual shrinkage itself.

10.3 Theoretical considerations

10.3.1 Basic principle of composites: rationale

The basic principle behind the production of a composite material is that the properties of the final mixture are determined by the properties and the proportions of the individual components. Composites are produced for a number of reasons, including cost reduction (often inexpensive fillers are added to expensive matrix materials to reduce costs), improved properties, altered thermal or optical effects, improved handling, and so on. Dental composites were developed to provide a tooth-coloured, direct restorative material that would have improved properties over existing unfilled polymer systems based on polymethylmethacrylate. While adding inorganic fillers to the cross-linked dimethacrylate matrix significantly enhances mechanical properties, other benefits derived from this addition include reduced thermal expansion coefficient, reduced shrinkage, enhanced optical properties and improved handling and placement characteristics.

10.3.2 Behaviour: rule of mixtures

As a first approximation, the properties of a composite material can be predicted using a simple rule of mixtures, as depicted by a Voigt 'isostrain' model where the strain on each component of the composite is equal (Darvell, 2000). To predict mechanical properties, this model assumes perfect bonding between the two components and the relationship between the mechanical property and the volume fraction of the filler is a straight line (Fig. 10.2). In general, dental composites do not follow the simple rule

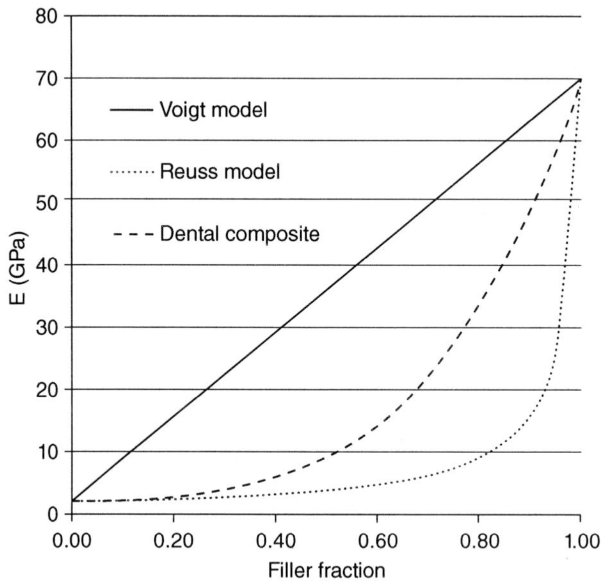

10.2 Graph showing the relationship between elastic modulus (*E*) and the filler volume fraction for dental composites compared to the Voigt model, which follows the simple rule of mixtures, and the Reuss model, which shows a much slower acquisition of elastic modulus as the filler fraction increases.

of mixtures (Braem *et al.*, 1986; Chantler, 1999). While they are typically isotropic, owing to the particulate and uniformly distributed nature of the filler reinforcement, dental composites require high filler volumes to achieve high strength and toughness. In contrast to the Voigt model, they typically follow more closely a Reuss 'isostress' model, which assumes that components are subjected independently to the same stress and are not perfectly linked together.

There are a variety of intermediate models available for predicting properties of different types of composite materials that have varied levels of interaction between their two components (Saffar *et al.*, 2010). This lack of conformity to the expected linear relationship between the specific mechanical property and the proportion of reinforcing fillers is due to the imperfect bond and stress distribution between the filler and the polymer matrix. In addition, incomplete polymerization of the polymer matrix and the existence of porosities contribute to this deviation from theory. Other properties, such as polymerization shrinkage, thermal expansion coefficient and water sorption, do generally follow this simple rule of mixtures and are more easily predicted based on a simple consideration of the proportion of the two components.

10.4 Types of fillers used in dental composites

10.4.1 Classification systems: particle size

The most common classifications of resin composite systems have been established using size, shape, volume fraction, chemical composition and manufacturing techniques of the filler, or combinations thereof (Lutz and Phillips, 1983; Marshall *et al.*, 1988; Willems *et al.*, 1992; Lang *et al.*, 1992; Kim *et al.*, 2002; Klapdohr and Moszner, 2005; Ardu *et al.*, 2010). Early classifications in terms of particle size were relatively straightforward. However, owing to the continuous introduction of many composite versions with subtle morphological differences and the use of innovative chemistry, creating a simple modern classification system is more problematic.

Resin composites have been commonly classified according to the mean size or volume percentage of the filler (Lang *et al.*, 1992; Willems *et al.*, 1992). Following the inception of resin-based composite (RBC) restoratives in the 1960s, it was soon recognised that conventional ('macrofilled') resin composites inherently suffered from poor aesthetic quality and inadequate wear resistance owing to large mean filler diameters ranging from 10–100 μm. The importance of a critical filler diameter and the separating distance between particles within the resin matrix led to the development of so-called 'microfillers' to obtain sufficient polishability and improved long-term aesthetic quality. However, the inclusion of very small particle diameters had a profound effect on composite rheology. A high surface area-to-volume ratio of microfillers precludes a high mass fraction within the resin matrix and therefore early homogeneous microfilled composites containing pyrogenic silica (~0.1 μm filler diameter) were unsuitable for use in load-bearing situations. In order to improve microfiller loading significantly, highly filled prepolymerised particles were included in the resin matrix with further addition of sub-micrometre sized particles. Degradation and premature clinical failure of so-called 'heterogeneous microfills' was recognised by reduced covalent bonding at the filler-resin interface (Ferracane, 1995) and the inability to achieve particularly high loading regardless of prepolymerised particle inclusions.

A compromise between adequate mechanical properties and wear resistance and aesthetic quality was pursued. This led to a reduction in particle size and the common classification of 'small particle hybrid' composites, or 'midifills' with a bimodal filler distribution, that is; a larger filler particle diameter ranging from ~1–10 μm and inclusion of ~0.05 μm 'microfiller' (Marshall *et al.*, 1988; Lang *et al.*, 1992). Subsequent improvements in filler manufacturing techniques resulted in further decreases in average particle sizes, typically in the region of 0.5–1 μm diameter that were coined 'minifills', or 'microhybrids', the latter phrase being routinely used today to describe many modern resin composites. The carefully graded distribution of filler sizes in modern microhybrids minimizes interparticulate spaces allowing them to fit together more efficiently and therefore maximizing packing. An acceptable combination of mechanical and aesthetic qualities of these materials indicated them for both anterior and posterior restorations and are termed 'universal' or 'all-purpose' resin composites.

The current strategy of dental resin composite marketing is bolstered by the prefix 'nano-', which has attracted particular consumer attention in recent years. Indeed, over the last decade, many manufacturers have increased numbers of sub-micrometre, 'nanofill' particles and prepolymers in order to create 'nanohybrid' composites. However, by definition, a 'nanomaterial' possesses components and/or structural features, such as fibres or particles, with at least one dimension less than 100 nm, which can demonstrate novel and distinct properties (Harris and Ure, 2006; Lui and Webster, 2007). Here, the morphological differences between nanofill/nanohybrid and microhybrids are not defined, which explains their general similarity in mechanical and physical material properties (Beun *et al.*, 2007; Ilie and Hickel, 2009). Considering the unremitting hype and often aggressive marketing of 'nano' composites, it is interesting to note that the size of fillers present in microfills do not differ vastly from that of nanohybrid materials. The terminology differs only because of the lack of recognition of the nano concept in the last century (Ferracane, 2011) and theoretically, nanotechnology has been used in dental composites for more than 40 years (Fig. 10.3)!

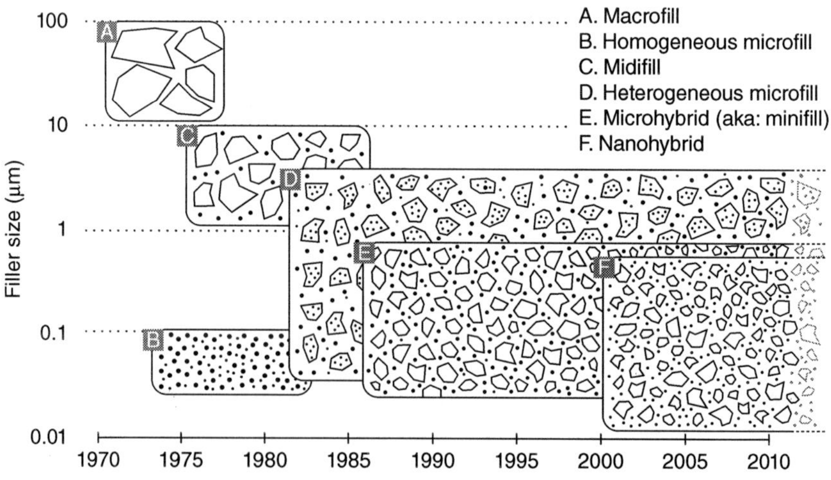

10.3 Diagram showing the chronological development of different types of dental composites with a representation of their particle sizes and distributions.

Methods of classification usually involve chemical or thermal decomposition of the filler from the uncured resin matrix using either solvent washing, thermogravimetric analysis or ashing followed by scanning electron microscopy to determine filler load and morphology and/or energy dispersive X-ray spectroscopy to determine filler composition (Marshall *et al.*, 1988; Hosoda *et al.*, 1990; Khan *et al.*, 1992; Lang *et al.*, 1992; Sabbagh *et al.*, 2004a; Beun *et al.*, 2007). In many cases, manufacturers do not disclose the exact composition of their composite materials and typically will only approximate filler percentage. Chemical and/or thermal decomposition therefore provides a useful tool for gathering the information required for appropriate filler classification. However, such techniques, which dissolve the resin matrix to reveal the inorganic portion may, in turn, affect filler morphology. Part organic, prepolymerized particles will decompose upon heating and aggressive solvents such as chloroform may defragment existing particle structures (Sabbagh *et al.*, 2004a; Leprince *et al.*, 2010).

Although different categories of modern dental resin composites remain unclear, classification by particle size remains the most useful: larger particles tend to increase wear rates, but allow higher filler loadings for increased strength, modulus and fracture toughness. Sub-micrometre fillers, that have diameters far less than the wavelength of visible light, provide superior polishability and durable surface gloss, but their vastly increased surface area prevents high particle loading. Discrete non-agglomerated nano-sized particles can reduce the thickening effect of traditional microfillers by efficient dispersion throughout the matrix (Bauer *et al.*, 2003). With the introduction of innovative resin chemistries that are either commercially available or under development (siloxane-oxirane, dimer acids, thiol-ene, silsesquioxane), new dental composite classification systems may be warranted in the near future (Ardu *et al.*, 2010).

10.4.2 Chemical composition

Generally, dental resin composites contain a mixture of at least two types of filler to provide adequate mechanical properties, wear resistance, radiopacity and coefficient of thermal expansion, and to minimize volumetric shrinkage (the direct effects of which are discussed later in this chapter). The filler mixtures can be composed of crystalline quartz, silicate glass (usually barium or strontium-silicates to provide some radiopacity), prepolymerized particles (usually based on methacrylate resin and fumed silica), fluorosilicates and ytterbium fluoride (for the release of fluoride ions), fumed silica and titanium dioxide (used as an opacifier).

In modern composites, larger fillers (usually greater than 1 μm but less than 5 μm) are mechanically prepared by grinding and milling quartz, glass and ceramic materials to the desired size and these purely inorganic particles exhibit irregular morphology owing to the method of preparation. By milling, particle agglomeration is inevitable below a specific diameter where interparticulate forces are greater than the weight of individual particles. Since nano-sized fillers cannot be produced by grinding, alternative methods such as flame-spraying and sol–gel techniques have been developed. Pyrogenic silica (such as Aerosil®, Cab-O-Sil®) is widely available and has been used since the inception of homogeneous and heterogeneous microfills with particle diameters less than 100 nm.

Chemical processing via the sol–gel method using mixtures of orthosilicates and metal alkoxides (titanium (IV) and zirconium (IV) ethoxide) produces primary particles with an average diameter of 5–100 nm (Klapdohr and Moszner, 2005). As the particle diameter decreases, the specific surface area increases considerably and filler loading is restricted by the increased viscosity associated with aggregated and agglomerated microfiller particles. Previous research and patent literature over the last decade feature the development of non-agglomerated nanoparticles (1–50 nm), which claim to reduce the thickening effect compared with pyrogenic silica (Rheinberger *et al.*, 1999; Zhang *et al.*, 2001; Bauer *et al.*, 2003). Improved dispersion following appropriate filler silanization prevents settling and the relatively lower viscosity achieved with discrete nanoparticles provides a composite material with higher filler loads and ultimately decreased shrinkage and improved mechanical properties. Examples of the chemical composition of discrete nanoparticles include silica organosols, which may be produced by condensation of silicic acid in water under appropriate conditions (Brinker and Scherer, 1990) or by a conventional Stöber method using alkoxysilane precursors (Stöber *et al.*, 1968; Park *et al.*, 2002).

Other hybrid materials have been processed to bridge the gap between dissimilarities in resin matrix and filler particle characteristics. Organic–inorganic components can be processed partially to replace the conventional organic phase of the composite. So-called polyhedral oligomeric silsesquioxane (POSS) chemistry offers isotropic nanoscale structures (~2 nm), which are suggested to improve mechanical properties and decrease polymerization shrinkage of POSS-containing methacrylate-based resins (Gao *et al.*, 2001; Wu *et al.*, 2010). These materials are produced from chemically modified silica particles that provide a cage-like structure containing copolymerizable methacrylate groups, which avoid the requirements of filler silanization (Fong *et al.*, 2005).

10.4.3 Particle shape: irregular, spherical, chopped fibres

Generally, filler particle shape is determined by the manufacturing process. Small quartz or glass particles produced by milling result in splintered or irregular morphology, whereas those produced by pyrogenic or sol–gel techniques normally provide near spherical particles. Filler geometry has been shown to affect the mechanical and physical properties of the composite significantly. Because of the differences in filler surface area of irregular and round geometries, varying interfacial effects between the filler and resin matrix might be expected. Indeed, it is known that specific spherical particle size distributions are more easily incorporated into the resin and can occupy more space than an irregular particle morphology (Miyasaka and Yoshida, 2000). Chopped fibres (Drummond *et al.*, 2009; Garoushi *et al.*, 2008) and whiskers (Xu *et al.*, 1999) have also been either tried or proposed as fillers for dental composites owing to the strong reinforcing effect obtained with particles of high aspect ratio (length to diameter).

10.4.4 Surface treatment: silanization

The weakest portion of a resin composite material is the filler–resin interface, and the filler surface must be modified to improve interfacial adhesion to the resin matrix. In conventional composites, organofunctional silanes are used to promote the chemical bond, which possesses amphiphilic properties consisting of a methoxysilane group at one end of the molecule and a methacrylate functional group at the other. In addition to enhancing the interfacial adhesion affecting reinforcing stress transfer to the stronger filler from the weaker matrix, other advantages of filler silanization include enhanced filler particle distribution (i.e. less agglomeration) and increased filler loading owing to more optimal wetting of the fillers by the monomers.

The most common silane agent used for dental resin composites is 3-methacryloxypropyltrimethoxysilane (γ-MPTS; Fig. 4(a)). Silanization usually involves coating filler particles by solution deposition techniques, where an interfacial layer is created between the filler and coupling agent through complex hydrolysis–condensation reactions. A simplified explanation involves the silane molecule becoming hydrolysed by an aqueous solvated solution forming silanol (Si–OH) groups and intermediate hydrogen bonds (Fig. 10.4(b)). Subsequent condensation reactions result in the formation of vertical covalent (oxane) bonds (Si–O–Si) between the silane molecule and the silica surface together with horizontal bonds forming a siloxane network. Ideally, more hydrogen bonds will occur between the –OH group at the silica surface and carbonyl group of MPTS to improve its parallel orientation (Fig. 10.4(c)). Following incorporation of the surface modified filler into the organic matrix, the methacryl functionality of the silane molecule allows copolymerization with the resin. In the absence of a silica substrate, these organosilanes may undergo hydrolysis and self-condensation reactions that produce the complex oligomers and polymers, known as silsesquioxanes, described in Section 10.4.2 (Antonucci *et al.*, 2005).

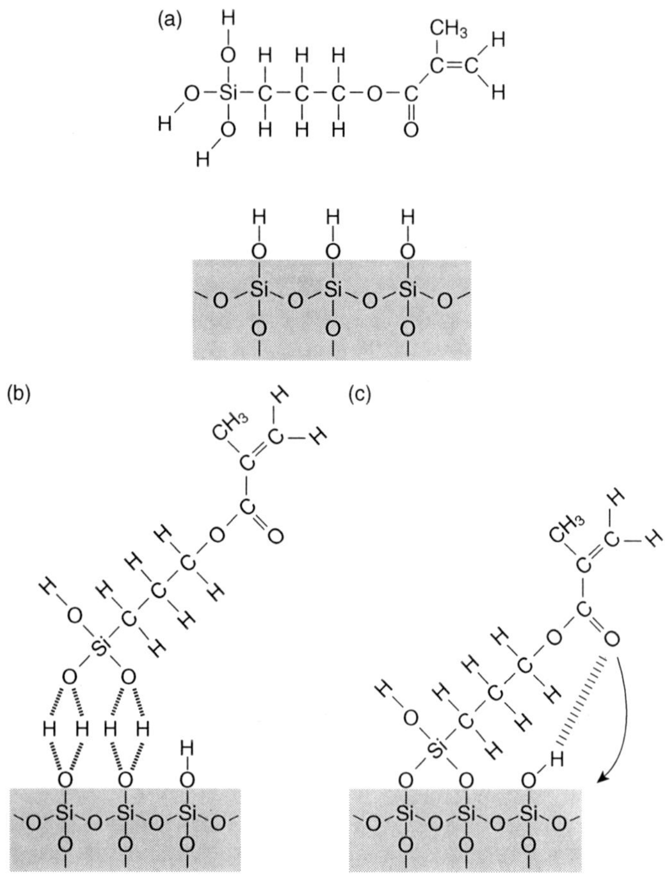

10.4 (a) Chemical structure of 3-methacryloxypropyltrimethoxysilane (γ-MPTS), the most common silane molecule used to couple the inorganic filler to the polymer matrix in dental composites. (b) Diagram showing how the silane molecule becomes hydrolysed by an aqueous solvated solution to form silanol (Si–OH) groups that make intermediate hydrogen bonds with the Si–OH groups on the filler surface. (c) Condensation reactions produce covalent (oxane) bonds (Si–O–Si) between the silane molecule and the silica surface, supplemented by additional hydrogen bonding.

The term 'interface' is commonly used to refer to the boundary layer between the filler and resin, however, as a result of this complex chemical process, a less sharp transition exists between the inorganic and organic parts and has been more accurately described as a multi-layered 'interphase' (Antonucci *et al.*, 2005). Ideally, the silane treatment should create a molecular monolayer on the filler surface; however, in practice it is known that the film is substantially thicker (50–100 nm) and randomly orientated

(Söderholm and Shang, 1993; Matinlinna *et al.*, 2004). Only the oxane groups closest to the filler surface form a chemical bond and as the layer thickness increases, physical adsorption and disorganization may result in weaker bonding. The processing conditions used to silanize filler particles (such as type and amount of silane, water content, solvent type, pH and temperature) will significantly affect the formation and nature of the interphase, which, in turn, will affect stress transfer under masticatory load and bond degradation between the resin and filler. The oxane bond between filler and resin is susceptible to hydrolytic degradation due to its ionic character and this, in combination with the plasticizing effect of water on the resin matrix, may result in decreased mechanical properties of resin composites over time (Drummond *et al.*, 2004; Ferracane and Berge, 1995).

In order to improve the hydrolytic stability of the filler–resin interphase, alternative silanes have been developed, such as 10-methacryloxydecyltrimethoxysilane (MDTS). This molecule exhibits a greater hydrocarbon content and is therefore more hydrophobic, providing improved durability following water immersion. A disadvantage of using a silane molecule with a longer hydrocarbon chain is increased flexibility, which has produced composites with inferior mechanical properties compared with those containing shorter propyl spacers (Klapdohr and Moszner, 2005).

The use of MPTS is considered the standard for commercial resin composites and there appears to be only limited success in using alternative trialkoxysilanes or other silane chemistries. However, some multifunctional organosilanes have been tested for their potential as coupling agents. The reaction of 3-isocyanatopropyltriethoxysilane and bis-GMA provided a silane agent that improved hydrolytic stability by an increased degree of crosslinking in the interphase (Antonucci *et al.*, 2005). The use of 3-styrylethyltrimethoxysilane and 3-acryloxypropyltrimethoxysilane have been reported to enhance filler–resin adhesion and blends of functional and cross-linking silanes show moderately improved flexural strengths compared with composites containing fillers silanized with conventional MPTS (Matinlinna *et al.*, 2011).

10.5 Effect of fillers on properties of dental composites

10.5.1 Mechanical properties

In general, the mechanical properties of dental composites are directly influenced by several characteristics: the filler volume fraction, the quality of the bonded interface between the filler and the resin matrix, and the monomer type, degree of conversion and cross-linking density of the polymer matrix. Other factors, such as porosity, also have a negative influence on the strength. Regarding the direct effects of the filler, previous research has implicated filler shape as being important in controlling the wear performance and degree of conversion (Turssi *et al.*, 2005) and shrinkage strain (Satterthwaite *et al.*, 2009) of resin composite materials. In terms of mechanical properties, an irregular morphology may result in increased stress concentrations at sharp line-angles of the filler–resin interface and decreased fracture strength compared with that of the smoother surfaces of spheroidal particles (Suzuki *et al.*, 1995; Sabbagh *et al.*, 2004a; Curtis *et al.*, 2009).

It was noted previously that the mechanical properties of dental composites increase with their filler volume, but not typically in a linear manner. This was attributed to an imperfect bond and stress transfer between the reinforcing filler and the polymer matrix. This bond is mediated by the silane coupling agent and there are many variables that may affect the quality of this interphase, as stated previously. The individual sections below provide specific information about how the characteristics of the filler itself directly affect the various mechanical properties of dental composites.

Strength and elastic modulus

As expected, the flexure strength and modulus of dental composites increases as their filler content increases (Ferracane *et al.*, 1998; Sabbagh *et al.*, 2002; Masouras *et al.*, 2008b), with one study showing a maximum being attained at about 60% by volume (Ilie and Hickel, 2009). The filler size is likely to be less important than the filler amount (Pick *et al.*, 2011) and a study comparing two commercial composites with three orders of magnitude difference in filler size but nearly equivalent filler loads showed them to have similar strengths (Rodrigues *et al.*, 2008). However, a recent study has shown that for comparable filler volumes, higher elastic modulus (as determined by nanoindentation) is achieved with larger and more irregular-shaped fillers compared with spherical fillers, possibly due to the enhanced interaction between tightly packed irregular fillers (Masouras, 2008a).

Silane coupling between the filler particles and the resin matrix enhances the strength of resin composites, but the amount of silane applied was not shown to have a highly significant effect in a recent study (Sideridou and Karabela, 2009). The presence of prepolymerized resin fillers, which is common in many nanohybrid dental composites, in part to reduce polymerization shrinkage, is likely to reduce the strength, as the overall inorganic filler level is less in these composites than in most microhybrid composites and the bond between the resin matrix and the prepolymerized filler is relatively weak (Blackham *et al.*, 2009).

Attempts to enhance the strength and elastic modulus of composites through altered particle shape have included the addition of short glass fibres (Garoushi *et al.*, 2008) and longer e-glass fibres (Abdulmajeed *et al.*, 2011). A recent study in which nanofibrillar silicate was added at relatively low concentrations of 1% and 2.5% significantly enhanced the elastic modulus of particulate-filled composites (Tian *et al.*, 2008). Other work reported the development of high-modulus thermal-cured dental composites by the addition of high modulus alumina nanopowder (Wang *et al.*, 2007). However, relatively opaque fillers, such as alumina, have a strong negative impact on the optical properties of dental composites and are not likely to be tried commercially.

Fracture toughness

The fracture toughness of dental composites is generally increased with filler volume fraction (Kim *et al.*, 1994; Ferracane and Berge, 1995; Zhao *et al.*, 1997)(Fig. 10.5(a)) owing to a variety of energy increasing mechanisms that have been summarized as: increasing crack surface area and crack blunting, plastic deformation of the resin matrix at the crack tip, crack bowing due to pinning of the crack between particles, microcrack formation and extension around the crack tip, and crack deflection by particles (Chan *et al.*, 2007; Kim and Okuno, 2002). Recent studies have shown that crack bridging is also an effective toughening mechanism in certain dental composites (Shah *et al.*, 2009). Here the crack appears discontinuous and seems to 'jump' from one site to another, bypassing a filler, for example, and expending more energy in the process, leading to toughening (Fig. 10.6). The strong correlation between filler content and toughness becomes limited once composites achieve approximately 55–60 vol% filler (Kim *et al.*, 2002; Ilie *et al.*, 2012), possibly caused by a reduction in the effectiveness of crack pinning once the interparticle spacing becomes too small (Ferracane *et al.*, 1987).

Efforts to enhance the toughness of dental composites further have come through the addition of alternative fillers. Xu *et al.* (2004, 2010) have shown that high toughness composites can be made by incorporating silicon carbide and silicon nitride whiskers into the composite. These materials are relatively opaque and must be self-cured or heat-cured; thus their usefulness as direct restorative materials is limited.

The fracture toughness of dental composites is significantly affected by the interfacial adhesion quality between the fillers and the polymer matrix. But in a study in which the total filler content was maintained constant and the proportion of silane treated fillers varied from 20–100%, the fracture toughness was not substantially increased once the percentage of silane-treated particles exceeded 60–80% (Ferracane *et al.*, 1998) (Fig. 10.5(b)).

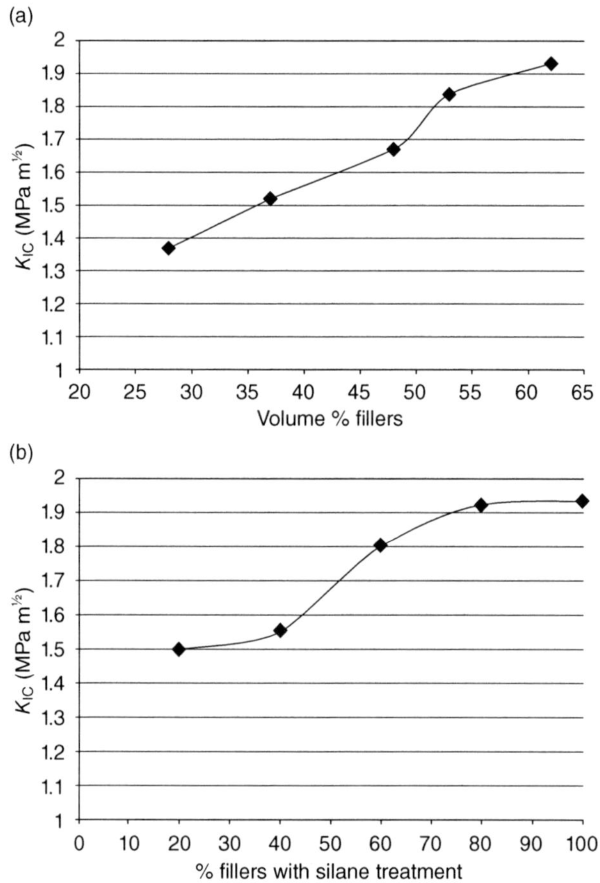

10.5 (a) Fracture toughness (K_{IC}) for dental composite showing increase in toughness with increase in filler volume fraction (from Ferracane *et al.*, 1998). (b) Fracture toughness (K_{IC}) for dental composite showing an increase in toughness with increase in percentage of total fillers that have been silane treated, but reaching a maximum near 80% (from Ferracane *et al.*, 1998).

The possibility that unbonded particles may provide sites for energy release during crack propagation has been previously suggested as an explanation for this phenomenon (Ferracane and Marker, 1992).

Hardness

The surface hardness of dental composites is a function of filler content (Xu *et al.*, 2002), as well as of the properties of the reinforcing filler itself. A recent study showed that filling dental composite with a harder filler

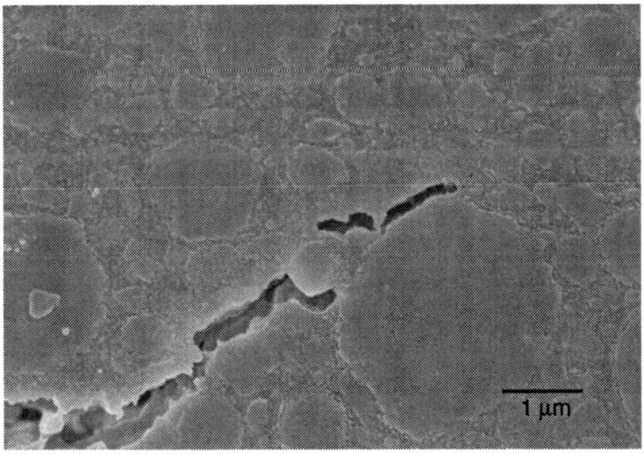

10.6 Scanning electron micrograph showing evidence of crack bridging as a toughening mechanism in a dental composite.

particle, that is a particulate lithium disilicate ceramic versus a particulate glass, produced a harder and more wear-resistant composite (Atai *et al.*, 2007). There is no strong correlation overall between wear and composite hardness (Hahnel *et al.*, 2011), but in general, harder surfaces are more desirable for resisting occlusal and abrasive forces. Hardness does not seem to be a function of particle size if composites with equal amounts of overall filler are compared (Schwartz and Soderholm, 2004).

Fatigue

There is a general trend of higher fatigue strength for dental composites with higher filler volumes (Lohbauer *et al.*, 2003; Drummond *et al.*, 2009). However, earlier studies suggested that there might be an optimum filler level for maximizing fatigue resistance, as composites with filler levels below 60% and above 80% by weight had reduced fatigue strength in a tooth cavity model (Htang *et al.*, 1995). Fatigue has also been shown to be related to the quality of the filler/matrix interfacial bond, with composites that have a silane treated filler having greater fatigue strength than those without a silanated filler (McCool *et al.*, 2001).

The fatigue strength of particulate-filled composite has been shown to be significantly improved by the addition of glass fibres (Bae *et al.*, 2004). Keulemans *et al.* (2009) also reported that fibre-reinforced composites had improved fatigue strength compared with particulate-reinforced composites. Drummond *et al.* (2009) reported that composites with larger filler particles, including fibre-reinforced materials, generally had higher fatigue strength, although in this particular study these composites also had the highest filler loads, making it difficult to isolate the two effects. Drummond (2008) has published an excellent article reviewing the effects of filler and overall composition on the fatigue and failure of dental resin composites.

Wear

Wear of dental composites cannot be directly correlated to one specific property, although theory suggests that it should be related to hardness. In studies in which composites with different filler sizes and shapes have been studied, wear seems to be somewhat less for composites with smaller fillers (Schwartz and Söderholm, 2004; Turssi *et al.*, 2005; Wonglamsam *et al.*, 2008). Söderholm *et al.* (2001) showed no difference in clinical wear rate for two composites with equivalent resins but either quartz or barium glass (both at 3 μm average size). Further in their study, two different methods of applying the silane surface treatment to the fillers did not affect clinical wear.

The relationships between wear and filler characteristics are most effectively studied using experimental composite materials in which variables can be controlled. Lim *et al.* (2002) studied the wear of composites containing silica nanoparticles and showed that the wear was reduced as filler volume fraction increased. This result was not unexpected and is in agreement with the 'protection hypothesis' of wear which states that wear is related to the resin spacing between the particles, because the polymer is less wear resistant than the filler, and that reducing the size of the space protects the resin and reduces wear (Bayne *et al.*, 1992). Venhoven *et al.* (1996) noticed a similar trend when subjecting composites of various filler sizes to abrasion in a wear machine. They also suggested that there is a minimal particle size needed to protect the matrix from the abrasive effects of the food bolus.

Lim *et al.* (2002) also demonstrated that good filler/matrix adhesion mediated by a functional silane coupling agent was needed to minimize wear. Turssi *et al.* (2005), when investigating two composites with the same amount and size of fillers, showed that the one with irregular fillers was more wear resistant, possibly owing to its enhanced surface area and adhesion to the resin matrix. Xu *et al.* (2004) produced dental composites with reduced wear compared to other commercial composites by virtue of the addition of nanosilica fused whiskers. While composites made with fibres greater than a micrometre in size have not been shown to be more wear resistant than particulate filled composites (Ferracane *et al.*, 1999), the use of whiskers has the advantage of a dramatically reduced size and greater polymer matrix reinforcement explaining the beneficial effect seen by Xu *et al.* (2004).

10.5.2 Other properties

Aesthetics: translucency

Resin composites can be manufactured to mimic the aesthetic quality of the surrounding tooth tissue and the level of translucency is an important factor. In smaller restorations, translucent materials tend to provide what in dentistry has been called 'chameleon' characteristics by reflection and transmission of light from neighbouring tooth structure (Sidhu *et al.*, 2006). Where there is limited underlying tooth structure in bulkier fillings or those with no tooth structure backing in Class III and IV cavities, a wide range of shades and opacities are available. Layering techniques are devised to place increasingly translucent materials in order to create an optical depth of field that will improve aesthetic quality. For optimum aesthetic quality of the final resin composite restoration, materials should exhibit similar optical properties to those of natural teeth. Specifically, similar translucency, light reflection, scattering, fluorescence and opalescence should be expected. Translucency is an important property of a resin composite, which provides an indication of the quality and quantity of reflected light (Winter, 1993) and, along with colour properties, has the greatest influence on the final visual effects of the restoration.

Opalescence in resin composites is important for optical mimicry of enamel and is also strongly dependent on the translucency of the material (Lee and Yu, 2005). Opalescence is created by scattering of shorter (blue) and transmission of longer (orange/red) wavelengths of light. The resin matrix must be translucent in order to observe the scattered light from the filler and the resulting opal effect to be observed. In order to attain opalescent properties similar to enamel it has been suggested that at least one component of the composite be in the size range 380–500 nm. A refractive index constant (the RI ratio between resin and filler) of more than 1.1 will result in brilliant opalescent colours (Egen *et al.*, 2004; Lee, 2008). Given the refractive index of a typical cured resin might range from ~1.534–1.554 (41 : 59 and 60 : 40, 2,2′-bis[4-(methacryloxypropoxy)-phenyl]-propane (bis-GMA): triethyleneglycol dimethacrylate) TEGDMA) (Shortall *et al.*, 2008), to achieve opalescence, the filler RI should range from ~1.40–1.70, although the extremes of this range may not be possible with conventional filler particle types. Other techniques have been explored, which include a significant increase in the opalescence parameter following the addition of small amounts of titanium dioxide nanoparticles, although a colour change and decreased translucency were also noted (Yu *et al.*, 2009). Although light scattering is of apparent importance to optically relevant parameters for high aesthetic quality of composite restorations, it is detrimental for deep curing, the factors associated with which will be discussed in more detail in Section 10.5.2, Depth of cure.

Radiopacity

The dental practitioner must be able to identify the resin composite material on radiographs in order to assess the integrity of the restoration following patient recall, and to differentiate between the composite and adjacent tissue and detect porosities, overhangs and marginal defects (Jandt *et al.*, 2002; Ergücü *et al.*, 2010). The radiopacity of the material is usually compared with that of enamel, dentine or aluminium and in order to detect secondary caries the filling must be more radiopaque than the surrounding dental tissue (Epselid *et al.*, 1991; Willems *et al.*, 1991).

The elemental composition of the organic dimethacrylate resin matrix includes carbon, oxygen and hydrogen with low electron density allowing X-ray photons to pass freely through, rendering the material radiolucent. Part of the inorganic fraction of the composite must therefore provide a radiopacifier, which usually consists of conventional glass fillers containing elements with a high atomic number such as barium and strontium silicates, silica–zirconia and silica–titania and tantalum–silica mixed oxides (Klapdohr and Moszner, 2005). Other non-silicate radiopacifying agents may include ytterbium and yttrium fluoride, non-agglomerated zirconia particles and barium and strontium sulphates, the latter of which cannot be surface modified with silanes (Moszner and Salz, 2007). Previous research has highlighted the wide differences in radiopacity between material types (Sabbagh *et al.*, 2004b; Amirouche *et al.*, 2007; Ergücü *et al.*, 2010), with a linear correlation between filler percentage by weight and X-ray film radiopacity (Sabbagh *et al.*, 2004b) where some 'flowable' composite types show radiopacity only similar to that of dentine (Attar *et al.*, 2003).

Radiopacifiers may also affect the aesthetic quality of the material by reducing translucency. However, incorporation of heavy metal oxides into conventional silicates (Ba, Sr-silicate, etc.) will increase the refractive index and this can be useful in achieving higher translucency in certain resin mixtures (Shortall *et al.*, 2008). If the particle size is less than 50 nm without agglomeration, translucency can be achieved owing to low light scattering independent of refractive index values, thus producing an optically translucent material that still exhibits radiopacity. Several companies have patented composite materials containing nanoparticles of mixed oxides to achieve this goal (Klapdohr and Moszner, 2005). Large proportions of radiopacifiers can also result in inferior composite material properties, such as decreased surface hardness (Amirouche *et al.*, 2007) and poor wear resistance (Watts, 1987), although the mixed oxide type and volume effect of radiopaque fillers has no significant effect on the degree of conversion and shrinkage strain (Amirouche-Korichi *et al.*, 2009).

Viscosity: handling

Not only do fillers play an important role in the final properties of the set composite, but also in the rheology and handling of the paste material prior to curing. Indeed, many practitioners will select commercial composites depending upon their perception of good handling: packability, stickiness and 'pull-back' potential, pseudoplastic and thixotropic properties and slump resistance, all of which may affect the ease of placement.

Historically, in an attempt to increase the ease of manipulation, high viscosity or 'packable' composites were developed, offering handling characteristics similar to amalgam (Leinfelder *et al.*, 1998). Several approaches have utilized alternative filler particle types and morphology to conventional microfilled and hybrid composites, although total filler levels do not vary from highly filled hybrid composites (Ferracane *et al.*, 1999). Commonly, filler loads within the resin matrix exceed 65% by volume. Other previous attempts have included the use of a wide particle size distribution of irregular shaped fillers from 0.04–10 μm within a highly filled matrix (Surefil; Dentsply, Surrey, UK), where it was suggested that the flow of smaller particles past or around the larger particles is prevented, allowing filler particles to move closer together to achieve a 'packable' characteristic of the monomer paste (Nash *et al.*, 2001). Other high viscosity formulations have included the use of porous fillers ranging from 2–20 μm diameter, into which the surrounding resin is allowed to flow (Solitaire; Heraeus Kulzer, Dormagen, Germany) and the incorporation of a highly filled (84% by weight) fibre and particulate-reinforced resin matrix where the fibres range from 40–60 μm in length and the fillers range from 6–10 μm in diameter (Alert; Jeneric-Pentron, Wallingford, CT, US). Perceived disadvantages in the handling properties of highly filled 'packable' type composites include less ability to conform to line angles and corners of the cavity and an increased likelihood of porosity and voids, especially between layers of the restoration following manipulation of the high viscosity paste.

A further concept derived from the clinicians demand for specific handling properties of composite materials has been the introduction of low viscosity or 'flowable' RBCs, which contain a resin of lower filler fraction and/or increased diluent resin to obtain an arbitrarily fluid material. These materials were designed for use in cavities which present difficult access, such as the marginal repair of amalgam or conventional composite restorations, pit and fissure sealants and as a lining material for Class I, II and III laminate restorations. The effect of decreasing the volume fraction of fillers to produce a 'flowable' restorative will inevitably result in decreased strength and elastic modulus and an increase in polymerization shrinkage, manifested by the increase in volume of the organic resin phase and/or use of lower molecular weight resins. The increased volumetric shrinkage produced by 'flowable' composites may lead to high stress levels being developed at the tooth/restoration interface, although dependent upon the number of bonded surfaces and compliance of surrounding tooth structure, a decreased elastic modulus may reduce interfacial stress and improve marginal integrity (Braga *et al.*, 2003).

The rheology of flowable composites varies considerably between product type (Lee *et al.*, 2006; Beun *et al.*, 2008) and the incorporation of fillers into the resin matrix results in a composite that exhibits non-Newtonian fluid dynamics, where an increase in shear rate reduces viscosity, a desirable material property for placement allowing for improved adaptation. Flowable composites are usually applied through a narrow gauge needle, which reduces the viscosity and increases flow because of the pseudoplastic nature of the material. Subsequently, when shearing forces are removed, there may be a time-dependent recovery of initial viscosity, which describes its thixotropic characteristic and ideally the material should retain its shape following application in order to avoid migration and marginal overhangs. However, previous work has suggested a wide variation in the ability of several flowable composite materials to withstand slumping after placement when the shear rate approaches zero (Lee *et al.*, 2010). A more recent attempt to alter the viscosity of composite is to use sonic energy placement methods with a heavily filled composite (Sonicfill, Kerr).

Comonomer composition and the complex, time-dependent interaction between the filler and resin matrix will affect the fluid dynamics and handling properties of the material. Nanoscale particles are known to have a much greater impact on the rheology of composite materials than larger micrometre-sized fillers, owing to the vastly increased surface area of the former (Lee and Bowman, 2006; Beun *et al.*, 2009). In fact, this interaction and change in viscoelastic properties may significantly affect the final properties of the cured material. Recently, significantly decreased polymer conversion was observed for some flowable composites cured with high intensity curing protocols. For similar radiant exposure (18 $\mathrm{J\,cm^{-2}}$), a reduced conversion under high irradiance for short exposure (3000 $\mathrm{mW\,cm^{-2}}$ for 6 s) was observed compared with those cured with lower irradiance and longer irradiation times (400 $\mathrm{mW\,cm^{-2}}$ for 45 s) (Hadis *et al.*, 2011).

Thermal expansion

The coefficient of thermal expansion (CTE) has been suggested to be an important property in the performance of resin composite restorations (Powers *et al.*, 1979; Xu *et al.*, 1989). If a large mismatch in the CTE exists

Table 10.1 Coefficient of thermal expansion for different types of dental composites compared with other natural and synthetic dental materials

Material	Product	Filler load (vol %)	CTE (linear) (10^{-6}/°C)	Temperature range (°C)
Pit/fissure sealants[1]	Kerr Sealant[a]		70.9 (3.9)	0–60
	Delton[b]		103.5 (2.0)	0–60
Microfill[2]	Heliomolar[c]	41.3	44.7 (1.2)	26–75
Microhybrid[3]	Z100[d]	66	23.2 (1.7)	0–60
	Z250[d]	60	33.0 (0.6)	0–60
Nanohybrid[4]	Grandio[e]	71.4	28.5 (0.7)	30–80
	Filtek Supreme[f]	59.5	50.8 (1.4)	30–80
Enamel[5]			17.0 (3.8)	10–80
Dentine[5]			11.0 (2.4)	10–80
Gold alloys[6]			~14–15.5	25–500
Dental amalgam[6]			~22–28.0	20–50

[1] Powers *et al.*, 1979; [2] Versluis *et al.*, 1996; [3] Sideridou *et al.*, 2004; [4] Park *et al.*, 2010; [5] Xu *et al.*, 1989; [6] O'Brien, 2008.
[a] Kerr Manufacturing Co; [b] Johnson & Johnson; [c] Vivadent; [d] 3M; [e] Voco; [f] 3M ESPE Dental Products.

between the restorative and surrounding tooth tissue, ingestion of hot or cold fluids will result in dissimilar expansion and contraction between the two materials. Any difference in dimensional change will impose stresses at the tooth–restoration interface, which may compromise its integrity and lead to sensitivity and/or marginal gaps and secondary infection. The CTE for enamel and dentine is compared with various restorative material types in Table 10.1.

The CTE of resin composites, as with many other material properties discussed in this chapter, is not entirely attributed to effects of filler inclusions. Generally, a significant inverse linear correlation between CTE and volume percentage of filler has been reported (Söderholm, 1984; Vaidyanathan *et al.*, 1992; Versluis *et al.*, 1996; Park *et al.*, 2010), whilst others highlight the effect of the thermal properties of the filler particles, the efficacy of their silanization treatment (Yamaguchi *et al.*, 1989; Kanie *et al.*, 2004) and the resin matrix composition (Sideridou *et al.*, 2004). Whilst temperature increases are greatly reduced in highly filled composites, the thermal effects on restorative materials that contain less filler (such as adhesives, sealants and flowables) become more significant. Recent studies have used interferometry techniques to highlight the inherent interplay between non-isothermal polymerization and the effects of temperature on thermal expansion and shrinkage strain (Mucci *et al.*, 2009; Hadis *et al.*, 2010).

Thermal diffusivity

At steady state, the material property that describes heat flow through a composite is thermal conductivity (λ: $W m^{-1} K^{-1}$), and materials with high values will transfer heat more quickly than those with low conductivity. Thermal diffusivity (α: $m^2 s^{-1}$) explains the transient heat flow through a material and is related to conductivity by: $\alpha = \lambda / \rho C_p$ where, ρ is the density and C_p is the specific heat capacity (and ρC_p is the volumetric heat capacity).

Enamel and dentine have relatively low thermal conductivity and are therefore good insulating materials, an important characteristic for pulp protection. Although enamel exhibits low conductivity, its diffusivity is significantly greater than that of dentine (4.7×10^{-6} and $1.8–1.9 \times 10^{-6}$ $m^2 s^{-1}$), which suggests that the temperature in enamel will increase at a greater rate when subjected to an external heat source and may form enamel microcracks if the temperature change is sufficiently high (Brown *et al.*, 1970).

With the development and ever-increasing popularity of high irradiance curing lights and the reaction exotherm of light-activated resin composites, heat transfer through the composite material to the surrounding tooth structure and its potential thermal gradient between enamel and dentine, and insult to the pulp, are therefore critical considerations. There has been much interest in the potential heating effects of curing lights and controversy remains regarding the upper limit of thermal insult prior to pulpal cell damage. Whilst, in recent history, it has been suggested that resin composites cannot be over-cured, with the advent of powerful curing lights, over-heating of the pulp chamber in certain situations may become a clinical concern. Consequently, an important role of the composite restorative is to exhibit appropriate thermal diffusivity. Previous work has highlighted the effect of filler type, size and loading on thermal properties of resin composites and the findings of many researchers suggest that even with the significant changes in composition, resin composites provide good thermal insulation. More traditional materials were reported to exhibit higher diffusivity owing to the incorporation of quartz fillers in contrast to the more favourable thermal properties of composites that contain silicate glass or microfine silica (Watts *et al.*, 1987). A more recent study has suggested that thermal conductivity could be reduced by using nano-sized fillers (~1–10 nm), although the decrease in temperature rise at the pulp–dentine junction was minimal compared with existing commercial resin composites (Jakubinek *et al.*, 2010).

As curing light irradiance decreases through composite thickness because of reflection, absorption and scattering, a thermal property gradient is expected as a function of depth. Photothermal radiometry techniques have been adopted to measure optical and thermal depth profiles. Increasing thermal diffusivity was observed through deeper composite layers and attributed to reduced polymerization (Martinez-Torres *et al.*, 2009, 2010). Such techniques may offer further insight into the spatial physical properties of thick composite layers rather than relying on bulk measurements alone.

Polymerization shrinkage

Volumetric contraction throughout and following polymerization remains a major drawback of modern resin composites. A plethora of research spanning five decades has examined the effects of filler morphology and resin chemistry on shrinkage. Although shrinkage is an important material property to consider, it is not wholly responsible for gap formation at the tooth–restoration interface and the clinical implication of lower shrinkage values for a particular resin composite may not necessarily be beneficial (Tantbirojn *et al.*, 2011). Essentially, a compromised margin is a result of the inferior bond strength of the adhesive layer to tooth tissue compared with the magnitude of polymerization shrinkage stress generated throughout and/or following cure. The manifestation of shrinkage stress is a multifactorial process and relies upon intrinsic material properties such as volumetric shrinkage and elastic modulus, and may be higher or lower as filler loading increases. Further considerations include the onset of gelation of the resin matrix and polymerization rate, configuration factor (the ratio of the surface area of the bonded to unbonded surfaces) and the compliance of the surrounding tooth structure.

There has been considerable success in reducing resin shrinkage by using higher molecular weight resins, chemistries that exhibit ring-opening mechanisms (Weinmann *et al.*, 2005) or those that delay the gel point such as thiol–ene reactions (Pfeifer *et al.*, 2011). Indeed, recent research suggests that the resin matrix has significantly more influence on polymerization shrinkage stress compared with filler content and has highlighted possibilities for reducing stress by modifying the resin chemistry without sacrificing filler content (Goncalves *et al.*, 2011).

In conventional resin composites when considering the effects of fillers on shrinkage characteristics, there is a compromise between filler load, shrinkage and stiffness. As filler volume increases, the reduced resin volume will reduce shrinkage values, while the elastic modulus increases. Conversely, less filler reduces elastic modulus (potentially beneficial as a stress-absorbing layer using 'flowable' composite types), although generally shrinkage is increased, which may negate any stress relief. For cavities where surrounding tissue compliance is high, it might be expected that shrinkage strain will govern the magnitude of polymerization shrinkage stress, whilst under lower compliance (stiffer cavities) elastic modulus and shrinkage of the composite are both influential in the generation of interfacial stress (Min *et al.*, 2010).

Filler particle size and shape may also affect polymerization shrinkage strain. Previous work has identified a reduction in shrinkage strain for resins containing spherical compared with irregular-shaped fillers and increasing spherical particle size (Satterthwaite *et al.*, 2009), although the former observation may be related to differences in degree of conversion. An innovative approach to reducing shrinkage and shrinkage stress was realized through the addition of nano-sized prepolymer ('nanogel') particles, where a 36% reduction in shrinkage was reported for resins containing 40 wt% nanogel compared with those without (Moraes *et al.*, 2011).

Depth of cure

Curing depth is a limiting factor in the use of light-activated resin composites and usually practitioners are advised not to cure increments of more than 2 mm thickness. However, this is an arbitrary value considering the need for a dentist to judge accurately the layer thickness and the wide variation in material composition and shade. Notwithstanding the effects of coloured photoinitiators (that may not fully bleach upon light irradiation) and pigments (usually iron oxide and/or titanium dioxide particles) used for different shades of composite, filler morphology and their optical characteristics will alter the translucency of the composite prior to, throughout and following cure, which ultimately reduces light transport and the extent of cure through deeper layers.

As the curing light irradiates the translucent resin matrix, it is reflected at the surface, transmitted, scattered and absorbed. Curing light transmission is affected by the change in optical path length caused by filler particle scattering. When the particle diameter is much greater than the wavelength of the curing light (3.3–15 μm), scattering is known to be inversely proportional to filler size (Campbell *et al.*, 1986; Lee, 2007). For particles with mean diameters that are in the region of the wavelength of incident light, it is has been reported that scattering will increase with larger particle diameters (1.81 μm compared with 0.78 μm) and that increased filler density and filler silanization also may result in greater light absorption (Emami *et al.*, 2005). As the mean particle diameter decreases and approaches half the wavelength of the curing light, scattering is increased (Ruyter and Øysaed, 1982). Therefore, it would be expected that filler diameters of approximately 0.2–0.35 μm (half the wavelength of the visible light spectrum) would result in the highest amount of scattering and a reduced translucency. However, the subtle differences in composition between the multitude of commercial resin composite types provides a complex interaction of light with filler morphology and between the filler and resin matrix and translucency is not determined by filler size alone. Even if particle morphologies present much smaller diameters than the wavelength of light (e.g. microfillers with an average diameter of ~50 nm) and therefore do not scatter light (Klapdohr and Moszner, 2005), particle agglomeration results in an effectively larger diameter, which may decrease translucency (Kawaguchi *et al.*, 1994).

For effective packing of fillers in resin composites, a range of filler sizes is used and this distribution will complicate scattering and may reduce light transmission rather than considering only the mean particle size. Light refraction also occurs at the interface between the resin and filler and scattering is reduced when the difference in refractive index between phases is small (Shortall *et al.*, 2008). Indeed, resin composites generally become more translucent throughout cure as the refractive index of the resin increases to approach that of the filler. Model composite systems may be designed that exhibit very high cure depths (>10 mm), although the aesthetic quality might be compromised (Shortall *et al.*, 2008; Leprince *et al.*, 2011). The transport of light necessary to cure the bulk material is affected by a complex interaction between material constituents, curing conditions (irradiance and temperature) and the optical properties of resin composites (Howard *et al.*, 2010).

Water sorption and solubility

Generally, water uptake and solubility are determined by the extent of conversion and cross-linking and the hydrophilic nature of the resin, and to less of an extent, filler composition, although predictable correlations between increasing filler load and decreasing water sorption and solubility have been reported (Yap and Wee, 2002). Many of the numerous studies on water uptake have used commercial composites and the lack of knowledge of their exact composition can lead to a difficult interpretation of results. The literature is also bereft of long-term *in vitro* studies (>6 months) and is further complicated by the choice of immersion media; de-ionized water and artificial saliva (and their composition) are known to affect the rate and quantity of water sorption and solubility significantly (Musanje *et al.*, 2001; Martin *et al.*, 2003).

Although the filler itself may play a less important role, the properties of silanization (Section 10.4.4) and formation of the silane layer are known to affect water diffusion significantly since the oxane bond between filler and resin is susceptible to hydrolytic degradation. Recent studies have highlighted the effect of filler size on sorption and solubility, where a decreasing average filler diameter results in an increase in the amount of water uptake

(Karabela and Sideridou, 2011; Curtis *et al.*, 2008). This may have future implications for the use of dental 'nanocomposites' since the greater surface area of nano-sized particulates inevitably results in a larger area of hydrophilic silane moieties available for water sorption (Curtis *et al.*, 2008).

10.6 Stability, degradation and clinical outcomes

10.6.1 Effect of solvents

There is a general softening and reduction in properties of dental composites when aged in good solvents, such as ethanol/water (Ferracane and Berge, 1995; Drummond *et al.*, 2004, 2009; Ravindranath *et al.*, 2007). The fatigue lifetime has also been shown to be reduced by ageing in ethanol/water (McCool *et al.*, 2001). But the effect of ageing in water is less clear and suggests minimal degradation of composite in this environment (Ferracane *et al.*, 1998). These effects are most likely to be due to a direct effect on the resin matrix and not the filler.

Silica and glass fillers have shown evidence of leaching ions into water in an almost linear fashion (Söderholm, 1983, 1990, 2000). Söderholm *et al.* (1984) have shown that quartz or pyrogenic silica (microfillers) release into water or artificial saliva less silicon than glass fillers containing barium or strontium, and that cracks within the composite surface develop due to osmotic pressures built up at the matrix–filler interface as the filler releases ions. However, there is little evidence that this causes significant degradation of the filler, or the filler/matrix interface, in the clinical situation. It may be that the typical glasses and silica-based fillers used in dental composites are relatively stable in the oral cavity, or at least stable enough to resist significant breakdown. Other fillers that have been experimented with for dental composites, such as nano-sized hydroxylapatite, are not stable in water and rapidly degrade owing to their small size and high surface area (Domingo *et al.*, 2003).

Acidulated phosphate fluoride (APF) gels have been shown to degrade the surface of dental composite, causing roughening and reduction in surface hardness caused by its erosive effect on the filler surface, although the effect varies based on the type of composite (Kula *et al.*, 1997; Papagiannoulis *et al.*, 1997). This effect appears to be dependent upon the type of APF gel as well, probably caused by the protective effects of certain additives to the gels and to their non-acidic nature (Yeh *et al.*, 2011). Studies of the degradation and release of components of dental composites when subjected to attack by enzymes from the oral cavity have shown that composites with a higher filler content, as long as the fillers are silane treated, are somewhat less affected, probably due to the reduced polymer phase in the composite (Finer and Santerre, 2007).

10.6.2 Thermal stresses affect filler/matrix interface

Studies have shown a reduction in strength of dental composites after thermal cycling (Hirabayashi *et al.*, 1990), presumably due to stress generation at or degradation of the filler/matrix interface. Others have shown similar results, but with little change in the elastic modulus (Rüttermann *et al.*, 2008). Any effect of thermal stress may be highly dependent upon specific composite formulation as a study of commercial and whisker reinforced experimental composites showed no reduction in strength, modulus or hardness for up to 10000 thermal cycles (Xu *et al.*, 2002).

10.6.3 Clinical outcomes related to specific filler systems

There are few published studies in which the filler formulation has been systematically varied for a series of composites in a clinical trial. In one comprehensive clinical evaluation of a series of composites with a varied resin matrix (bis-GMA vs. urethane dimethacrylate (UDMA) as the base monomer), filler type (quartz vs. less stable barium glass) and silane application to the fillers (with or without a heat treatment to enhance adhesion), the resin matrix significantly influenced the main outcome, which was wear, with the UDMA materials performing more optimally (Söderholm *et al.*, 2001). In contrast, filler type and silane application method did not have a significant influence on clinical wear.

Composites tend to fail because of secondary caries formation and fracture. Fracture would be expected to be related to the mechanical properties of the material and at least one study has shown a direct correlation between the fracture toughness of composites (two hybrids and two microfills, the latter being significantly less tough than the former) and the clinical failure rate from fracture-related phenomena (Tyas, 1990). Similarly, some microfill composites have been shown to undergo more chipping and fracture in posterior teeth than hybrid composites (Lambrechts *et al.*, 1987; Tyas *et al.*, 1989).

Despite dramatic differences in the physical properties of dental composites, there is little indication from clinical studies that the *in vivo* performance can be directly related to filler characteristics. For example, some microfilled composites, such as Heliomolar (Ivoclar Vivadent) typically show very low strength, elastic modulus and fracture toughness when compared with most hybrid composites, yet the results of clinical evaluations show excellent success for this material in anterior or posterior applications both in the published literature (Rasmussen and Lundin, 1995) and anecdotally. Perhaps the reason for this lack of effect is that most clinical studies are not of long enough duration. A recent study of the clinical evaluation of two hybrid composites, P-50 (midifill, 3M ESPE) and Herculite (minifill,

Kerr) in a private practice showed a better performance for the more heavily filled hybrid composite (a midifill) compared with the less filled hybrid (minifill) after 22 years (da Rosa Rodolpho *et al.*, 2011), while the study concluded that there was no difference between the two composites when they were evaluated after 17 years (da Rosa Rodolpho *et al.*, 2006). One might argue, however, that these success rates are clinically acceptable in either case and therefore the subtle difference between the two materials is of little overall significance. It is also possible that the differences between materials may only become apparent when tested under the most stringent situations. A recent study evaluating the use of two microfill composites, one being Heliomolar HB and the other an experimental microfill for use as a light/heat-cured inlay/onlay material, to restore severely worn dentition showed unacceptably high failure rates owing to wear or complete loss of material after three years (Bartlett and Sunderam, 2006). It is unclear how a more heavily filled microhybrid type composite would have fared under these conditions.

10.7 Current and future trends

10.7.1 Antibacterial fillers

Conventional resin composites exhibit little antibacterial activity and it is well known that surface plaque formation and the accumulation of micro-organisms at the restoration margins can be greater than those of other restorative material types (Hahn *et al.*, 1993; Beyth *et al.*, 2007). A number of adhesive systems with antibacterial agents have been introduced in an attempt to reduce the incidence of secondary caries resulting from bacterial invasion at the dentine–restoration interface. There appears to be recent interest in improving the antimicrobial properties of bulk resin composites in order to inhibit biofilm formation, although significant problems such as deterioration of mechanical properties, short-lived antibacterial action and discoloration have been reported in the past (Yamamoto *et al.*, 1996; Syafiuddin *et al.*, 1997; Xu and Burgess, 2003; Leung *et al.*, 2005).

Examples of antibacterial components include acidified monomers (Imazato *et al.*, 1998), gluteraldehyde (Meiers and Miller, 1996), chlorohexidine diacetate (Mehdawi *et al.*, 2009) and filler modification with silver ions, zinc oxide and polyethyleneimine nanoparticles. The use of microparticulate silver and a novel process for synthesizing silver nanoparticles *in situ* using the polymerization process of methacrylate-based monomers shows promise in terms of antimicrobial properties, although discoloration and potential cytotoxicity may remain a concern (Bürgers *et al.*, 2009; Fan *et al.*, 2011). Other attempts of including antibacterial fillers studied the addition of 5% tetrapod-like zinc oxide whiskers (T-ZnOw) to methacrylate-based resin composites, which exhibit long-term antibacterial effectiveness (three months' inhibition of *Streptococcus mutans*) and improved mechanical properties compared with resin composites without T-ZnOw. A recent study has highlighted the potential of hydrophobic quaternized polyethyleneimine nanoparticles to modify the surface of resin composites by preventing surface alterations caused by bacterial adherence and inhibiting their growth (Beyth *et al.*, 2010).

10.7.2 Remineralizing fillers

Modification of conventional glass filler types with an appropriate ion-releasing capability has shown significant promise in developing composite materials that can remineralize carious lesions. The main drawback of replacing fillers with those that must leach into the surrounding environment to provide any therapeutic effect remains a substantial reduction in mechanical properties, especially if the remineralizing filler is not tethered to the resin matrix by silanization. Recent work has developed a whisker-reinforced fluoride-containing calcium phosphate-based resin composite, which exhibits significantly higher remineralization in natural dentine carious lesions than a resin-modified glass ionomer cement (Yang *et al.*, 2011). No strength data were provided for the experimental system and the ion-releasing fillers were not silanized (which may otherwise negate or at least slow down ion dissolution). However, given the proposed application of this material for atraumatic restorative treatment and the adhesive nature of the resin matrix, strength characteristics may not be as critical as they would be for a stress-bearing restoration.

Research and development of resin composite-containing amorphous calcium phosphate (ACP) fillers show great potential since ACP is a precursor for the formation of apatite and, as such, has been successful in effective remineralization (Skrtic *et al.*, 1996, 2000; Langhorst *et al.*, 2009). Other calcium phosphate-releasing composites with enhanced mechanical properties have been developed which use ACP particles that approach the nanoscale (~120 nm) (Xu *et al.*, 2011) at lower filler loading (20%) than similar fillers used previously (Skrtic *et al.*, 1996; Dickens *et al.*, 2003), although ion release was comparable. The ability to incorporate a higher amount of reinforcing, non-leachable fillers affords significantly improved mechanical properties without sacrificing remineralization potential and may lead to a successful commercial bulk restorative material in the near future.

10.7.3 Enhanced reinforcement

Fibre-based technology and the use of nanoscale filler components have been used frequently in an attempt to enhance reinforcement and improve the mechanical properties of resin composites. The use of fibres offers several advantages including significantly improved mechanical and physical properties. Based on fibre morphology (uni- or bi-directional, chopped) and orientation, properties such as anisotropic strength (Dyer *et al.*, 2004), shrinkage strain (Tezvergil *et al.*, 2006) and thermal expansion are affected (Tezvergil *et al.*, 2003). Small quantities of nano-sized fibres (1–2 wt%) containing highly aligned fibrillar silicate crystals substantially improved the flexural strength, elastic modulus and fracture toughness of resin composites (Tian *et al.*, 2008). The use of single-walled carbon nanotubes (SWCNT) in resin composite materials has also attracted some attention owing to their high surface area to volume ratio and enhanced interfacial interaction with the matrix. The incorporation of SWCNT as a secondary filler in an existing composite material resulted in superior flexural strengths compared with the unmodified material, although the aesthetic quality was compromised (Zhang *et al.*, 2008). Nanotubes are hollow structures and, as such, provide interfacial interlocking between the resin and the exterior and interior surfaces of the tubes (Khaled *et al.*, 2010). However, because of their high surface area and chemical reactivity, the use of SWCNTs may present cytotoxic characteristics (Lam *et al.*, 2004). A recent study has investigated the use of titania nanotubes within an acrylic composite material, which provide enhanced fracture toughness, strength and modulus without altering the rheological characteristics or reducing cell viability (Khaled *et al.*, 2010). Although such systems may enhance mechanical and physical properties, many still rely on two-component mixing and chemical polymerization regimes since increased opacity negates effective depth of cure for light curing mechanisms. Current and future challenges for direct photo-cured resin composites that contain enhanced fibre reinforcement may focus on improved translucency to optimize aesthetic quality and bulk curing.

10.8 Sources of further information and advice

The following references are suggested as further reading, providing reviews of specific topics covered in this chapter, but to a greater extent. The first two provide reviews of current dental composite materials and address future trends. The third and fourth references review factors affecting the mechanical properties of composites. The last provides a review of the silane treatment of surfaces for enhanced bonding.

Chen MH (2010) 'Update on dental nanocomposites'. *Journal of Dental Research*, **89**, 549–60.

Ferracane JL (2011) 'Resin composite – State of the art'. *Dental Materials*, **27**, 29–38.

Drummond JL (2008) 'Degradation, fatigue and failure of resin dental composite materials'. *Journal of Dental Research*, **87**, 710–19.

Ilie N and Hickel R (2009) 'Investigations on mechanical behaviour of dental composites'. *Clinical Oral Investigation*, **13**, 427–38.

Matinlinna JP, Lassila LV, Ozcan M, Yli-Urpo A and Vallittu PK (2004) 'An introduction to silanes and their clinical applications in dentistry'. *International Journal of Prosthodontics*, **17**, 155–64.

10.9 References

Abdulmajeed AA, Närhi TO, Vallittu PK and Lassila LV (2011) 'The effect of high fiber fraction on some mechanical properties of unidirectional glass fiber-reinforced composite'. *Dental Materials*, **27**, 313–21.

Amirouche A, Mouzali M and Watts DC (2007) 'Radiopacity evaluation of bisGMA/TEGDMA/opaque mineral filler dental composites'. *Journal of Applied Polymer Science*, **104**, 1632–9.

Amirouche-Korichi A, Mouzali M and Watts DC (2009) 'Effects of monomer ratios and highly radiopaque fillers on degree of conversion and shrinkage-strain of dental resin composites'. *Dental Materials*, **25**, 1411–8.

Antonucci JM, Dickens SH, Fowler OB, Xu HHK and McDonough (2005) 'Chemistry of silanes: interfaces in dental polymers and composites'. *Journal of Research of the National Institute of Standards and Technology*, **110**, 541–58.

Ardu S, Braut V, Uhac, I, Benbachir N, Feilzer A and Krejci I (2010) 'A new classification of resin-based aesthetic adhesive materials'. *Collegium Antropologicum*, **3**, 1045–50.

Atai M, Yassini E, Amini M and Watts DC (2007) 'The effect of a leucite-containing ceramic filler on the abrasive wear of dental composites'. *Dental Materials*, **23**, 1181–7.

Attar N, Tam LE and McComb D (2003) 'Flow, strength, stiffness and radiopacity of flowable resin composites'. *Journal of the Canadian Dental Association*, **69**, 516–21.

Bae JM, Kim KN, Hattori M, Hasegawa K, Yoshinari M, Kawada E and Oda Y (2004) 'Fatigue strengths of particulate filler composites reinforced with fibers'. *Dental Materials Journal*, **23**, 166–74.

Bartlett D and Sundaram G (2006) 'An up to 3-year randomized clinical study comparing indirect and direct resin composites used to restore worn posterior teeth'. *International Journal of Prosthodontics*, **19**, 613–17.

Bauer F, Sauerland V, Ernst H, Glasel H-J, Naumov S and Mehnert R (2003) *Macromolecular Chemistry and Physics*, **204**, 375.

Bayne SC, Taylor DF and Heymann HO (1992) 'Protection hypothesis for composite wear'. *Dental Materials*, **8**, 305–9.

Beun S, Glorieux T, Devaux J, Vreven J and Leloup G (2007) 'Characterization of nanofilled compared with universal and microfilled composites'. *Dental Materials*, **23**, 51–9.

Beun S, Bailly C, Devaux J and Leloup G (2008) 'Rheological properties of flowable resin composites and pit and fissure sealants'. *Dental Materials*, **24**, 548–55.

Beun S, Bailly C, Dabin A, Vreven J, Devaux J and Leloup G (2009) 'Rheological properties of experimental Bis-GMA/TEGDMA flowable resin composites with various macrofiller/microfiller ratio'. *Dental Materials*, **25**, 198–205.

Beyth N, Domb AJ and Weiss EI (2007) 'An *in vitro* quantitative antibacterial analysis of amalgam and composite resins'. *Journal of Dentistry*, **35**, 201–6.

Beyth N, Yudovin-Fearber I, Domb AJ and Weiss EI (2010) 'Long-term antibacterial surface properties of composite resin incorporating polyethyleneimine nanoparticles'. *Quintessence International*, **41**, 827–35.

Blackham JT, Vandewalle KS and Lien W (2009) 'Properties of hybrid resin composite systems containing prepolymerized filler particles'. *Operative Dentistry*, **34**, 697–702.

Braem M, Lambrechts P, Van Doren V and Vanherle G (1986) 'The impact of composite structure on its elastic response'. *Journal of Dental Research*, **65**, 648–53.

Braga RR, Hilton TJ and Ferracane JL (2003) 'Contraction stress of flowable composite materials and their efficacy as stress-relieving layers'. *Journal of the American Dental Association*, **134**, 721–8.

Brinker CJ and Scherer GW (1990) *Sol–gel Science: The Physics and Chemistry of Sol–gel Processing*, Academic Press, San Diego.

Brown WS, Dewey WA and Jacobs HR (1970) 'Thermal properties of teeth'. *Journal of Dental Research*, **49**, 752–55.

Bürgers R, Eidt A, Frankenberger R, Rosentritt M, Schweikl H, Handel G and Hahnel S (2009) 'The anti-adherence activity and bactericidal effect of microparticulate silver additives in composite resin materials'. *Archives of Oral Biology*, **54**, 595–601.

Campbell PM, Johnston WM and O'Brien WJ (1986) 'Light scattering and gloss of an experimental quartz-filled composite'. *Journal of Dental Research*, **65**, 892–94.

Chan KS, Lee YD, Nicolella DP, Furman BR, Wellinghoff S and Rawls HR (2007) 'Improving fracture toughness of dental nanocomposites by interface engineering and micromechanics'. *Engineering Fracture Mechanics*, **74**, 1857–71.

Chantler PM, Hu X and Boyd NM (1999) 'An extension of a phenomenological model for dental composites'. *Dental Materials*, **15**, 144–9.

Curtis AR, Shortall Ac, Marquis PM and Palin WM (2008) 'Water uptake and strength characteristics of a nanofilled resin-based composite'. *Journal of Dentistry*, **36**, 186–193.

Curtis AR, Palin WM, Fleming GJP, Shortall ACC and Marquis PM (2009) 'The mechanical properties of nanofilled resin-based composites: The impact of dry and wet cyclic pre-loading on bi-axial flexure strength'. *Dental Materials*, **25**, 188–97.

da Rosa Rodolpho PA, Cenci MS, Donassollo TA, Loguércio AD and Demarco FF (2006) 'A clinical evaluation of posterior composite restorations: 17-year findings'. *Journal of Dentistry*, **34**, 427–35.

da Rosa Rodolpho PA, Donassollo TA, Cenci MS, Loguércio AD, Moraes RR, Bronkhorst EM, Opdam NJ and Demarco FF (2011) '22-year clinical evaluation of the performance of two posterior composites with different filler characteristics'. *Dental Materials*, **27**, 955–63.

Darvell, BW (2000) *Materials Science for Dentistry*, 6th edn, Darvell, Hong Kong.

Dickens SH, Flaim GM and Takagi S (2003) 'Mechanical properties and biochemical activity of remineralizing resin-based Ca-PO_4 cements'. *Dental Materials*, **19**, 558–66.

Domingo C, Arcís RW, Osorio E, Osorio R, Fanovich MA, Rodríguez-Clemente R and Toledano M (2003) 'Hydrolytic stability of experimental hydroxyapatite-filled dental composite materials'. *Dental Materials*, **19**, 478–86.
Drummond JL (2008) 'Degradation, fatigue and failure of resin dental composite materials'. *Journal of Dental Research*, **87**, 710–9.
Drummond JL, Andronova K, Al-Turki LI and Slaughter LD (2004) 'Leaching and mechanical properties characterization of dental composites'. *Journal of Biomedical Materials Research, Part B*, **71**, 172–80.
Drummond JL, Lin L, Al-Turki LA and Hurley RK (2009) 'Fatigue behaviour of dental composite materials'. *Journal of Dentistry*, **37**, 321–30.
Dyer SR, Lassila LV, Jokinen M and Vallittu PK (2004) 'Effect of fiber position and orientation on fracture load of fiber-reinforced composite'. *Dental Materials*, **20**, 947–55.
Egen M, Braun L, Zentel R, Tännert K, Frese P and Reis O (2004) 'Artificial opals as effect pigments in clear coating'. *Macromolecular Materials Engineering*, **289**, 158–63.
Emami N, Sjödahl M and Söderholm K-JM (2005) 'How filler properties, filler fraction, sample thickness, and light source can affect light attenuation in particulate filled resin composites'. *Dental Materials*, **21**, 721–30.
Epselid I, Tveit AB, Erickson RL, Keck SC and Glasspoole EA (1991) 'Radiopacity of restorations and detection of secondary caries'. *Dental Materials*, **7**, 144–17.
Ergücü Z, Türkün LS, Önem E and Güneri P (2010) 'Comparative radiopacity of six flowable resin composites'. *Operative Dentistry*, **35**, 436–40.
Fan C, Chu L, Rawls R, Norling BK, Cardenas HL and Whang K (2011) 'Development of an antibacterial resin – a pilot study'. *Dental Materials*, **27**, 322–28.
Ferracane JL (1995) 'Current trends in dental composites'. *Critical Reviews in Oral Biological Medicine*, **6**, 302–18.
Ferracane JL (2011) 'Resin composite – State of the art'. *Dental Materials*, **27**, 29–38.
Ferracane JL and Berge HX (1995) 'Fracture toughness of experimental dental composites aged in ethanol'. *Journal of Dental Research*, **74**, 1418–23.
Ferracane JL and Marker VA (1992) 'Solvent degradation and reduced fracture toughness in aged composites'. *Journal of Dental Research*, **71**, 13–9.
Ferracane JL, Antonio RC and Matsumoto H (1987) 'Variables affecting the fracture toughness of dental composites. *Journal of Dental Research*, **66**, 1140–5.
Ferracane JL, Berge HX and Condon JR (1998) '*In vitro* aging of dental composites in water–effect of degree of conversion, filler volume, and filler/matrix coupling'. *Journal of Biomedical Materials Research*, **42**, 465–72.
Ferracane JL, Choi KK and Condon JR (1999) '*In vitro* wear of packable dental composites'. *Compendium of Continuing Education in Dentistry Supplement*, **25**, S60–6.
Finer Y and Santerre JP (2007) 'Influence of silanated filler content on the biodegradation of bisGMA/TEGDMA dental composite resins'. *Journal of Biomedical Materials Research, Part A*, **81**, 75–84.
Fong H, Dickens SH and Flaim GM (2005) 'Evaluation of dental restorative composites containing polyhedral oligomeric silsesquioxane methacrylate'. *Dental Materials*, **21**, 520–9.
Gao F, Tong Y, Schricker SR and Culbertson BM (2001) 'Evaluation of neat resins based on methacrylates modified with methacryl-POSS, as potential

organic-inorganic hybrids for formulating dental restoratives'. *Polymers for Advanced Technologies*, **12**, 355–60.

Garoushi S, Vallittu PK and Lassila LV (2008) 'Short glass fiber reinforced restorative composite resin with semi-inter penetrating polymer network matrix'. *Dental Materials*, **23**, 1356–62.

Goncalves F, Azevedo CL, Ferracane JL and Braga RR (2011) 'BisGMA/TEGDMA ratio and filler content effects on shrinkage stress'. *Dental Materials*, **27**, 520–6.

Hadis MA, Tomlins PH, Shortall AC and Palin WM (2010) 'Dynamic monitoring of refractive index change through photoactive resins'. *Dental Materials*, **26**, 1106–12.

Hadis M, Leprince JG, Shortall AC, Devaux J, Leloup G and Palin WM (2011) 'High irradiance curing and anomalies of exposure reciprocity law in resin-based materials'. *Journal of Dentistry*, **39**, 549–57.

Hahn R, Weiger R, Netuschil L and Brüch M (1993) 'Microbial accumulation and vitality on different restorative materials'. *Dental Materials*, **9**, 312–16.

Hahnel S, Schultz S, Trempler C, Ach B, Handel G and Rosentritt M (2011) 'Two-body wear of dental restorative materials'. *Journal of the Mechanical Behavior of Biomedical Materials*, **4**, 237–44.

Harris J and Ure D (2006) 'Exploring whether "nano" is always necessary'. *Nanotechnology Perceptions*, **2**, 1–15.

Hirabayashi S, Nomoto R, Harashima I and Hirasawa T (1990) 'The surface degradation of various light-cured composite resins by thermal cycling'. *Shika Zairyo Kikai*, **9**, 53–64.

Hosoda H, Toshimoto Y and Shigeshisa I (1990) 'SEM and elemental analysis of composite resins'. *Journal of Prosthetic Dentistry*, **64**, 669–76.

Howard B, Wilson ND, Newman SM, Pfeifer CS and Stansbury JW (2010). 'Relationships between conversion, temperature and optical properties during composite photopolymerization'. *Acta Biomaterialia*, **6**, 2053–9.

Htang A, Ohsawa M and Matsumoto H (1995) 'Fatigue resistance of composite restorations: effect of filler content'. *Dental Materials*, **11**, 7–13.

Ilie N and Hickel R (2009) 'Investigations on mechanical behaviour of dental composites'. *Clinical Oral Investigation*, **13**, 427–38.

Ilie N, Hickel R, Valceanu AS and Huth KC (2012) 'Fracture toughness of dental restorative materials.' *Clinical Oral Investigations*, **16**, 489–98.

Imazato S, Imai T and Ebisu S (1998) 'Antibacterial activity of proprietary self-etching primers'. *American Journal of Dentistry*, **11**, 106–8.

Jakubinek MB, Price, R and White MA (2010) 'Thermal conductivity of light-cured dental composites: importance of filler particle size'. *Advances in Bioceramics and Porous Ceramics II, Ceramic Engineering and Science Proceedings*, **30**, 159–67.

Jandt KD, Al-Jasser AMO, Al-Ateeq K, Vowles RW and Allen GC (2002) 'Mechanical properties and radiopacity of experimental glass-silica-metal hybrid composites'. *Dental Materials*, **18**, 429–35.

Kanie T, Arikawa H, Fujii K and Inoue K (2004) 'Physical and mechanical properties of PMMA resins containing gamma-methacryloxypropyltrimethoxysilane'. *Journal of Oral Rehabilitation*, **31**, 161–71.

Karabela MM and Sideridou ID (2011) 'Synthesis and study of properties of dental resin composites with different nanosilica particle sizes'. *Dental Materials*, **27**, 825–35.

Kawaguchi M, Fukushima T and Miyazaki K (1994) 'The relationship between cure depth and transmission coefficient of visible-light-activated resin composites'. *Journal of Dental Research*, **73**, 516 21.

Keulemans F, Palav P, Aboushelib MM, van Dalen A, Kleverlaan CJ and Feilzer AJ (2009) 'Fracture strength and fatigue resistance of dental resin-based composites'. *Dental Materials*, **25**, 1433–41.

Khaled SMZ, Miron RJ, Hamilton DW, Charpentier PA and Rizkalla AS (2010) 'Reinforcement of resin based cement with titania nanotubes'. *Dental Materials*, **26**, 169–78.

Khan AM, Suzuki H, Nomura Y, Taira M, Wakasa K, Shintani H and Yamaki M (1992) 'Characterization of inorganic fillers in visible-light cured dental composites'. *Journal of Oral Rehabilitation*, **19**, 361–70.

Kim KH and Okuno O (2002) 'Microfracture behaviour of composite resins containing irregular-shaped fillers'. *Journal of Oral Rehabilitation*, **29**, 1153–9.

Kim KH, Park JH, Imai Y and Kishi T (1994) 'Microfracture mechanisms of dental resin composites containing spherically-shaped filler particles'. *Journal of Dental Research*, **73**, 499–504.

Kim KH, Ong JL and Okuno O (2002) 'The effect of filler loading and morphology on the mechanical properties of contemporary composites'. *Journal of Prosthetic Dentistry*, **87**, 642–9.

Klapdohr S and Moszner N (2005) 'New inorganic components for dental filling composites'. *Monatshefte fur Chemie*, **136**, 21–45.

Kula K, McKinney JE and Kula TJ (1997) 'Effects of daily topical fluoride gels on resin composite degradation and wear'. *Dental Materials*, **13**, 305–11.

Lam CW, James CT, McCluskey R and Hunter RL (2004) 'Pulmonary toxicity of single-wall carbon nanotubes in mice 7 and 90 days after intratracheal instillation'. *Toxicological Sciences*, **77**, 126–34.

Lambrechts P, Braem M and Vanherle G (1987) 'Buonocore memorial lecture. Evaluation of clinical performance for posterior composite resins and dentin adhesives'. *Operative Dentistry*, **12**, 53–78.

Lang BR, Jaarda M and Wang RF (1992) 'Filler particle size and composite resin classification systems'. *Journal of Oral Rehabilitation*, **19**, 569–84.

Langhorst SE, O'Donnell JNR and Skrtic D (2009) '*In vitro* remineralization of enamel by polymeric amorphous calcium phosphate composite: quantitative microradiographic study'. *Dental Materials*, **25**, 884–91.

Lee IB Cho BH, Son HH and Um CM (2006) 'Rheological characterization of composites using a vertical oscillation rheometer'. *Dental Materials*, **23**, 425–32.

Lee IB, Min SH, Kim SY and Ferracane JL (2010) 'Slumping tendency and rheological properties of flowable composites'. *Dental Materials*, **26**, 443–8.

Lee TY and Bowman CN (2006) 'The effect of functionalized nano-particles on thiol-ene polymerization kinetics'. *Polymer*, **47**, 6057–65.

Lee YK (2007) 'Influence of scattering/absorption characteristics on the color of resin composites'. *Dental Materials*, **23**, 124–31.

Lee YK (2008) 'Influence of filler on the difference between the transmitted and reflected colors of experimental resin composites'. *Dental Materials*, **24**, 1243–7.

Lee YK and Yu B (2005) 'Measurement of opalescence of tooth enamel'. *Journal of Dentistry*, **35**, 690–4.

Leinfelder KF, Radz GM and Nash RW (1998) 'A report on a new condensable composite resin'. *Compendium of Continuing Education in Dentistry*, **19**, 230–7.

Leprince JG, Palin WM, Mullier T, Devaux J, Vreven J and Leloup G (2010) 'Investigating filler morphology and mechanical properties of new low-shrinkage resin composite types'. *Journal of Oral Rehabilitation*, **37**, 364–76.

Leprince JG, Hadis M, Shortall AC, Ferracane JL, Devaux J, Leloup G and Palin WM (2011) 'Photoinitiator type and applicability of exposure reciprocity law in filled and unfilled photoactive resins'. *Dental Materials*, **27**, 157–64.

Leung D, Spratt DA, Pratten J, Gulabivala K, Mordan NJ and Young AM (2005) 'Chlorohexidine-releasing methacrylate dental composite materials'. *Biomaterials*, **26**, 7145–53.

Lim BS, Ferracane JL, Condon JR and Adey JD (2002) 'Effect of filler fraction and filler surface treatment on wear of microfilled composites'. *Dental Materials*, **18**, 1–11.

Lohbauer U, von der Horst T, Frankenberger R, Kramer N and Petschelt A (2003) 'Flexural fatigue behavior of resin composite dental restoratives'. *Dental Materials*, **19**, 435–40.

Lui H and Webster TJ (2007) 'Nanomedicine for implants: A review of studies and necessary experimental tools'. *Biomaterials*, **28**, 354–69.

Lutz F and Philips RW (1983) 'A classification and evaluation of composite resin systems'. *Journal of Prosthetic Dentistry*, **50**, 480–8.

Marshall GW, Marshall SJ and Bayne SC (1988) 'Restorative dental materials: Scanning electron microscopy and X-ray microanalysis'. *Scanning Microscopy*, **2**, 2007–28.

Martin N, Jedynakiewicz NM and Fisher AC (2003) 'Hygroscopic expansion and solubility of composite restoratives'. *Dental Materials*, **19**, 77–86.

Martinez-Torres P, Mandelis A and Alvarado-Gil JJ (2009) 'Photothermal determination of thermal diffusivity and polymerization depth profiles of polymerized dental resins'. *Journal of Applied Physics*, **106**, 114906.

Martinez-Torres P, Mandelis A and Alvarado-Gil JJ (2010) 'Optical and thermal depth profile reconstructions of inhomogeneous photopolymerization in dental resin using photothermal waves'. *Journal of Applied Physics*, **108**, 054902.

Masouras K, Akhtar R, Watts DC and Silikas N (2008a) 'Effect of filler size and shape on local nanoindentation modulus of resin-composites'. *Journal of Materials Science Materials in Medicine*, **19**, 3561–6.

Masouras K, Silikas N and Watts DC (2008b) 'Correlation of filler content and elastic properties of resin-composites'. *Dental Materials*, **24**, 932–9.

Matinlinna JP, Lassila LVJ, Ozcan M, Yli-Urpo A and Vallittu PK (2004) 'An introduction to silanes and their clinical applications in dentistry'. *International Journal of Prosthodontics*, **17**, 155–64.

Matinlinna JP, Vallittu PK and Lassila LV (2011) 'Effects of different silane coupling agent monomers of flexural strength of an experimental filled resin composite'. *Journal of Adhesion Science and Technology*, **25**, 179–92.

McCool JI, Boberick KG and Baran GR (2001) 'Lifetime predictions for resin-based composites using cyclic and dynamic fatigue'. *Journal of Biomedical Materials Research*, **58**, 247–53.

Mehdawi I, Abou Neel EA, Valappil SP, Palmer G, Salih V, Prateen J, Spratt DA and Young AM (2009) 'Development of remineralizing, antibacterial dental materials'. *Acta Biomaterialia*, **5**, 2525–39.

Meiers JC and Miller GA (1996) 'Antibacterial activity of dentin bonding systems, resin modified glass ionomers and polyacid modified composite resins'. *Operative Dentistry*, **21**, 257–64.

Min SH, Ferracane JL and Lee IB (2010) 'Effect of shrinkage strain, modulus, and instrument compliance on polymerization shrinkage stress of light-cured composites during the initial curing stage'. *Dental Materials*, **26**, 1024–33.

Miyasaka T and Yoshida T (2000) 'Effect of binary and ternary filler mixtures on the mechanical properties of composite resins'. *Dental Materials Journal*, **19**, 229–44.

Moraes RR, Garcia JW, Barros MD, Lewis SH, Pfeifer CS, Liu J and Stansbury JW (2011) 'Control of polymerization shrinkage and stress in nanogel-modified monomer and composite materials'. *Dental Materials*, **27**, 509–19.

Moszner N and Salz U (2007) 'Recent developments of new components for dental adhesive and composites'. *Macromolecular Materials Engineering*, **292**, 245–71.

Mucci V, Arenas G, Duchowicz R, Cook WD and Vallo C (2009) 'Influence of thermal expansion on shrinkage during photopolymerization of dental resins based on bis-GMA/TEGDMA'. *Dental Materials*, **25**, 103–14.

Musanje L, Shu M and Darvell BW (2001) 'Water sorption and mechanical behaviour of cosmetic direct restorative materials in artificial saliva'. *Dental Materials*, **17**, 394–401.

Nash RW, Lowe RA and Leinfelder KF (2001) 'Using packable composites for posterior restorations'. *Journal of the American Dental Association*, **132**, 1099–104.

O'Brien WJ (2008) *Dental Materials and their Selection*, Quintessence Publishing, Chicago, IL, USA.

Papagiannoulis L, Tzoutzas J and Eliades G (1997) 'Effect of topical fluoride agents on the morphologic characteristics and composition of resin composite restorative materials'. *Journal of Prosthetic Dentistry*, **77**, 405–13.

Park JK, Hur B, Ko CC, Garcia-Godoy F, Kim HI and Kwon YH (2010) 'Effect of light curing units on the thermal expansion of resin nanocomposites'. *American Journal of Dentistry*, **23**, 331–4.

Park SK, Kim KD and Kim HT (2002) 'Preparation of silica nanoparticles: determination of the optimal synthesis conditions for small and uniform particles'. *Colloid and Surfaces A: Physiochemical Engineering Aspects*, **197**, 7–17.

Pfeifer CS. Wilson ND, Shelton ZR and Stansbury JW (2011) 'Delayed gelation through chain-transfer reactions: Mechanisms for stress reduction in methacrylate networks'. *Polymer*, **52**, 3295–303.

Pick B, Pelka M, Belli R, Braga RR and Lohbauer U (2011) 'Tailoring of physical properties in highly filled experimental nanohybrid resin composites'. *Dental Materials*, **27**, 664–9.

Powers JM, Hostetler RW and Dennison JB (1979) 'Thermal expansion of composite resins and sealants'. *Journal of Dental Research*, **58**, 584–7.

Rasmusson CG and Lundin SA (1995) 'Class II restorations in six different posterior composite resins: five-year results'. *Swedish Dental Journal*, **19**, 173–82.

Ravindranath V, Gosz M, De Santiago E, Drummond JL and Mostovoy S (2007) 'Effect of cyclic loading and environmental aging on the fracture toughness of dental resin composite'. *Journal of Biomedical Materials Research, Part B*, **80**, 226–35.

Rheinberger V, Moszner N and Fischer UK (1999) *Filled and Polymerizable Dental Material*, US Patent: 5.936.006; Ivoclar-Vivadent.

Rodrigues SA Jr, Ferracane JL and Della Bona A (2008) 'Flexural strength and Weibull analysis of a microhybrid and a nanofill composite evaluated by 3- and 4-point bending tests'. *Dental Materials*, **24**, 426–31.

Rüttermann S, Wandrey C, Raab WH and Janda R (2008) 'Novel nano-particles as fillers for an experimental resin-based restorative material'. *Acta Biomateriala*, **4**, 1846–53.

Ruyter IE and Øysaed H (1982) 'Conversion in different depths of ultraviolet and visible light activated composite materials'. *Acta Odontologica Scandinavica*, **40**, 179–92.

Sabbagh J, Vreven J and Leloup G (2002) 'Dynamic and static moduli of elasticity of resin-based materials'. *Dental Materials*, **18**, 64–71.

Sabbagh J, Ryelandt L, Bacherius L, Biebuyck JJ, Vreven J, Lambrechts P and Leloup G (2004a) 'Characterization of the inorganic fraction of resin composites'. *Journal of Oral Rehabilitation*, **31**, 1090–101.

Sabbagh J, Vreven J and Leloup G (2004b) 'Radiopacity of resin-based materials measured in thin film radiographs and storage phosphor plate (Digora)'. *Operative Dentistry*, **29**, 677–84.

Saffar, KP, Arshi, AR, JamilPour, N, Najafi, AR, Rouhi, G and Sudak, L (2010) 'A cross-linking model for estimating Young's modulus of artificial bone tissue grown on carbon nanotube scaffold'. *Journal of Biomedical Materials Research Part A*, **94**, 594–602.

Satterthwaite JD, Vogel K and Watts DC (2009) 'Effect of resin composite filler particle size and shape on shrinkage-strain'. *Dental Materials*, **25**, 1612–15.

Schwartz JI and Söderholm KJ (2004) 'Effects of filler size, water, and alcohol on hardness and laboratory wear of dental composites'. *Acta Odontologica Scandinavica*, **62**, 102–6.

Shah MB, Ferracane JL and Kruzic JJ (2009) 'R-curve behavior and micromechanisms of fracture in resin based dental restorative composites'. *Journal of the Mechanical Behavior of Biomedical Materials*, **2**, 502–11.

Shortall AC, Palin WM and Burtscher P (2008) 'Refractive index mismatch and monomer reactivity influence composite curing depth'. *Journal of Dental Research*, **87**, 84–8.

Sideridou ID and Karabela MM (2009) 'Effect of the amount of 3-methacyloxypropyltrimethoxysilane coupling agent on physical properties of dental resin nanocomposites'. *Dental Materials*, **25**, 1315–24.

Sideridou I, Achilias DS and Kyrikou E (2004) 'Thermal expansion characteristics of light-cured dental resins and resin composites'. *Biomaterials*, **25**, 3087–97.

Sidhu SK, Ikeda T, Omata Y, Fujita M and Sano H (2006) 'Change of colour and translucency by light curing in resin composites'. *Operative Dentistry*, **31**, 598–603.

Skrtic D, Antonucci JM and Eanes ED (1996) 'Improved properties of amorphous calcium phosphate fillers in remineralizing dental composites'. *Dental Materials*, **12**, 295–301.

Skrtic D, Antonucci JM, Eanes ED, Eichmiller FC and Schumacher GE (2000) 'Physiological evaluation of bioactive polymeric composites based on hybrid amorphous calcium phosphates'. *Journal of Biomedical Materials Research*, **53B**, 381–91.

Söderholm KJ (1983) 'Leaking of fillers in dental composites'. *Journal of Dental Research*, **62**, 126–30.
Söderholm KJ (1984) 'Influence of silane treatment and filler fraction on thermal expansion of composite resins;. *Journal of Dental Research*, **63**, 1321–6.
Söderholm KJ (1990) 'Filler leachability during water storage of six composite materials'. *Scandinavian Journal of Dental Research*, **98**, 82–8.
Soderhölm KJ and Shang SW (1993) 'Molecular orientation of silane at the surface of colloidal silica'. *Journal of Dental Research*, **72**, 1050–54.
Söderholm KJ, Zigan M, Ragan M, Fischlschweiger W and Bergman M (1984) 'Hydrolytic degradation of dental composites'. *Journal of Dental Research*, **63**, 1248–54.
Söderholm KJ, Yang MC and Garcea I (2000) 'Filler particle leachability of experimental dental composites'. *European Journal of Oral Science*, **108**, 555–60.
Söderholm KJ, Lambrechts P, Sarrett D, Abe Y, Yang MC, Labella R, Yildiz E and Willems G (2001) 'Clinical wear performance of eight experimental dental composites over three years determined by two measuring methods'. *European Journal of Oral Science,* **109**, 273–81.
Stöber W, Fink A and Bohn E (1968) 'Controlled growth of monodisperse silica spheres in the micron size range'. *Journal of Colloidal Interface Science*, **26**, 62–9.
Suzuki S, Leinfelder KF, Kawai K and Tsuchitani Y (1995) 'Effect of particle variation on wear rates of posterior composites'. *American Journal of Dentistry*, **8**, 173–8.
Syafiuddin T, Hisamitsu H, Toko T, Igarashi T, Goto N, Fujishima A and Miyazaki T (1997) '*In vitro* inhibition of caries around a resin composite restoration containing an antibacterial filler'. *Biomaterials*, **18**, 1051–7.
Tantbirojn D, Pfeifer CS, Braga RR and Versluis A (2011) 'Do low-shrink composites reduce polymerization shrinkage effects?' *Journal of Dental Research*, **90**, 596–601.
Tezvergil A, Lassila LV and Vallittu PK (2003) 'The effect of fiber orientation on the thermal expansion coefficients of fiber-reinforced composites'. *Dental Materials*, **19**, 471–7.
Tezvergil A, Lassila LV and Vallittu PK (2006) 'The effect of fibre orientation on the polymerization shrinkage strain of fiber-reinforced composites'. *Dental Materials*, **22**, 610–16.
Tian M, Gao Y, Liu Y, Liao Y, Hedin NE and Fong H (2008) 'Fabrication and evaluation of Bis-GMA/TEGDMA dental resins/composites containing nano fibrillar silicate'. *Dental Materials,* **24**, 235–43.
Turssi CP, Ferracane JL and Vogel K (2005) 'Filler features and their effects on wear and degree of conversion of particulate dental resin composites'. *Biomaterials*, **26**, 4932–7.
Tyas MJ (1990) 'Correlation between fracture properties and clinical performance of composite resins in Class IV cavities'. *Australian Dental Journal*, **35**, 46–9.
Tyas MJ, Truong VT, Goldman M and Beech DR (1989) 'Clinical evaluation of six composite resins in posterior teeth'. *Australian Dental Journal,* **34**, 147–53.
Vaidyanathan J, Vaidyanathan TK, Wang Y and Viswanadhan T (1992) 'Thermoanalytical characterization of visible light cure dental composites'. *Journal of Oral Rehabilitation*, **19**, 49–64.

Venhoven BA, de Gee AJ, Werner A and Davidson CL (1996) 'Influence of filler parameters on the mechanical coherence of dental restorative resin composites'. *Biomaterials*, **17**, 735–40.

Versluis A, Douglas WH and Sakaguchi RL (1996) 'Thermal expansion of dental composites measured with strain gauges'. *Dental Materials*, **12**, 290–4.

Wang Y, Lee JJ, Lloyd IK, Wilson OC Jr, Rosenblum M and Thompson V (2007) 'High modulus nanopowder reinforced dimethacrylate matrix composites for dental cement applications'. *Journal of Biomedical Materials Research, Part A*, **82**, 651–7.

Watts DC (1987) 'Radiopacity versus composition of some barium and strontium glass composites'. *Journal of Dentistry*, **15**, 38–43.

Watts DC, McAndrew R and Lloyd CH (1987) 'Thermal diffusivity of composite restorative materials'. *Journal of Dental Research*, **66**, 1576–8.

Weinmann W, Thalacker C and Guggenberger R (2005) 'Siloranes in dental composites'. *Dental Materials*, **21**, 68–74.

Willems G, Noack MJ, Inokoshi S, Lambrechts P, Van Meerbeek B, Braem M, Roulet JF and Vanherle G (1991) 'Radiopacity of composites compared with human enamel and dentine'. *Journal of Dentistry*, **19**, 362–5.

Willems G, Lambrechts P, Braem M, Celis JP and Vanherle G (1992) 'A classification of dental composites according to their morphological and mechanical characteristics'. *Dental Materials*, **8**, 310–19.

Winter R (1993) 'Visualizing the natural dentition'. *Journal of Esthetic Dentistry*, **5**, 102–17.

Wonglamsam A, Kakuta K and Ogura H (2008) 'Effects of occlusal and brushing cycles on wear of composite resins in combined wear test'. *Dental Materials Journal*, **27**, 243–50.

Wu X, Sun Y, Xie W, Liu Y and Song X (2010) 'Development of novel dental nanocomposites reinforced with polyhedral oligomeric silsesquioxanes (POSS)'. *Dental Materials*, **26**, 456–62.

Xu HC, Liu WY and Wang T (1989) 'Measurement of thermal expansion coefficient of human teeth'. *Australian Dental Journal*, **34**, 530–5.

Xu HH, Martin TA, Antonucci JM and Eichmiller FC (1999) 'Ceramic whisker reinforcement of dental resin composites'. *Journal of Dental Research*, **78**, 706–12.

Xu HH, Eichmiller FC, Smith DT, Schumacher GE, Giuseppetti AA and Antonucci JM (2002) 'Effect of thermal cycling on whisker-reinforced dental resin composites'. *Journal of Materials Science Materials in Medicine*, **13**, 875–83.

Xu HH, Quinn JB and Giuseppetti AA (2004) 'Wear and mechanical properties of nano-silica-fused whisker composites'. *Journal of Dental Research*, **83**, 930–5.

Xu HH, Weir MD, Sun L, Moreau JL, Takagi S, Chow LC and Antonucci JM (2010) Strong nanocomposites with Ca, PO(4), and F release for caries inhibition'. *Journal of Dental Research*, **9**, 19–28.

Xu HH, Moreau JL, Sun L and Chow LC (2011) 'Nanocomposite containing amorphous calcium phosphate nanoparticles for caries inhibition'. *Dental Materials*, **27**, 762–9.

Xu X and Burgess JO (2003) 'Compressive strength, fluoride release and recharge of fluoride releasing materials'. *Biomaterials*, **24**, 2451–61.

Yamaguchi R, Powers JM and Dennison JB (1989) 'Thermal expansion of visible light cured composite resins'. *Operative Dentistry*, **14**, 64–7.

Yamamoto K, Ohashi S, Aono M, Kokubo T, Yamada I and Yamamoto K (1996) 'Antibacterial activity of silver ions implanted in SiO_2 filler on oral streptococci'. *Dental Materials*, **12**, 227–9.

Yang B, Flaim G and Dickens SH (2011) 'Remineralization of human natural caries and artificial caries-like lesions with an experimental whisker-reinforced ART composite'. *Acta Biomaterialia*, **7**, 2303–9.

Yap AU and Wee KE (2002) 'Effects of cyclic temperature changes on water sorption and solubility of composite restoratives'. *Operative Dentistry*, **27**, 147–53.

Yeh ST, Wang HT, Liao HY, Su SL, Chang CC, Kao HC and Lee BS (2011) 'The roughness, microhardness, and surface analysis of nanocomposites after application of topical fluoride gels'. *Dental Materials*, **27**, 187–96.

Yu B, Ahn JS, Lim JI and Lee YK (2009) 'Influence of TiO_2 nanoparticles on the optical properties of resin composites'. *Dental Materials*, **25**, 1142–7.

Zhang X, Kolb B, Hanggi D and Craig B (2001) *Radiopaque Dental Materials with Nano-sized Particles*, WO Patent: 01/30309; 3M

Zhang F, Xia Y, XU L and Gu N (2008) 'Surface modification and microstructure of single-walled carbon nanotubes for dental resin-based composites'. *Journal of Biomedical Materials Research, Part B*, **86**, 90–7.

Zhao D, Botsis J and Drummond JL (1997) 'Fracture studies of selected dental restorative composites'. *Dental Materials*, **13**, 198–207.

11
Composite-based oral implants

TIMO O. NÄRHI, University of Turku, Finland,
AHMED M. BALLO, Gothenburg University, Sweden and
King Saud University, Saudi Arabia and
PEKKA K. VALLITTU, University of Turku, Finland

DOI: 10.1533/9780857096432.3.336

Abstract: This chapter describes the background of the need for non-metallic implants and provides an example of using fiber-reinforced composite as an oral implant material. The chemical composition and mechanical properties of fiber-reinforced composite implants are presented. The chapter also provides information on the biological aspects of fibre reinforced composite implants in cell culture conditions and *in vivo*. Clinical considerations are discussed based on current knowledge of use of polymers in regenerative medicine.

Key words: bioactive glass, bis-GMA, bone, composite, e-glass, osteoblast, polymer, TEGDMA.

11.1 Introduction

Biocompatibility is a descriptive term which indicates the ability of the material to perform with an appropriate host response, in a specific application (Black and Hasting, 1998). This definition has been extended and distinguishes between the surface and structural compatibility of an implant (Wintermantel and Mayer, 1995). Surface compatibility expresses chemical, biological and physical (including surface morphology) suitability of an implant surface for a host tissue. Structural compatibility, on the other hand, is the optimum adaptation to the mechanical behavior of the host tissues. Therefore, structure compatibility refers to the mechanical properties of the implant material, such as elastic modulus, strength, implant design and optimal load transmission (minimum interfacial strain mismatch) at the implant/tissue interface.

Among metallic biomaterials, titanium and its alloys exhibit the most suitable properties for biomedical applications because of their high biocompatibility, mechanical strength and corrosion resistance (Palmqvist *et al.*, 2010). Titanium implants have been successfully used to retain fixed and removable dental prostheses (Albrektsson, 1995). The survival rates of titanium oral implants are currently very high, more than 90% of the implants survive for over 10 years (Wennerberg and Albrektsson, 2011). In compromised bone conditions implant survival is lower, although various surface treatments have improved their longevity (Wennerberg and Albrektsson, 2010). The success of an oral implant is primarily based on good osseointegration, which depends on the biocompatibility of the implant material and implant surface properties, as well as on bone quantity and quality (Roynesdal *et al.*, 1998; Porter and Fraunhofer, 2005).

The survival of an implant does not mean that treatment itself has been successful. Marginal bone loss and gingival retraction occur frequently, decreasing the final success rates. As a result, the implant surface can be exposed in the oral cavity, which may create esthetic complications in visible regions.

Until now, none of the commercially available oral implants have been able to attach to bone tissue with a periodontal ligament-like structure that might reduce the impact of the occlusal loads transmitted to the bone (Misch *et al.*, 1999). In poor bone conditions, the mismatch of stiffness between bone and metallic implant may lead to implant failure (Lemons, 1998). This occurs when the tensile or compressive load exceeds the physiological limit of bone tolerance and causes microfracture at the bone-to-implant interface, or initiates bone resorption (Brunski, 1999).

Composite resin has been used for nearly 50 years as a restorative material in dentistry (Stein *et al.*, 2005). Carbon fiber-reinforced composites have been developed for many applications including oral implants (Adams *et al.*, 1978). In medicine, fiber-reinforced composites have been tested in orthopedics as bone cements, implants, osseous screws and joint-bearing articular surfaces, and most recently in calvarial bone implants (Tuusa *et al.*, 2008).

Bone can be considered to be a natural fiber-reinforced composite (FRC) material composed of collagen fibers and an inorganic hydroxyapatite matrix. Therefore, FRCs can be considered interesting materials for oral implants. The use of FRCs is increasing in dentistry. Initially, FRCs have been used in the automobile industry and in weight critical aerospace components. Later, the domain enlarged to infrastructure applications with additional performance requirements like environmental stability, moldability, damage resistance, and so on. Nowadays, with biocompatible fibers and matrix systems, FRCs are also used as biomaterials in reconstructive medicine and dentistry (Ramakrishna *et al.*, 2001).

FRCs are durable materials with a lower elastic modulus than metals (Cheal *et al.*, 1992). In fact, FRCs have properties that closely mimic those of the bone (Goldberg and Burstone, 1992). There is growing interest in using FRC in dental applications and surgical implants for orthopedic and craniofacial surgery involving some degree of structural performance under load-bearing conditions (Freilich *et al.*, 2002; Behr *et al.*, 2001; Tuusa *et al.*, 2007; Aho *et al.*, 2004), which also makes FRC an interesting material for oral implants. This chapter provides an overview of mechanical, biomechanical and biological properties of FRC materials focusing on their potential use as oral implants.

11.2 Composition and structure

The reinforcement in a composite material is fundamentally used for increasing the mechanical properties of the neat resin system, while the resin combines the fibers together and protects the fibers from moisture in the external environment (Vallittu, 1995).

Since FRCs combine a resin system and reinforcing fibers, the properties of the resulting composite material will combine some of the properties of the resin on its own with those of the fibers on their own. Overall, the properties of the composite are determined by: (1) The properties of the fiber; (2) the properties of the resin; (3) the ratio of fiber to resin in the composite (fiber volume fraction (FVF)); and (4) the geometry and orientation of the fibers in the composite. All of the different fibers (such as glass, carbon and aramid) used in composites have different properties which also affect the properties of the composite in different ways. It is also necessary to specify the geometry of the reinforcement, its concentration, distribution and orientation (Alexander, 1996).

11.2.1 Chemical composition

The only substances that harmonize completely in the body are those produced by the body itself (autogenous) and any other substance that is recognized as foreign, initiates some type of host–tissue response. Many different cell types may attach to the surface of the implants after insertion into the bone. Under favorable conditions osseointegration is achieved.

Polymers may contain various additives, traces of catalysts, inhibitors and other chemical compounds needed for their synthesis. Over time in the physiological environment, these compounds can leach from the polymer surface. As is the case with corrosion by-products released from metallic implants, the chemicals released from the polymers may induce adverse local and systemic host reactions that cause clinical complications. This is of concern for materials, such as bone cement, that are polymerized *in situ*.

The release of residual monomers from bisphenol A-glycidyl methacrylate–triethylene glycol dimethacrylate (bis-GMA-TEGDMA) polymer may influence the biocompatibility of polymer implants (MacDougall *et al.*, 1998). Residual monomer can also cause allergic reactions if there is sensitization for the monomers, as has been noticed in clinical dental practice (Pfeiffer and Rosenbauer, 2005). Because of this, the FRC implants should have an optimum degree of monomer conversion. This can be obtained by lengthening the photopolymerization time in combination with heat-induced post-curing (Ferracane and Condon, 1992).

Only a few *in vitro* studies of cell response to bis-GMA-TEGDMA have been reported (Engelmann *et al.*, 2004; Lin *et al.*, 2007), even though the *p*-bis-GMA-*p*TEGDMA copolymer is already used clinically as bone cement (Andreassen *et al.*, 2004; Evans *et al.*, 2002; Palussière *et al.*, 2005).

It has been shown that the degree of monomer conversion (DC%) of approximately 90% of the polymer could be achieved by photopolymerization in a vacuum and post-curing for 24 h at 120°C. This temperature is close to the glass transition temperature (T_g) of *p*-bis-GMA-*p*TEGDMA-copolymer (Ballo *et al.*, 2008a). With further storage in water the residual monomers are leached out from the FRC implants, which improves the biocompatibility of the polymer.

11.2.2 Mechanical properties

Glass-fiber reinforcements were produced for the first time in 1893. E-glass fiber takes its name from its electrical properties. Now it is one of the most attractive reinforcements owing to its high performance, good properties and wide range stability in different pH conditions. The composition of E-glass fiber is: 55% SiO_2, 15% Al_2O_3, 22% CaO, 6% B_2O_3, 0.5% MgO and >1.0% Fe + Na + K. The good properties of glass fibers include high tensile strength, excellent compression and impact properties, relatively high E-modulus, resistances to high temperatures and corrosive environments, and also good esthetic appearance.

Fibers are mechanically more effective in achieving a durable and stiff composite than particulate fillers, and with the aid of fibers, the load-bearing capacity of the material can be increased. However, the loading and direction of the fibers influences the stiffness and strength of the composite. Unidirectional FRC has relative strength and stiffness comparable to metal when loading along the fibers, but with much less weight. Because of the anisotropic nature of unidirectional FRC, the material has different physical properties in different directions.

The efficiency of the fiber reinforcement (Krenchel's factor) varies in FRC laminates with different fiber orientations in relation to direction of stress (Fig. 11.1). For this reason, designing an FRC device should be done carefully. This is especially important in the oral environment as the implant can be under varying mechanical loading. Unidirectional fibers can most effectively reinforce the composite when positioned on the tension side (Dyer *et al.*, 2004). The strength and modulus of elasticity of the composite improves when the fiber content of the composite increases (Vallittu, 1998). Fibers can be oriented in two directions when using woven fibers if stiffness and strength are needed in several directions.

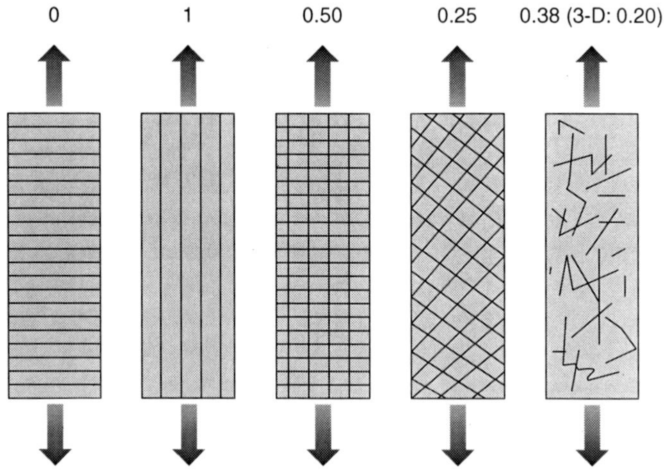

11.1 Reinforcing efficiency (Krenchel's factor) of fibers with different fiber orientations in the plane.

Effective wetting of fibers by the resin matrix, also called resin impregnation, is a prerequisite for their effective use (Vallittu, 1995, 1998, 2007). With good impregnation, optimal reinforcement and transfer of stresses from the polymer matrix to the reinforcing fibers may be achieved. An improper degree of impregnation causes increasing water sorption through voids, leading to reduced mechanical properties of the FRC (Miettinen and Vallittu, 1997). In the case of photopolymerization of FRC, the light intensity, exposure time and the polymerization temperature have an effect on flexural properties and monomer conversion (Loza-Herrero *et al.*, 1998).

Experimental screw-type FRC implants have been evaluated previously (Ballo *et al.*, 2007a, 2008a). Fibers were aligned in a uniaxial or longitudinal direction and impregnated with a bis-GMA-TEGDMA resin system that produced a semi-interpenetrating polymer network in the polymer matrix. The resin matrix contained 1 wt% camphorquinone and DMAEMA (*N*,*N*-dimethyl aminoethyl methacrylate) as the photo-initiator.

A bundle of E-glass fibers were passed through an appropriate molding and the implants were polymerized by light curing with an Optilux 501 (Kerr-Have., I, USA) hand light-curing unit, in a light curing oven at 80°C (LicuLite, Dentsply De Trey GmbH, Dreieich, Germany) and post-cured at 120°C, at the temperature close to the glass transition temperature (T_g) of *p*-bis-GMA-*p*TEGDMA-copolymer.

Experimental FRC implants were tested in laboratory conditions (Ballo *et al.*, 2007a, 2008a) and in preclinical environment (Ballo *et al.*, 2009, 2011). The mechanical properties of FRC implants were found to be dependent on polymerization conditions, fiber architecture (unidirectional with, or

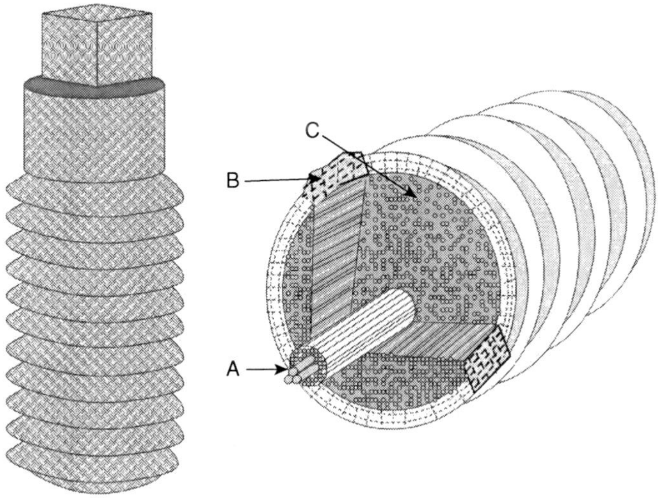

11.2 Schematic and simplified picture of structural design of a threaded fiber reinforced composite implant. A, Unidirectional (E-glass) fibers; B, bidirectional fiber weaves; C, polymer matrix.

without woven support) and quality of impregnation of fibers by resin. The different fiber architectures offer flexibility in shaping and designing the composite implant. Complete interlocking of the weave structure to the outer surface of the FRC thread increases the structural integrity (Figs 11.2 and 11.3), reduces the risk of delamination, and smoothens the progress of load transfer. An increase in the fiber volume of 10% improves significantly the modulus of elasticity, toughness and above all the load-bearing capacity of an FRC implant (Abdulmajeed *et al.*, 2011). Therefore, fiber composition, concentration and orientation can be tailored to provide strength or stiffness closer to that of human bone and isotropic mechanical properties.

The failure force in bending the experimental FRC specimens with an average dental implant diameter is 1400 N, which exceeds maximum static human bite forces (Kloostra, 2002). A push-out test in a simulated bone model has also shown that the threads of FRC implants can withstand static loading values up to the maximal human bite without fracture. These values were almost twice as high as the values achieved with identical threaded titanium implants. Fracture always occurred in the simulated bone and no thread failures were observed (Ballo *et al.*, 2007a). The reason for the higher push-out force of FRC specimens is probably related with good matching of the modulus of elasticity of FRC (40 GPa) and the surrounding artificial bone (Yuehuei, 2000). Under a vertical load, the stress distributes more evenly in the FRC structure and to the surrounding bone compared to the titanium which is a significantly stiffer material than bone.

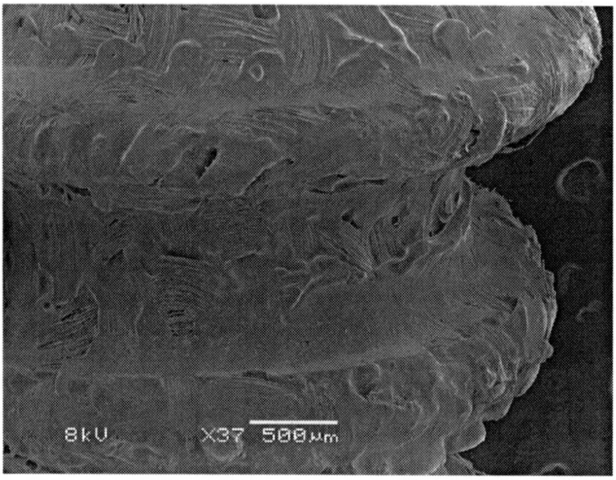

11.3 SEM micrograph illustrating the fiber-reinforced thread structure of a fiber-reinforced composite implant.

11.3 Surface modification

The same techniques can be used for the surface texturing of FRC materials as have been used for titanium implants. Air abrasion, for example, allows fabrication of micro rough surfaces. On the other hand, the fabrication of an apatite coating that requires sintering at high temperatures is not possible with polymer composites. Composites offer alternative routes for producing bioactive surfaces since bioactive particles can be embedded within the resin matrix or applied directly to the surface during the fabrication process. Bioactive glasses (BAG) are well-known biocompatible and osteoconductive materials, which makes them an interesting component for FRC implants. BAG provides a favorable environment for human osteoblast proliferation and function (Price *et al.*, 1997; Stanley *et al.*, 1976, 1981). BAG implant coatings have been shown to improve osseointegration of titanium implants in both *in vitro* and *in vivo* conditions (Aldini *et al.*, 2002; Moritz *et al.*, 2004). BAG particles have been used as a bioactive component in FRC implants.

11.4 Biological response

11.4.1 Cell response

The long-term stability of an implant prosthesis depends on the integration between the bone tissue and the implanted biomaterials, which requires the availability of preosteoblasts and their differentiation into the osteoblastic phenotype. Classically, these interactions are tested in cell culture conditions using osteoblast-like cells isolated and expanded from bone marrow.

Currently, data concerning *in vitro* interaction of mammalian cells with FRC substrates are sparse. The proliferation and osteogenic potential of bone marrow-derived osteoblast like cells were investigated on FRC substrates (Ballo *et al.*, 2008b) and the study showed that osteoblast attachment, proliferation and differentiation on the bis-GMA-TEGMA polymer with E-glass fiber reinforcement is comparable to that observed on titanium.

A SEM investigation revealed that the cultured cells proliferated on all experimental FRC surfaces and eventually formed multicellular layers that entirely covered the specimens. After 21 days of culture, no visible differences could be noted between different FRC substrates and titanium, indicating that the tested FRC specimens were cytocompatible showing a similar cellular response to that of titanium.

The normal cell differentiation process of osteogenic cells includes a reciprocal relationship between proliferation and differentiation (Malaval *et al.*, 1994; Stein *et al.*, 1990). Accordingly, the cells seeded on FRC–BAG substrates have been shown to stop expanding when their ALP activity reaches peak value during the second week of culture (Ballo *et al.*, 2008b). Furthermore, their gene expression profiles increased to levels similar to those on the titanium surface and the cells started to mineralize more rapidly than the cells seeded on titanium. The enhanced differentiation cascade with FRC–BAG is probably related to Ca, PO_4, and Si ions initially released from the BAG (Hench *et al.*, 2004; Radin *et al.*, 2005). The Ca and Si ions released from the bioactive glasses are known to stimulate the osteoblastic function and maturation (Yao *et al.*, 2005). Hench and West (1996) have proposed that the release of soluble silica from the surface of bioactive glasses might be at least partially responsible for stimulating the proliferation of bone-forming cells on bioactive glass surfaces.

11.4.2 *In vivo* behavior

Only a few *in vivo* studies of tissue response to FRC have been reported (Tuusa *et al.*, 2007, 2008; Hautamäki *et al.*, 2008). It is accepted that FRC is biocompatible and well tolerated by local tissues and induces neither toxic nor inflammatory reactions.

Residual monomers (MMA) leaching from PMMA-based fiber-reinforced polymers have even been associated with cytotoxic effects, but this has been proven to be clinically irrelevant after adequate processing and preoperative storage (Vallittu *et al.*, 1995; Miettinen and Vallittu 1997).

The porous surface structure of FRC implants enhances appositional bone growth on the implant surface (Ballo *et al.*, 2009, 2011). Under load-bearing conditions the implant appears to function like an osteoconductive prosthesis, enabling direct mobilization and rapid return to full weight bearing (Hautamäki *et al.*, 2008). It has been shown that the polymer surface can guarantee equal bone formation after 4 and 12 weeks of healing with titanium (Ballo *et al.*, 2009). Neither grit-blasted FRC implants nor BAG-coated FRC implants showed toxicity to the pig bone tissue during the 12-week healing period. The direct attachment of osseous tissue to the bis-GMA-TEGMA polymer with E-glass fiber reinforcement indicates that the FRC implant is biocompatible in the bone environment.

Grit-blasted FRC and BAG-coated FRC implants have shown extensive bone growth along the entire implant surface (Figs 11.4 and 11.5). The bone

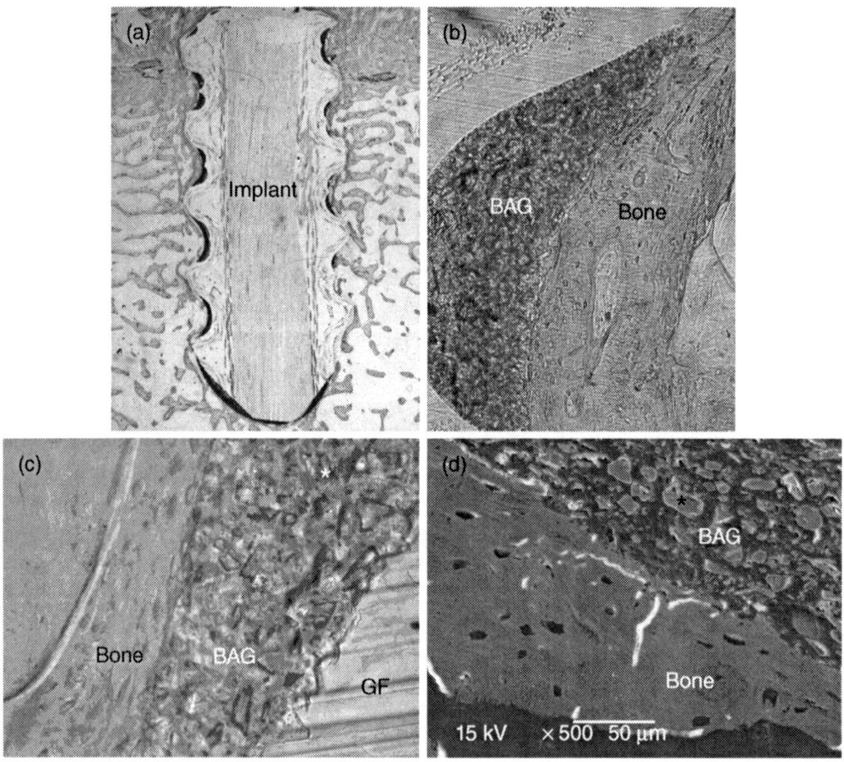

11.4 Histology and scanning electron microscopy pictures of BAG-coated FRC implant after 12 weeks of implantation in the pig femur: (a) bone growth along and in direct contact with the implant surface, using the implant as template (magnification × 100), and (b, c) detail of figure (magnification × 200 and 400, respectively). (d) Backscattered electron microscopy image of bone interface to BAG-coated FRC implant. The implant is seen to be well osseointegrated, as most of the implant surface was in tight contact with mature lamellar bone and regular osteons were recognizable at the bone-implant interface. * indicates BAG granules and GF indicates glass fiber.

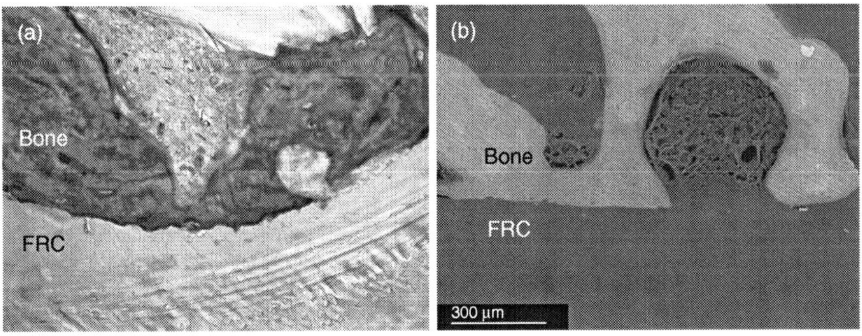

11.5 Histology and pictures of bone growth in direct contact with FRC surfaces after 12 weeks of implantation in the pig femur: (a) bone growth along and in direct contact with the grit-blasted FRC surface (magnification × 400) and (b) backscattered electron microscopy image of a bone–FRC surface.

was found to be in direct contact with the exposed BAG particles (Ballo *et al.*, 2009, 2011). The significantly greater percentage of bone implant contact (BIC) adjacent to BAG-containing FRC (46.9%) than in micro rough FRC (40.2%) or titanium implants (41.8%) at 12 weeks of implantation is clearly related to the reactivity of BAG (Fig. 11.5).

Thus, the addition of BAG significantly improves the performance of FRC implants: the bone bonding surface area is larger and bonding strength higher than with sand–blasted FRC or control titanium implants. Delamination of BAG does not challenge osseointegration as BAG particles are embedded beneath the polymer surface. A mechanical bone bonding study has shown that push-out failure takes place within the bone tissue but not in the bone-to-implant interface (Ballo *et al.*, 2007b).

The fact that the BAG will eventually be resorbed completely is non-essential, as when the implant is integrated into bone, long-term fixation will be achieved through bone ingrowth into the porous surface structure of the FRC implant.

11.5 Clinical considerations and future trends

The mechanical properties of FRC implants can be optimized to meet clinical requirements in different bone conditions. According to a finite element analysis, mechanical stress distributes to the surrounding bone more evenly from FRC implants than from titanium (Shinya *et al.*, 2011). This may improve implant survival especially in situations where bone quality and volume is questionable.

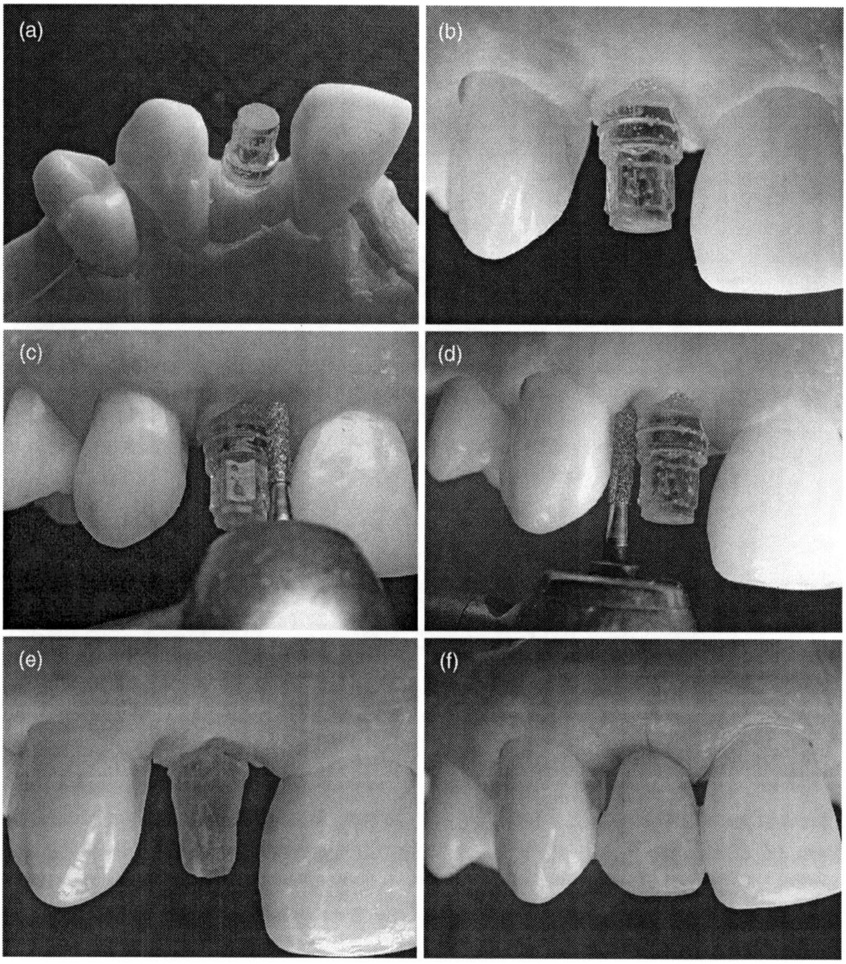

11.6 Illustration simulating the clinical preparation of an abutment portion of FRC implant. (a) Palatal view of an abutment portion of FRC implant, (b) labial view of an abutment portion of FRC implant, (c) and (d) intra-oral preparation of an abutment portion of FRC implant, (e) finished preparation, (f) composite crown on FRC implant.

One shortcoming of titanium as an oral implant material is that it does not allow intraoral preparations. Some attempts at doing this have been made with poor results. Intraoral preparation would let the clinician determine the location of the preparation margins individually (Fig. 11.6). This is important in situations where marginal gingiva retracts after implant placement and upon renewal of prosthetic superstructures. FRC material is normally radiolucent and virtually invisible to X-ray inspection. However,

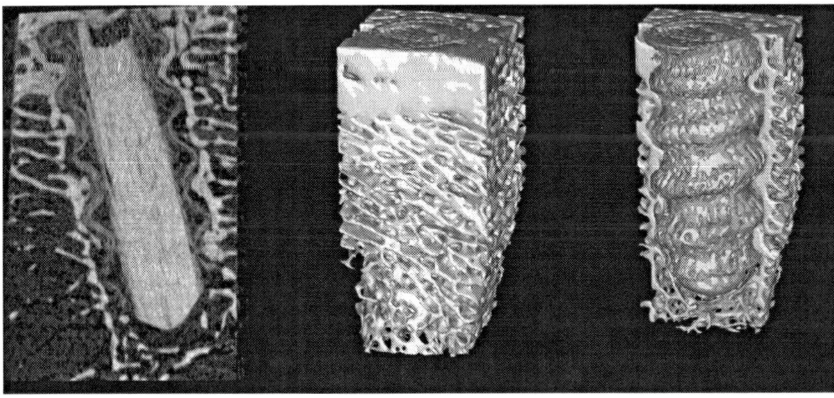

11.7 Micro-CT images and three-dimensional visualization of the bone growth around and between the threads of experimental FRC implants.

implants can be made visible by adding radiopaque filler materials, such as barium. The composition of FRC materials is relatively easy to adjust to give clear computed tomography (CT) and magnetic resonance imaging (MRI) images (Fig. 11.7). This is important as the imaging techniques are set to develop quickly in the near future. The possibility of staining FRC implants is another important aspect. Esthetical demands are increasing and gingival appearance is playing an increasing role in implant dentistry. Tooth-colored implants and implant abutments may facilitate good results in esthetic zone treatments. The possibility of adjusting the mechanical behavior, color and surface properties of FRC implants open new horizons in implant treatments.

Although there are some promising results with FRC in preclinical studies, many questions remain to be answered before FRC implants can be introduced into clinical use. In the future, flexural fatigue studies of the implant-bone system are needed to simulate the dynamic loading conditions of the masticatory system. Further studies are needed to evaluate the bone remodeling process and the mechanical strength of the FRC implant under loading conditions. Also, the designing principles of the FRC implants–crown system need to be considered in relation to materials' properties.

11.6 References

Abdulmajeed AA, Närhi TO, Vallittu PK and Lassila LV (2011) 'The effect of high fiber fraction on some mechanical properties of unidirectional glass fiber-reinforced composite'. *Dent Mater*, **27** (4), 313–21.

Adams D, Williams DF and Hill J (1978) 'Carbon fiber-reinforced carbon as a potential implant material'. *J Biomed Mater Res*, **12**, 35–42.

Aho AJ, Hautamäki M, Mattila R, Alander P, Strandberg N, Rekola J, Gunn J, Lassila LV and Vallittu PK (2004) 'Surface porous fiber-reinforced composite bulk bone substitute'. *Cell Tissue Bank*, **5**, 213–21.

Albrektsson, T (1995) 'Principles of osseointegration'. In: *Dental and Maxillofacial Implantology*, Hobkirk JA and Watson K, (eds), 1st edn, Mosby-Wolfe, London, p. 9.

Aldini NN, Fini M, Giavaresi G, Torricelli P, Martini L, Giardino R, Ravaglioli A, Krajewski A, Mazzocchi M, Dubini B, Ponzi-Bossi MG, Rustichelli F and Stanic V (2002) 'Improvement in zirconia osseointegration by means of a biological glass coating: An *in vitro* and *in vivo* investigation'. *J Biomed Mater Res*, **61**, 282–9.

Alexander H (1996) 'Composites'. In: *Biomaterials Science*. Ratner BD, Hoffman AS, Schoen FJ and Lemons JE (eds), Academic Press, San Diego.

Andreassen GS, Hoiness PR, Skraamm I, Granlund O and Engebretsen L (2004) 'Use of a synthetic bone void filler to augment screws in osteopenic ankle fracture fixation'. *Arch Orthop Trauma Surg*, **124**, 161–5.

Ballo, AM, Lassila L, Vallittu PK and Närhi TO (2007a) 'Load bearing capacity of bone anchored fiber-reinforced composite device'. *J Mater Sci: Mater Med*, **18**, 2025–31.

Ballo AM, Akca EA, Ozen T Moritz N, Lassila L, Vallittu PK and Närhi TO (2007b) 'Biomechanical measurements of bioactive fiber-reinforced composite as bone anchored device'. *IADR-Continental European Division Annual Meeting*, Thessaloniki, Greece, September 2007, p 164.

Ballo AM, Lassila L, Närhi TO and Vallittu PK (2008a) '*In vitro* mechanical testing of glass fiber-reinforced composite as dental implants'. *J Contemp Dent Practi*, **9**, 41–8.

Ballo AM, Kokkari AK, Meretoja VV, Lassila L, Vallittu PK and Närhi TO (2008b) 'Osteoblast proliferation and maturation on fiber-reinforced composite surface'. *J Mater Sci: Mater Med*, **19**, 3169–77.

Ballo AM, Akca EA, Ozen T, Lassila L, Vallittu PK and Närhi TO (2009) 'Bone tissue responses to glass fibre-reinforced composite implants – a histomorphometric study'. *Clin Oral Implants Res*, **20**(6), 608–15.

Ballo AM, Närhi TO, Akca EA, Ozen T, Syrjänen SM, Lassila LV and Vallittu PK (2011) 'Prepolymerized vs. *in situ*-polymerized fiber-reinforced composite implants – a pilot study'. *J Dent Res*, **90**(2), 263–7.

Behr M, Rosentritt M, Lang R and Handel G (2001) 'Glass fiber-reinforced abutments for dental implants'. *Clin Oral Implants Res*, **12**, 174–8.

Black J, Hasting GW (1998) *Handbook of Biomaterials Properties*, Chapman and Hall, London, UK.

Brunski JB (1999) '*In vivo* bone response to biomechanical loading at the bone/dental-implant interface'. *Adv Dent Res*, **13**, 99–119.

Cheal EJ, Spector M and Hayes WC (1992) 'Role of loads and prosthesis material properties on the mechanics of the proximal femur after total hip arthroplasty'. *J Orthop Res*, **10**, 405–22.

Dyer SR, Lassila LV, Jokinen M and Vallittu PK (2004) 'Effect of fiber position and orientation on fracture load of fiber-reinforced composite'. *Dent Mater*, **20**, 947–55.

Engelmann J, Janke V, Volk J, Leyhausen G, von Neuhoff N, Schlegelberger B and Geurtsen W (2004) 'Effects of BisGMA on glutathione metabolism andapoptosis in human gingival fibroblasts *in vitro*'. *Biomaterials*, **25**, 4573–80.

Evans SL, Hunt CM and Ahuja S (2002) 'Bone cement or bone substitute augmentation of pedicle screws improves pullout strength in posterior spinal fixation'. *J Mater Sci-Mater Med*, **13**, 1143–5.

Ferracane, JL and Condon, JR (1992) 'Post-cure heat treatments for composites: Properties and fractography'. *Dent Mater*, **8**, 290–95.

Freilich MA, Duncan JP, Alarcon EK and Eckrote KA (2002) 'The design and fabrication of fiber-reinforced implant prostheses'. *J Prosthet Dent*, **88**, 449–54.

Goldberg AJ and Burstone CJ (1992) 'The use of continuous fiber reinforcement in dentistry'. *Dent Mater*, **8**, 197–202.

Hautamäki MP, Aho AJ, Alander P, Rekola J, Gunn J, Strandberg N and Vallittu PK (2008) 'Repair of bone segment defects with surface porous fiber-reinforced polymethyl methacrylate (PMMA) composite prosthesis: histomorphometric incorporation model and characterization by SEM'. *Acta Orthop*, **79**, 555–64.

Hench LL and West JK (1996) *In Life Chemistry Reports*, Harwood Academic Publishers, Amsterdam, The Netherlands.

Hench LL, Xynos ID and Polak JM (2004) 'Bioactive glasses for *in situ* tissue regeneration'. *J Biomater Sci Polym Ed*, **15**, 543–62.

Koolstra JH (2002) 'Dynamics of the human masticatory system'. *Crit Rev Oral Biol Med*, **13**(4), 366–76.

Lemons JE (1998) 'Unanticipated outcomes: dental implants'. *Implant Dent*, **7**, 351–4.

Lin NJ, Bailey LO, Becker ML, Washburn NR and Henderson LA (2007) 'Macrophage response to methacrylate conversion using a gradient approach'. *Acta Biomater*, **3**, 163–73.

Loza-Herrero MA, Rueggeberg FA, Caughman WF, Schuster GS, Lefebvre CA and Gardner FM (1998) 'Effect of heating delay on conversion and strength of a post-cured resin composite'. *J Dent Res*, **77**, 426–31.

MacDougall, M, Selden, JK, Nydegger, JR and Carnes, DL (1998) 'Immortalized mouse odontoblast cell line MO6-G3 application for *in vitro* biocompatibility testing'. *Am Jo Dent*, **11**, 11–6.

Malaval L, Modrowski D, Gupta AK and Aubin JE (1994) 'Cellular expression of bone-related proteins during *in vitro* osteogenesis in rat bone marrow stromal cell cultures'. *J Cell Physiol*, **158**, 555–72.

Miettinen VM and Vallittu PK (1997) 'Release of residual methyl methacrylate into water from glass fiber-poly (methyl methacrylate) composite used in dentures'. *Biomaterials*, **16**, 181–5.

Misch CE, Qu Z and Bidez MW (1999) 'Mechanical properties of trabecular bone in the human mandible: implications for dental implant treatment planning and surgical placement'. *J Oral Maxillofac Surg*, **57**, 700–8.

Moritz N, Rossi S, Vedel E, Tirri T, Ylänen H, Aro H and Närhi T (2004) 'Implants coated with bioactive glass by CO_2-laser, an *in vivo* study'. *J Mater Sci: Mater Med*, **15**, 795–802.

Palmquist A, Omar OM, Esposito M, Lausmaa J and Thomsen P (2010). 'Titanium oral implants: surface characteristics, interface biology and clinical outcome'. *J R Soc Interface*, 6; 7 Suppl **5**, S515–27.

Palussière J, Berge J, Gangi A, Cotten A, Pasco A, Bertagnoli R, Jaksche H, Carpeggiani P and Deramond H (2005) 'Clinical results of an open prospective study of a bis-GMA composite in percutaneous vertebral augmentation'. *Eur Spine J*, **14**, 982–91.

Pfeiffer, P and Rosenbauer, EU (2005) 'Residual methyl methacrylate monomer, water sorption and water solubility of hypoallergic denture base materials'. *J Prosthet Denti*, **1**, 72–8.

Porter JA and von Fraunhofer JA (2005) 'Success or failure of dental implants? A literature review with treatment considerations'. *Gen Dent*, **53**(6), 423–32; quiz 433, 446.

Price N, Bendall SP, Frondoza C, Jinnah RH and Hungerford DS (1997) 'Human osteoblast-like cells (MG63) proliferate on a bioactive glass surface'. *J Biomed Mater Res*, **37**, 394–400.

Radin S, Reilly G, Bhargave G, Leboy PS and Ducheyne P (2005) 'Osteogenic effects of bioactive glass on bone marrow stromal cells'. *J Biomed Mater Res A*, **73**, 21–9.

Ramakrishna S, Mayer J, Wintermantel E and Leong KW (2001) 'Biomedical applications of polymer-composite materials: a review'. *Comp Sci Technol*, **61**, 1189–224.

Roynesdal AK, Ambjornsen E, Stovne S and Haanaes HR (1998) 'A comparative clinical study of three different endosseous implants in edentulous mandibles'. *Int J Oral Maxillofac Implant*, **13**, 500–5.

Shinya A, Ballo AM, Lassila LV, Shinya A, Närhi TO and Vallittu PK (2011) 'Stress and strain analysis of the bone–implant interface: a comparison of fiber-reinforced composite and titanium implants utilizing 3-dimensional finite element study'. *J Oral Implantol*, **37**, 133–40.

Stanley HR, Hench L, Going R, Bennett C, Chellemi SJ, King C, Ingersoll N, Ethridge E and Kreutziger K (1976) 'The implantation of natural tooth form bioglasses in baboons'. A preliminary report. *Oral Surg, Oral Med, Oral Pathol*, **42**, 339–56.

Stanley HR, Hench LL, Bennett CG Jr, Chellemi SJ, King CJ 3rd, Going RE, Ingersoll NJ, Ethridge EC, Kreutziger KL, Loeb L and Clark AE (1981) 'The implantation of natural tooth form bioglass in baboons – long term results'. *Implantologist*, **2**, 26–36.

Stein GS, Lian JB and Owen TA (1990) 'Relationship of cell growth to the regulation of tissue-specific gene expression during osteoblast differentiation'. *FASEB J*, **4**, 3111–23.

Stein PS, Sullivan J, Haubenreich JE and Osborne PB (2005) 'Composite resin in medicine and dentistry'. *J Long Term Effect Med Implants*, **15**, 641–54.

Tuusa SM, Peltola MJ, Tirri T, Lassila LV and Vallittu PK (2007) 'Frontal bone defect repair with experimental glass-fiber-reinforced composite with bioactive glass granule coating'. *J Biomed Mater Res, Part B*, **82**, 149–55.

Tuusa SM, Peltola MJ, Tirri T, Puska MA, Röyttä M, Aho H, Sandholm J, Lassila LV and Vallittu PK (2008) 'Reconstruction of critical size calvarial bone defects in rabbits with glass-fiber-reinforced composite with bioactive glass granule coating'. *J Biomed Mater Res, Part B*, **84**, 510–19.

Vallittu PK (1995) 'The effect of void space and polymerization time on transverse strength of acrylic-glass fiber composite'. *J Oral Rehabil*, **22**, 257–61.

Vallittu PK (1998) 'Some aspects of the tensile strength of unidirectional glass fiber-polymethymethacrylate composite used in dentures'. *J Oral Rehabil*, **25**, 100–5.

Vallittu PK (2007) 'Effect of 10 years of *in vitro* aging on the flexural properties of fiber-reinforced resin composites'. *Int J Prosthodont*, **20**, 43–5.

Vallittu PK, Miettinen VM and Alakuijala P (1995) 'Residual monomer content and its release into water from denture base materials'. *Dent Mater*, **11**, 338–42.

Wennerberg A and Albrektsson T (2010) 'On implant surfaces: a review of current knowledge and opinions'. *Int J Oral Maxillofac Implant*, **25**(1), 63–74.

Wennerberg A and Albrektsson T (2011) 'Current challenges in successful rehabilitation with oral implants'. *J Oral Rehabil*, **38**, 286–94.

Wintermantel E and Mayer J (1995) 'Anisotropic biomaterials strategies and developments for bone implants', in *Encyclopedic Handbook of Biomaterials and Bioengineering, Part B-1*, D. Wise LD, Trantolo DJ, Altobelli DE, Yaszemiski JD, Gresser JD and Schwartz ER (eds), Marcel Dekker, New York, 3–42.

Yao J, Radin S, Reilly G, Leboy PS and Ducheyne P (2005) 'Solution-mediated effect of bioactive glass in poly (lactic-co-glycolic acid)-bioactive glass composites on osteogenesis of marrow stromal cells'. *J Biomed Mater Res, Part A*, **75**, 794–801.

Yuehuei H (2000) 'Mechanical properties of bone'. *Mechanical Testing of Bone and the Bone–Implant Interface*, CRC Press, New York, 41–64.

12
Fibre-reinforced composites (FRCs) as dental materials

PEKKA K. VALLITTU, University of Turku, Finland

DOI: 10.1533/9780857096432.3.352

Abstract: Fibre-reinforced composites (FRCs) are a novel group of dental materials characterized by fibrous fillers. The function of the fibres is to transfer loads from the weaker polymer phase to the more durable reinforcing fibres. In dentistry, the use of glass fibres is justified because of their good cosmetic–aesthetic properties and because they can be correctly bonded to the resins using silane coupling agents, which is impossible with polyethylene fibres. The quality of the FRC used is particularly critical in small dental appliances. Factors influencing FRCs that should be considered, include: fibre properties versus polymer matrix properties, impregnation of fibres in the resin, adhesion of fibres to the polymer matrix, quantity and direction of fibres, and location of the fibre-rich phase in construction. The most commonly used applications of FRCs are in removable dentures, minimally invasive fixed partial dentures, periodontal splints, root canal posts and orthodontic devices. Minimally invasive prosthodontics aims to preserve the remaining tooth substance. Certain design principles must be followed when minimally invasive fixed partial dentures are constructed, including occlusal rests against vertical forces, pontic reinforcements against veneer delamination, and additional bonding wings against dislodgement of the fixed partial denture. The use of large amounts of FRC in the coronal part of the root canal opening creates a highly durable post-and-core system which cannot be obtained by the current prefabricated and standard-sized fibre posts.

Key words: biomechanics, dentures, fibre-reinforced composites, fixed dental prostheses, root canal posts, strength.

12.1 Introduction to fibre-reinforced composites (FRCs) as dental materials

Fibre-reinforced composites (FRCs) are a new group of non-metallic dental biomaterials that were first tested as a means of reinforcing denture bases in the early 1960s.[1] In principal, by combining FRC with Bowen's resin, a durable and tough tooth-coloured material could have been produced for use in several applications even at those early stages. However, because there were some problems associated with combining resin systems with reinforcing fibres and with the technical and clinical handling of FRC, the material has not been available until recently. The development of FRCs with a new type of resin system, combined with a better understanding of the design principles governing device construction, has led to the use of FRCs in a variety of disciplines and applications: in removable prosthodontics,[2–7] fixed prosthodontics,[8–26] restorative dentistry,[27–30] periodontology,[31,32] orthodontics[33,34] and in repairs of fractured porcelain veneers.[35,36] The most recent application of FRCs is in tooth fillings. A critical evaluation of the available FRC materials and the correct patient selection is very important in ensuring the successful use of the material.

Why use FRCs in dentistry? Although there are several proven dental materials and treatment options based on conventional dental materials, a large number of partially edentulous patients are not treated using fixed dental prostheses to replace their missing teeth. This is often due to the high cost of the current generation of fixed prosthesis treatments and to the irreversible damage that the treatment causes during the grinding of abutment teeth to create space for metal and ceramic crowns. Other non-metallic alternative materials, such as zirconia, have become available; unfortunately, however, the use of zirconia requires just as much reduction of abutment tooth substance as restorations involving the fusion of porcelain and metal, and sometimes even more. At the moment, the only materials suitable for use by the direct technique for applications requiring high load-bearing capacity, such as for fixed dental prostheses, are FRCs. The use of FRCs in clinical dentistry is part of a value-based medicine, which integrates evidence-based medicine with improvement in quality of life, as viewed by the patient.[37]

12.2 Structure and properties of fibre-reinforced composites

FRC is a combination of polymer matrix and reinforcing fibres (Fig. 12.1). The fibres in the composite are the reinforcing phase when a load is applied to the composite[38]: the load is transferred to be carried by the fibres. The reinforcing fibres can be continuous unidirectional (rovings), continuous bidirectional (weaves), continuous random oriented (mat) or short random oriented fibres.

Of the many types of fibres available, those that have proved most clinically suitable are glass fibres that can be silanized and adhered to the resin matrix of the FRC.[39–41] Glass fibres vary according to their composition: the most commonly used are E-glass and S-glass, which offer chemically stable and durable glass in the pH range 4–11.[42] Carbon/graphite fibres have also been tested, but their black colour limited their clinical use.[43] Attempts to use ultra-high-molecular weight polyethylene fibres (UHMWP) have also been made,[3–7,44–47] but there are problems involved in bonding the fibres to the resin matrix.[48,49] Moreover, the high affinity of proteins and oral microbes

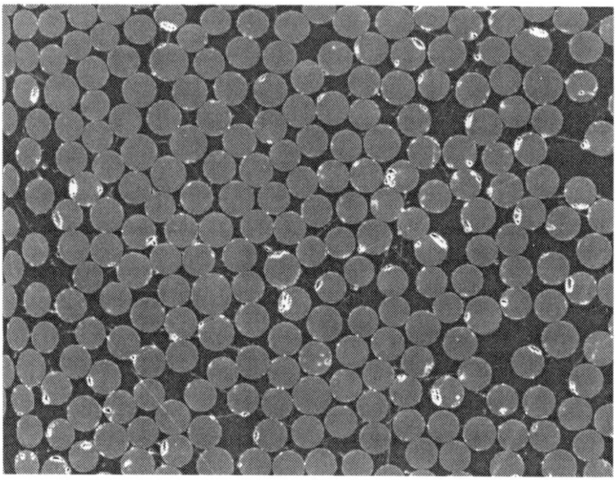

12.1 Cross-sectional view of glass fibre-reinforced composite showing good impregnation of the fibres with the resin matrix.

to adhere to the UHMWP FRC may limit their use as a dental material, as concluded by Tanner and co-workers.[50–52] The strength and rigidity of constructions made from FRC are dependent on the polymer matrix of the FRC and the type of fibre reinforcement.

In dental appliances of relatively small size, the quality of the load-bearing FRC sub-structure is very important. All factors influencing the properties of the FRC must therefore be carefully taken into consideration. This is especially important because the masticatory system produces cyclic loads on dental appliances. The appliance must therefore not only have adequate static strength, but also adequate dynamic (fatigue) strength. It should also be noted that dental constructions are multiphase in nature: for example, the FRC reinforced root-canal-post-system consists of dentine, composite resin cement, core build-up composite resin and, as a load-bearing material, the FRC root canal post. All of these phases need to have adequate strength and the must be well adhered to each other.

An important parameter governing the strength of the FRC is the impregnation of the fibres with resin. Reinforcing fibres are difficult to impregnate with resin systems of high viscosity[53–55] such as those mixed from polymer powder and monomer liquid which are used in denture bases, provisional FPDs and removable orthodontic appliances, or those made of light curing resins and particulate fillers. For dentistry applications, it is recommended that fibres should be impregnated with resin made by the fibre manufacturer, in order to ensure complete impregnation,[56] thereby allowing the resin to come into the contact with every fibre. If complete impregnation is not achieved because of high viscosity or polymerization shrinkage of the resin, the mechanical properties of FRC will not reach the optimal values calculated on the basis of the laws of mixture.[55]

Two types of resins can be used in FRCs, resulting in either a cross-linked (thermoset) polymer matrix, or a linear (thermoplastic) polymer matrix. The cross-linked matrix is formed from multifunctional or dimethacrylate resins, whereas monofunctional methacrylates form a linear (non-cross-linked) polymer matrix. Some impregnation methods have also been developed based on a combination of thermoset and thermoplastic resins. In that case, the polymer matrix is multiphase in nature and it is by definition a semi-interpenetrating polymer network (semi-IPN), with a cross-linked polymer and linear polymer mixed together.[57–59] In polymerization the dimethacrylate monomers form a predominantly cross-linked semi-IPN structure with phases of the linear polymer polymethyl methacrylate (PMMA). Cross-linked polymer matrix forms FRC with a higher modulus of elasticity than that obtained by thermoplastic or semi-IPN polymers.[61–63] On the other hand, thermoplastic and semi-IPN polymer matrices provide greater toughness than FRCs made from highly cross-linked thermosets. The semi-IPN polymer matrix of FRC offers advantages over cross-linked dimethacrylate and the epoxy type of polymer matrices in terms of its handling properties and the bonding of indirectly made restorations and root canal posts to resin luting cements and veneering composites.[27,58,64]

12.2.1 Mechanical strength

The static strength (ultimate flexural strength) of the FRC is dependent on the quantity of fibre to a level of approximately 70 vol%. A high quality glass FRC material with a high quantity of fibre provides good flexural properties (with E-glass at 1250 MPa).[61,62] Water sorption of the polymer matrix reduces the strength and modulus of elasticity of FRC made from semi-IPN polymer matrix by approximately 15% after 30 days' storage in water at 37°C.[64] A positive correlation exists between the water sorption of the polymer matrix and the reduction of flexural properties.[62] For instance, the high water sorption shown by a polyamide (nylon) matrix causes a strength reduction of over 50% in the FRC. The reduction of the flexural properties was reversible, that is dehydration of the FRC recovered these mechanical properties.[62] No significant reduction of flexural strength and modulus occurred even after long-term water storage (up to 10 years).[65,66]

The strength of FRC is also dependent on the direction of the fibre. The efficiency of fibre reinforcement (Krenchel's factor) varies in FRC laminates with different fibre orientations.[67] Continuous unidirectional fibres provide the highest strength and modulus of elasticity for the FRC, but this property is only available when the direction of stress is the same as that of the fibres. The anisotropic behaviour of unidirectional FRCs can also be observed in other properties, such as thermal expansion or polymerisation shrinkage.[68,69] A novel filling composite resin has been used to control polymerization shrinkage by fibres; this improves the adaptation of the filling to the axial walls of the cavity and increases the toughness of the restored tooth. The fibres can be classified according to whether the reinforcing effect applies in two or more directions, and FRCs are called orthotropic and isotropic with regard to their thermal and physical properties, respectively.

There are several studies that have dealt with the strength of FRC, but which may have shown misleading results. Testing specimens with small dimensions, such as root canal posts, can lead to incorrect calculated results in megapascals. In the three-point bending test, the commonly used mathematical formulas for calculating the flexural strength and modulus of elasticity of test specimens are dependent on the diameter (height) of the specimen and the span length of the test set-up.[70] With a constant span length, thinner specimens reveal a higher flexural strength and modulus of elasticity values than those observed for larger specimens of the same material. Thus, it is important to compare specimens of exactly the same diameter and span length in test set-up in order to achieve an accurate interpretation of the results obtained, for example, from root canal posts.

12.2.2 Bonding of cements and veneering composites to FRC

The adhesion of particulate filler composite (PFC) resin (resin luting cement, veneering composite) plays an important role in the load transfer from the surface of the device to the FRC framework and tooth. FRC as a bonding substrate contains different types of materials, from polymers to inorganic glass fibres and even particulate fillers.

Adhesion between the fibres and the polymer matrix enables load transfer from the weaker matrix to the reinforcing fibres. In both of the resin types (cross-linked and linear) the bonding is typically based on the silanation of glass fibres by methacrylated silanes and its polymerization reaction with the monomers of the resin system. If the fibre surface is not reactive with silanes, as is the case with polyethylene fibres (UHMWP), adequate bonding is not achieved and the composite is not durable enough for long-term use. Furthermore, if the impregnation of fibres by the resin system is carried out by melting a thermoplastic polymer, the covalent bond obtained between the polymer matrix and the fibres is less stable than when the monomeric resin system is used. Thus, the cohesional strength of the FRC is based on bonding the fibres to the matrix polymer. In this respect, the most suitable fibres are those in the OH-group, including glass and silica fibres which can be silanated to obtain adequate adhesion to the polymer matrix.[38–41] Less suitable fibres are ultra-high molecular weight polyethylene fibres (UHMWP), as it has been shown that suitable adhesion between these fibres and the resins can be difficult to achieve, even when the fibre surface has been activated by, for example, various types of high energy treatments.[48,49]

In the process of bonding a new resin to FRC, fibres and polymer matrix are the substrates for adhesion. If the fibres of the FRC are exposed on the bonding surface, the adhesional properties of the fibres themselves play a role in adhering the adhesive resin and composite resin luting cement to the FRC: glass fibres can be adhered to PFR by silanation, although bonding results have been quite poor. Owing to the cross-linked nature of the polymer matrix of most dental FRC materials, there are two possible means of achieving adhesion of the PFR to the FRC: mechanical interlocking, and adhesion based on ongoing polymerization of the resin matrix of the FRC soon after curing. If the FRC contains non-cross-linked polymer phases (i.e. thermoplastics or semi-IPN polymers), adhesion can also be based on the diffusion of monomers of the new resin or resin composite into the non-cross-linked polymer matrix.[58,59] This requires the solubility parameter of the linear polymer to be close to that of the monomer system of the FRC. Solubility parameters have been developed to provide a method of predicting and correlating the cohesive and adhesive properties of materials. The numerical value of the solubility parameter illustrates the amount of energy required to separate molecules. Two materials with similar solubility parameter values gain sufficient energy on mutual dispersion to permit mixing, which is essential for the interdiffusion of monomers. During polymerization of the resin, an adhesive bond based on the so-called secondary semi-IPN structure is formed. A well-known example of this type of structure is found in repairs of fractured denture bases using repair acrylic resin. The repair acrylic resin monomers dissolve and swell the surface, forming a durable secondary semi-IPN bond.[60,71,72]

Adhesion of PFC to FRC that is made directly or made at the chair-side differs from its adhesion to FRC made indirectly in a dental laboratory. It has been established that in the polymerization of resins and resin-based composites or FRC in air, a non-polymerized surface layer is formed, known as the oxygen inhibited layer.[73] PFCs can adhere to this layer by free radical polymerization of the PFR and form a durable bond.

12.3 Applications of fibre-reinforced composites in dentistry

12.3.1 Removable dentures

Research on dental FRCs began in the early 1960s when the first experiments were carried out into the use of glass fibres in denture base polymers.

In addition to glass fibres, some tests were also carried out on the use of carbon/graphite fibres for the same purpose. At the time, little attention was paid to the low reinforcing effect of any fibres when they were used with powder–liquid type denture base resins. In the 1990s studies were published that showed that a highly viscous resin mixture of PMMA powder and monomer liquid was not able to impregnate the fibres adequately.[53,54] The use of an excess of the monomer liquid to lower the viscosity of the resin mixture did not resolve the problem: instead, the higher quantity of monomer liquid in the resin mixture caused void formation in the composite owing to polymerization contraction.[53] This led to the development of a system of pre-impregnating the reinforcing fibres with porous PMMA.[74] Porous PMMA between the silanized glass fibres behaves as a polymer powder in the acrylic resin mixture, lowering the polymerization shrinkage of the resin between the fibres.

The fibre reinforcements used in denture bases are divided into two categories. Ladizesky and co-workers reported a method in which fibres were distributed throughout the entire denture base.[6,7] On the other hand, an approach by Vallittu is based on the fibre reinforcement of only the weakest part of the denture base (the location of fracture initiation). The two concepts are known as total fibre reinforcement (TFR) and partial fibre reinforcement (PFR), respectively (Fig. 12.2).[2] Clinical studies have been performed with FRC reinforced removable dentures,[2,75] which suggested that PFR offers an effective method of eliminating fractures in denture bases, as demonstrated by Narva.[76]

The successful use of PFR requires the correct positioning of the fibres in the denture base.[77–79] The fibres of the PFR should be placed at the region of the denture base where the fracture is most likely to begin (Fig. 12.2).

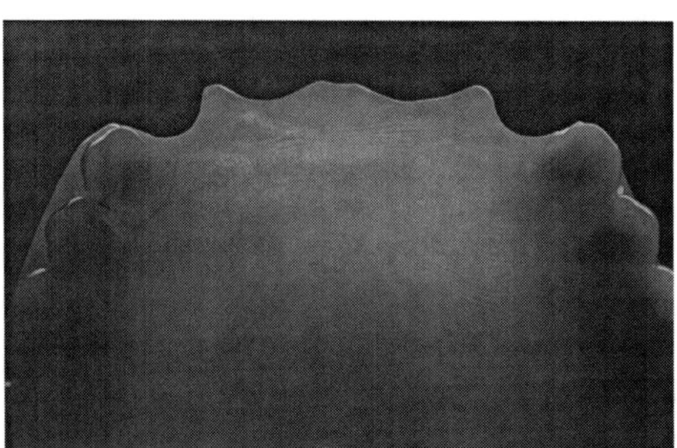

12.2 Removable partial denture with partial fibre reinforcement of woven glass fibres in the anterior part of the base plate.

The correct location for the fibres in upper complete dentures is close to the denture teeth and fibres should be directed along the ridge lap in a horseshoe shape. Continuous unidirectional fibres offer the highest resistance against mid-line fractures. In removable partial dentures, where the fracture is likely to occur in the anterior margin of the denture, fibres in the form of woven fabric are preferred. An FRC reinforced region with woven glass fibres, about 10 mm wide on average, eliminates denture fracture initiations and propagation. Overdentures are also reinforced with woven fibres to eliminate fractures in the denture base polymer close to the precision attachments of the dentures. It has been suggested that FRC could also lead to a reduction in loosening of the parts of these precision attachments.

12.3.2 Fixed dental prostheses (FDPs)

FRCs can be used to produce definitive fixed partial prostheses.[80] Based on current clinical results, it is reasonable to expect FRC fixed partial prostheses (FDP) to attain a good longevity.[80] FDPs made from FRC are classified in several different categories: surface retained FDPs, inlay/onlay retained FDPs, full coverage crown retained FDPs and hybrid FDPs.[81] The last of these is a combination of various retaining elements according to the requirement of the specific dentition. FRC FDPs can be made directly or indirectly. Implant supported FDPs have been fabricated from carbon/graphite FRC and glass FRC.[82–84] All permanent type, indirectly made tooth supported FRC FDPs must be luted with composite resin luting cements, although there are studies on the use of conventional luting cements.[20] Direct FRC FDPs can be bonded to teeth through the polymerization of restorative composite resins. The adhesive properties of FRC bonded directly to the dentine and enamel have been studied by Tezvergil *et al.*, who showed that only minor differences could be found between the adhesive properties of FRC and PFC.[85,86] In the FRC FDPs, the framework between the abutments is made of continuous unidirectional fibres which offer high flexural strength.[69,87] The crowns can be reinforced with woven fibres or, in some fabrication designs, by making a fibre loop of unidirectional fibres to surround the abutment.[14] Recent clinical studies have shown that the FRC framework needs to provide support for the veneering composite resin and, therefore, additional fibres need to be placed inside the pontic.[15] There are also studies that emphasize the importance of the fibre geometry of the FRC framework for the strength of the FDP construction.[88,89]

Surface-retained resin bonded FDPs made of metals are normally supported and bonded from one end only in order to reduce the number of debondings. In the case of surface-retained FRC FDPs, the bridgework can be supported from both ends thanks to the improved bonding characteristics and slight flexibility of the FRC framework.[81] The flexibility allows abutment teeth movement to occur to some extent without causing loosening of the FDP.[90] In the surface-retained FRC FDPs, the location of the bonding wing in the vertical dimension of the abutment is important. The fibres of the bonding wing should be placed close to the incisal edge to eliminate the momentary forces of dislodgement. On the other hand, the bonding wing needs to cover the bonding surface. The bonding wing is most frequently placed on the oral surfaces of abutments, but labial and buccal surfaces can also be used. To protect the fibres of the bonding wings, a layer of PFR is used to cover the wings. Good interfacial adhesion between the FRC framework and the particulate filler composite resin is important to avoid chipping of the latter.

In connectors, continuous unidirectional fibres should have a cross-sectional design which offers good resistance against occlusal forces. It has been shown that the thickness of the connector is a more important parameter than the width of the connector, when stiffness and strength are optimized. The cross-section of the connector normally has maximum quantity of fibre, but if there is excess space, the greatest strength can be achieved by placing the fibres at the tension side.[87] Surface-retained FRC FDPs are used in the anterior and premolar regions. Recent laboratory investigations have suggested that optimally designed FRC FDPs made on non-prepared abutments can provide an even higher load-bearing capacity than conventional FDPs based on porcelain fused to metal.[91]

Inlay/onlay-retained FDPs are made by filling the cavities of the abutments with continuous unidirectional fibres (Fig. 12.3 (a)–(e)). The FDP can be made indirectly or directly. In the case of indirect FDPs, cementation is carried out with composite resin luting cements, which contain regular adhesive resin, used to activate the bonding surface for secondary-IPN bonding. Self-adhesive cement adhesives do not provide optimal bonding. For canines, the addition of an additional bonding wing, either buccally or palatinally, to the framework is recommended, in order to avoid loosening of the inlay in cuspid protected articulation. In the case of existing old fillings, the complete or partial removal of the filling provides space for the FRC framework and veneering composite resin. Vertical support against occlusal loads is required: in intact teeth, an approximal box preparation of more than 1 mm in depth provides support for the FDP if the fibres are accurately placed into the box.[91] The load-bearing capacity of this type of FDP is higher than the maximal biting forces in the molar region.[92] Veneering of the FRC framework is carried out using laboratory veneering composite resin or restorative composite resin. The optimal thickness of the veneering composite resin on the occlusal surface of the FRC framework is more than 1.5 mm.[93,94]

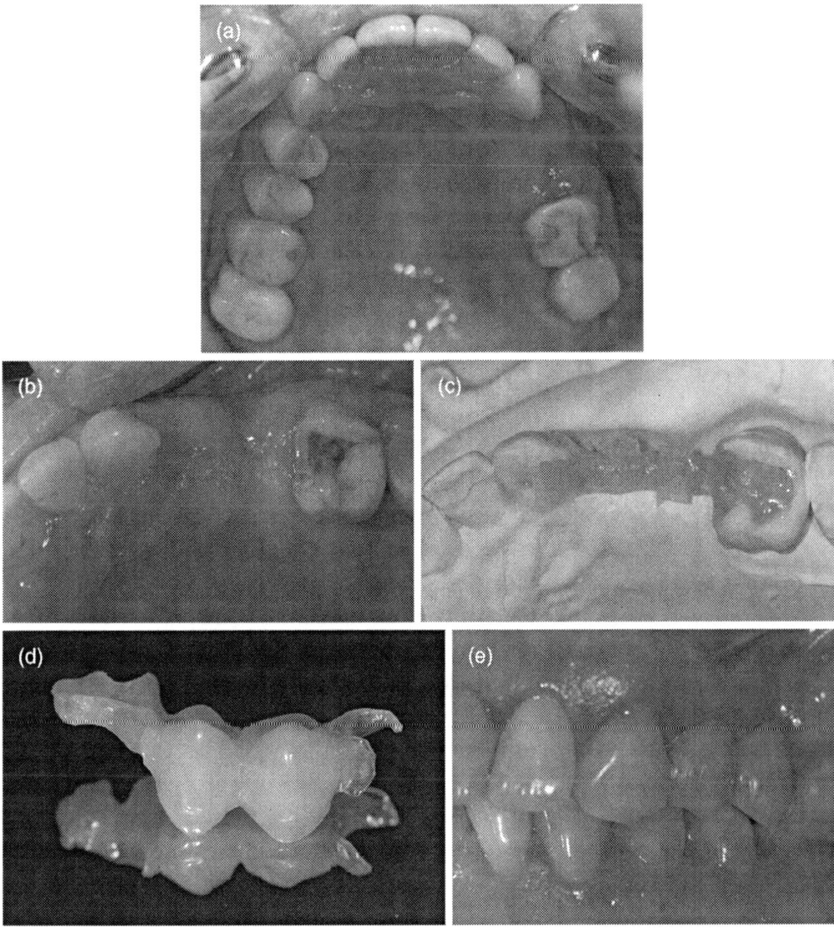

12.3 Indirectly made glass fibre-reinforced composite fixed dental prosthesis. (a) Occlusal view of the dental arch before treatment, (b) cavity preparation by the minimal invasive concept, (c) framework of a dental cast, (d) finished FDP and (e) FDP after being cemented with composite resin luting cement.

Full coverage crown-retained FPDs are made by layering woven FRC on prepared abutments. Abutments are connected by continuous unidirectional fibres, with additional pieces of FRC added to support the cusps of the pontics. Veneering is carried out using laboratory particulate filler composite resin. The FRC framework is intended to be fully covered by veneering composite resin in order to obtain a polishable and tooth-coloured surface. Special attention needs to be paid to the interproximal regions. If the FRC framework is not properly covered by the veneering composite resin, or preferably by opaque paint, the darkness of the oral cavity can be transmitted through the connectors, thereby causing cosmetic/aesthetic problems.

CAD-CAM (computer-aided design – computer-aided manufacturing) processed FRC blocks made from short random fibre-oriented FRC in a polyamide matrix (nylon) are also available for FRC framework fabrication. The mechanical properties of short FRC are considerably lower than those of continuous unidirectional FRC.[67] The water sorption of polyamide causes a reduction of the FRC by up to 60% after 30 days.[95] The use of full coverage crowns as retaining elements for FPDs goes against the principles of minimal invasiveness. FRCs can also be used as reinforcements of provisional FDPs during the fabrication of conventional FDPs.[96–100]

12.3.3 Root canal posts

The use of FRC in root canal posts to anchor cores and crowns has rapidly increased.[27,29,30,62,98] FRC can be used in root canal as both prefabricated solid posts and individually formed posts.

Prefabricated posts are made of reinforcing fibres (carbon/graphite, glass, quartz), with polymerized resin matrix between the fibres forming a solid post with a predetermined diameter. Individually formed posts are made from non-polymerized fibre-resin prepregs, typically consisting of glass fibres and a light-curing resin matrix (Fig. 12.4(a)). The purpose of the individually formed FRC post is to fill the entire space of the root canal with FRC material (Fig. 12.4(b)).[101–105] The increased fibre quantity, especially in the coronal part of the root canal, increases the load-bearing

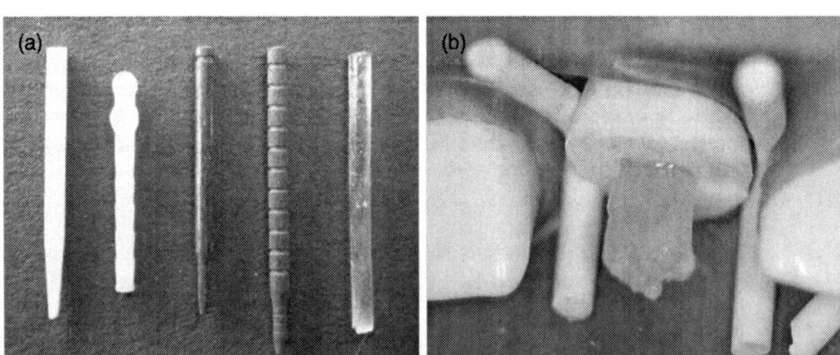

12.4 (a) Fibre-reinforced root canal posts, on the left are four prefabricated posts and on the right is a post material used for an individually formed post fabrication. (b) In the individually formed post, the FRC material fully fills the opening of the coronal root canal enabling a construction of high strength.

capacity of the system and the biomechanics of a tooth can be better simulated because the fibres are located closer to the dentine, where the highest stresses occur.[106]

A tooth restored with a root canal post system should be able to withstand cyclic loading of high magnitude for a long period of time without catastrophic failure or even marginal breakdown of the crown, which can cause a tooth to be predisposed to secondary caries. The load-bearing phase of the root canal post system, that is the FRC root canal post, should withstand the loads and maintain the crown margins intact. Repeated stress cycles cause microscopic cracks, mainly at the tension side of the construction and, after a period of time, a number of cracks can increase to such a size that a sudden fracture can occur even with a low stress level. Clinically, the material-based weakness in terms of fatigue resistance is compensated by the correct design and sizing of the cast metal or FRC post-and-core, thus increasing the quantity of reinforcing fibres in the cervical part of the tooth. This approach can be employed by fabricating individually formed posts instead of using prefabricated posts (Fig. 12.4(b)).

The fabrication of prefabricated FRC root canal posts is based on the impregnation of fibres with thermoset resins, such dimethacrylate or epoxy resins. If thermoset resins are used to form cross-linked polymer between the fibres, good bonding of the post to the resin cement cannot be achieved. To overcome the problem of adhesion, some manufacturers have added serrations to the post for mechanical retention of the cement. On the other hand, if the semi-IPN polymer matrix is used between the fibres, as is possible with individually formed posts, the adhesion of the post to cement is good.[27,101] It has been shown by radioactive labelled resins that monomers of an adhesive resin diffused to the semi-IPN polymer matrix of the post at a depth of 25 μm in only a few minutes. The resins should also allow the complete impregnation of fibres. There are some prefabricated FRC root canal posts on the market that do not entirely fulfil the requirement of complete impregnation and thus the strength of the post is lower than expected from the constituents.[61,63]

12.4 Fibre-reinforced filling composites

The use of fibres in filling composites has long been the subject of extensive research.[94,107,108] The reasons for its relative lack of success have been selection of fibres that were too short, and thus unable to increase the strength and toughness of the composite resin, and the use of bulky filling material which resulted in a filling surface that was not easily polishable. The current use of FRC in fillings relies on an FRC base with relatively long cut fibres which is then veneered with a conventional particulate filling composite resin (Fig. 12.5). It has been shown that if the fibre orientation is

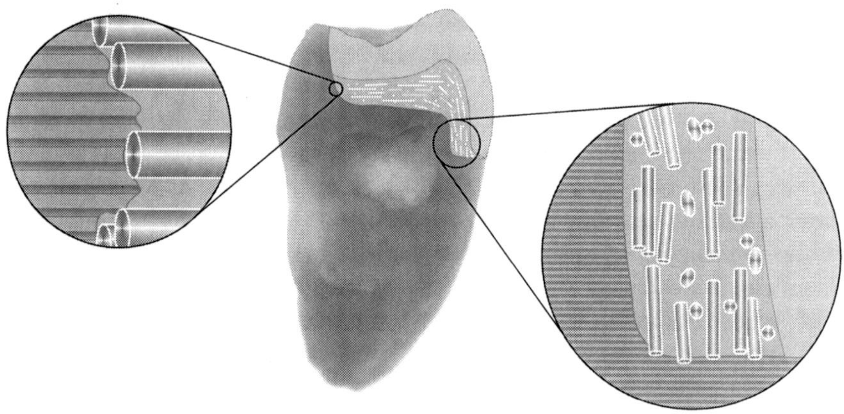

12.5 Illustration of the concept of using glass fibre-reinforced composite as base material for composite fillings to reduce marginal leakage and increase the toughness of the restoration.

perpendicular to the axial walls of a cavity, polymerization contraction of the composite is reduced. In dental fillings, the concept of using fibre-controlled polymerization contraction is based on using cut fibres 1–3 mm in length.[109] Packing the fibres into the cavity forces the fibres to be randomly oriented and thus perpendicular to the axial walls of the cavity. Based on the three-dimensional anisotropicity of the FRC, polymerization contraction occurs in the vertical direction rather than horizontally.

Another benefit of using an FRC base for filling composites is the increase in toughness of the composite filling. The toughness and other physical properties of the FRC base are better than those of conventional filling composites.[110–119] The function of the FRC base in filling composites is to support the filling composite layer and to serve as a crack prevention layer.

12.5 Future trends

A variety of dental FRC materials are available and they provide improvements in the mechanical strength of the resins and particulate filler composites. Continuous unidirectional FRC materials impregnated with light curing resin can provide bending strength values comparable to those observed of cast cobalt–chromium alloy or yttrium-stabilized zircomium dioxide. However, the properties are often anisotropic, which means the reinforcing effect is available only in one direction of the material. This means that dental professionals need to acquire a better understanding of the biomechanics of the dentition and of the design principles of the

FRC devices. If the reinforcing effect of the fibres is divided into several directions, the maximum values of strength are considerably lower, although the toughness of the material is increased.

There has been critical discussion among prosthodontists with regard to whether FRC devices are permanent, semi-permanent, long-term temporary or temporary in nature. Current expertise in materials science and recent clinical experience suggest that FRC devices, if they are made of high quality materials and designed correctly, fulfil the requirements for a device for long-term use. Therefore, FRC FPDs can be defined as definitive solutions. Furthermore, if we consider that the fabrication of many of the fixed FRC devices requires only minimal, if any, tooth preparation, FRCs can also be said to provide a modern adhesive alternative to single and multiple tooth replacements. The use of FRC FPDs is not limited to single tooth replacements, but is appropriate for the fabrication of multiple unit restorations of inlay, complete coverage crown or hybrid FPD design. Of these, the hybrid FPDs provide the greatest benefit to the patient by lowering the biological price of the treatment and also making it more economical. The long-term cost–benefit ratio of FRC FPDs versus conventional FPDs or implant retained FPDs requires further evaluation.

Current expertise in biomechanics of teeth and clinical experience since the early 1990s suggest that the use of FRC root canal posts provides an alternative to cast metal posts, which are more technique-sensitive in fabrication. However, the load-bearing capacity of FRC root canal posts with a small diameter has been criticized: thin FRC posts do not necessarily provide sufficient strength for the crown–core–post–root–bone complex, which can lead to the breakdown of the adhesive interface of the core-build-up composite into dentine and thus to marginal secondary caries. In principal, the alternative FRC post design using individually formed posts provides a solution to this problem.

Future developments in FRCs are focused on the optimization of the design of the sub-structures in FRC devices. Attempts have been made to employ a semi-IPN polymer matrix short glass FRC in filling material applications. Another field where FRCs are starting to be used is implantology. The use of FRC modified by bioactive glass has shown promising results in oral, orthopaedic and head-and-neck implants (Fig. 12.6).[120–125]

12.6 Conclusions

FRCs have been introduced in a variety of clinical applications. FRC is composed of reinforcing fibres which are embedded in a resin matrix. Currently, continuous unidirectional glass FRC provides the highest strength and is the most appropriate for dental use. Several parameters, including the fibre volume fraction and fibre direction have a substantial impact on

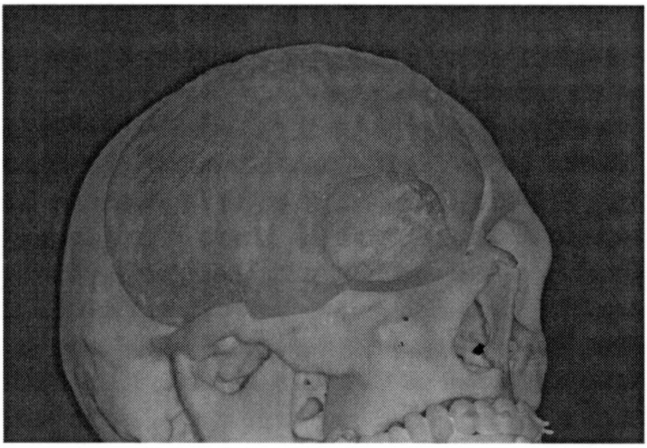

12.6 New applications for glass fibre-reinforced composites include implants used in head-and-neck surgery and as oral implants.

the properties of FRC, which can be anisotropic, orthotropic or isotropic. Clinically, FRC material is used in removable dentures, fixed partial dentures, periodontal splints, orthodontic retainers and root canal posts, and FRCs are currently claimed to be suitable for definitive, rather than provisional, prostheses. The longest and most encouraging clinical experience has been obtained with removable dentures and prefabricated root canal posts, but other applications also seem to benefit from the use of FRC material as an alternative to metal alloys and ceramics. The correct use and understanding of FRC device design principles allows minimally invasive long-term restorations, even for multiple tooth replacement.

12.7 References

1. Smith DC. 'Recent developments and prospects in dental polymers'. *Journal of Prosthetic Dentistry* 1962, **12**, 1066–78.
2. Vallittu PK. 'Glass fiber reinforcement in repaired acrylic resin removable dentures: preliminary results of a clinical study'. *Quintessence International* 1997, **28**, 39–44.
3. Cheng YY and Chow TW. 'Fabrication of complete denture bases reinforced with polyethylene woven fabric'. *Journal of Prosthodontics* 1999, **8**, 268–72.
4. Ladizesky NH. 'The integration of dental resins with highly drawn polyethylene fibres'. *Clinical Materials* 1990, **6**, 181–92.
5. Ladizesky NH, Chow TW and Ward IM. 'The effect of highly drawn polyethylene fibres on the mechanical properties of denture base resins'. *Clinical Materials* 1990, **6**, 209–25.
6. Ladizesky NH, Ho CF and Chow TW. 'Reinforcement of complete denture bases with continuous high performance polyethylene fibers'. *Journal of Prosthetic Dentistry* 1992, **68**, 934–9.

7. Ladizesky NH, Chow TW and Cheng YY. 'Denture base reinforcement using woven polyethylene fiber'. *International Journal of Prosthodontics* 1994, **7**, 307–14.
8. Körber HK and Körber S. 'Experimentelle Untersuchungen zur Passgenauigkeit con GFK-Bruckengerusten "Vectris"'. *Quintessenze Zahntechik* 1998, **24**, 43–53.
9. Kolbeck C, Rosentritt M, Behr M, Lang R and Handel G. '*In vitro* examination of the fracture strength of 3 different fiber composite and 1 all-ceramic posterior inlay fixed partial denture systems'. *Journal of Prosthodonics* 2002, **11**, 248–53.
10. Loose M, Rosentritt M, Leibrock A, Behr M and Handel G. '*In vitro* study of fracture strength and marginal adaptation of fiber-reinforced-composite versus all ceramic fixed partial dentures'. *European Journal of Prosthodontics and Restorative Dentistry* 1998, **6**, 55–62.
11. Göhring TN, Schmidlin PR and Lutzt F. 'Two-year clinical and SEM evaluation of glass-fiber-reinforced inlay fixed partial dentures'. *American Journal of Dentistry* 2002, **15**, 35–40.
12. Behr M, Rosentritt M, Lang R and Handel G. 'Flexural properties of fiber reinforced composite using a vacuum/pressure or a manual adapatation manufacturing process'. *Journal of Dentistry* 2000, **28**, 509–14.
13. Freilich MA, Karmarker AC, Burstone CJ and Goldberg AJ. 'Development and clinical applications of a light-polymerized fiber-reinforced composite'. *Journal of Prosthetic Dentistry* 1998, **80**, 311–8.
14. Freilich MA, Duncan JP, Alarcon EK, Eckrote KA and Goldberg AJ. 'The design and fabrication of fiber-reinforced implant prostheses'. *Journal of Prosthetic Dentistry* 2002, **88**, 449–54.
15. Freilich MA, Meiers JC, Duncan JP, Eckrote KA and Goldberg AJ. 'Clinical evaluation of fiber-reinforced fixed bridges'. *Journal of American Dental Association* 2002, **133**, 1524–34.
16. Freilich MA, Duncan JP, Meiers JC and Goldberg AJ. 'Preimpregnated, fiber-reinforced prostheses. Part I. Basic rationale and complete coverage and intracoronal fixed partial denture design'. *Quintessence International* 1998, **29**, 689–96.
17. Ahlstrand WM and Finger WJ. 'Direct and indirect fiber-reinforced fixed partial dentures: case reports'. *Quintessence International* 2002, **33**, 359–65.
18. Behr M, Hindelang U, Rosentritt M, Lang R and Handel G. 'Comparison of failure rates of adhesive-fixed partial dentures for *in vivo* and *in vitro* studies'. *Clinical Oral Investigations* 2000, **4**, 25–30.
19. Behr M, Rosentritt M and Handel G. 'Fiber-reinforced composite crowns and FPDs: a clinical report'. *International Journal of Prosthodontics* 2003, **15**, 239–43.
20. Behr M, Rosentritt M, Ledwinsky E and Handel G. 'Fracture resistance and marginal adaptation of conventionally cemented fiber-reinforced composite three unit FPDs'. *International Journal of Prosthodontics* 2002, **15**, 467–72.
21. Göhring TN, Mormann WH and Lutz F. 'Clinical and scanning electron microscopic evaluation of fiber-reinforced inlay fixed partial dentures: preliminary results after one year'. *Journal of Prosthetic Dentistry* 1999, **82**, 662–8.

22. Göhring TN, Schmidlin PR and Lutz F. 'Two-year clinical and SEM evaluation of glass-fiber-reinforced inlay fixed partial dentures'. *American Journal of Dentistry* 2002, **15**, 35–40.
23. Meiers JC, Duncan JP, Freilich MA and Goldberg AJ. 'Preimpregnated, fiber-reinforced prostheses: Part II. Direct applications: splints and fixed partial dentures'. *Quintessence International* 1998, **29**, 761–8.
24. Meiers JC and Freilich MA. Conservative anterior tooth replacement using fiber-reinforced composite. *Operative Dentistry* 2000, **25**, 239–43.
25. Meiers JC and Freilich MA. 'Chairside prefabricated fiber-reinforced composite fixed partial dentures'. *Quintessence International* 2001, **32**, 99–104.
26. Rosentritt M, Behr M, Lang R and Handel G. 'Experimental design of FPD made of all-ceramics and fibre-reinforced composite'. *Dental Materials* 2000, **16**, 159–65.
27. Mannocci F, Sheriff M, Watson TF and Vallittu PK. 'Penetration of bonding resins into fiber posts: a confocal microscopic study'. *Endodontic Journal* 2005, **38**, 46–51.
28. Fennis WMM, Tezvergil A, Kuijs RH, Lassila LVJ, Kreulen CM, Creugers NHJ and Vallittu PK. '*In vitro* fracture resistance of fiber reinforced cusp-replacing composite restorations'. *Dental Materials* 2005, **21**, 565–72.
29. Mannocci F, Ferrari M and Watson TF. 'Intermittent loading of teeth restored using quartz fiber, carbon-quartz fiber, and zirconium dioxide ceramic root canal posts'. *Journal of Adhesive Dentistry* 1999, **1**, 153–8.
30. Qualthrough AJ, Chandler NP and Purton DG. 'A comparison of the retention of tooth coloured posts'. *Quintessence International* 2003, **34**, 199–201.
31. Friskopp J and Blomlof L. 'Intermediate fibreglass splints'. *Journal of Prosthetic Dentistry* 1984, **51**, 334–7.
32. Sewón LA, Ampula L and Vallittu PK. 'Rehabilitation of a periodontal patient with rapidly progressing marginal alveolar bone loss. A case report'. *Journal of Clinical Periodontology* 2000, **27**, 615–19.
33. Kirzioglu Z and Erturk MS. 'Success of reinforced fiber material space maintainer'. *Journal of Dentistry for Children* 2004, **71**, 158–62.
34. Rantala LI, Lastumaki TM, Peltomaki T and Valliuttu PK. 'Fatigue resistance of removable orthodontic appliance reinforced with glass fibre weave'. *Journal of Oral Rehabilitation* 2003, **30**, 501–6.
35. Özcan M, van der Sleen JM, Kurunmäki H and Vallittu PK. 'Comparison of repair methods for ceramic-fused-to-metal crowns'. *Journal of Prosthodontics* 2006, **15**, 283–8.
36. Vallittu PK. 'Use of woven glass fibres to reinforce a composite veneer. A fracture resistance and acoustic emission study'. *Journal of Oral Rehabilitation* 2002, **29**, 423–9.
37. Quek SY. 'Value-based dentistry: Will it provide the best care for our patients' needs'. *Quintessence International* 2011, **42**, 363.
38. Murphy J. *The Reinforced Plastics Handbook*, Elsevier Advanced Technology, 1998, Oxford, UK, 11–26.
39. Rosen MR. 'From treating solution to filler surface and beyond. The life history of a silane coupling agent'. *Journal of Coating Technology* 1978, **50**, 70–82.
40. Matinlinna JP, Areva S, Lassila LVJ and Vallittu PK. 'Characterization of siloxane films on titanium substrate derived from three aminosilanes'. *Surface and Interfacial Analysis* 2004, **36**, 1314–22.

41. Vallittu PK. 'Comparison of two different silane compounds used for improving adhesion between fibers and acrylic denture base material'. *Journal of Oral Rehabilitation* 1993, **20**, 533–9.
42. Norström A, Watson H, Engström B and Rosenholm J. 'Treatment of E-glass fibres with acid, base and silanes'. *Colloids and Surfaces* 2001, **194**, 143–57.
43. Schreiber CK. 'Polymethylmethacrylate reinforced with carbon fibres'. *British Dental Journal* 1971, **130**, 29–30.
44. Chow TW, Ladizesky NH and Clarke DA. 'Acrylic resins reinforced with woven highly drawn linear polyethylene fibres. 2. Water sorption and clinical trials'. *Australian Dental Journal* 1992, **25**, 214–17.
45. Gutteridge DL. 'The effect of including ultra-high-modulus polyethylene fibre on the impact strength of acrylic resin'. *British. Dental Journal* 1988, **164**, 177–80.
46. Gutteridge DL. 'Reinforcement of poly(methylmethacrylate) with ultra-high-modulus polyethene fibre'. *Journal of Dentistry* 1992, **20**, 50–4.
47. Braden M, Davy KWM, Parker S, Ladizesky NH and Ward IM. 'Denture base poly(methylmethacrylate) reinforced with ultrahigh-modulus polyethylene fibres'. *British Dental Journal* 1998, **164**, 109–13.
48. Vallittu PK. 'Ultra-high-modulus polyethylene ribbon as reinforcement for denture polymethyl methcarylate. A short communication'. *Dental Materials* 1997, **13**, 381–2.
49. Takagi K, Fujimatsu H, Usami H and Ogasawara S. 'Adhesion between high strength and high modulus polyethylene fibers by use of polyethylene gel as an adhesive'. *Journal of Adhesion Science Technology* 1996, **9**, 869–82.
50. Tanner J, Vallittu PK and Söderling E. 'Adherence of Streptococcus mutans to an E-glass fiber-reinforced composite and conventional restorative materials used in prosthetic dentistry'. *Journal of Biomedical Materials Research* 2000, **49**, 250–6.
51. Tanner J, Vallittu PK and Söderling E. 'Effect of water storage of E-glass fiber-reinforced composite on adhesion of Streptococcus mutans'. *Biomaterials* 2001, **22**, 1613–18.
52. Tanner J, Carlén A, Söderling E and Vallittu PK. 'Adsorption of parotid saliva proteins and adhesion of *Streptococcus mutans* ATCC 21752 to dental fiber-reinforced composites'. *Journal of Biomedical Materials Research* 2003, **15**, 391–8.
53. Vallittu PK. 'The effect of void space and polymerisation time on transverse strength of acrylic-glass fiber composite'. *Journal of Oral Rehabilitation* 1995, **22**, 257–61.
54. Vallittu PK. 'Impregnation of glass fibers with polymethylmethacrylate using powder-coating method'. *Applied Composite Materials* 1995, **2**, 51–8.
55. Vallittu PK. 'Some aspects of the tensile strength of unidirectional glass fiber-polymethyl methacrylate composite used in dentures'. *Journal of Oral Rehabilitation* 1998, **25**, 100–5.
56. Goldberg AJ, Burstone CJ, Hadjinikolaou I and Jancar J. 'Screening of matrices and fibers for reinforced thermoplastics intended for dental applications'. *Journal of Biomedical Materials Research* 1994, **28**, 167–73.
57. Sperling LH. 'Over view of IPNs. Interpenetrating polymer networks'. *Advances in Chemistry Series*, 239, Klempner D, Sperling LH, Utracti LA (eds), American Chemical Society, Washington, DC 1994, 4–6.

58. Kallio TT, Lastumäki TM and Vallittu PK. 'Bonding of restorative and veneering composite resin to some polymeric composites'. *Dental Materials* 2001, **17**, 80–6.
59. Lastumäki T, Lassila LVJ and Vallittu PK. 'The semi-interpenetrating polymer network matrix of fiber-reinforced composite and its effect on the surface adhesive properties'. *Journal of Materials Science Materials in Medicine* 2003, **14**, 803–9.
60. Vallittu PK. 'Interpenetrating polymer networks (IPNs) in dental polymers and composites'. *Journal of Adhesion Science and Technology* 2009, **23**, 961–72.
61. Lassila LVJ, Tanner J, LeBell A-M, Narva K and Vallittu PK. 'Flexural properties of fiber reinforced root canal posts'. *Dental Materials* 2004, **20**, 29–36.
62. Lassila LVJ, Nohrström T and Vallittu PK. 'The influence of short-term water storage on the flexural properties of unidirectional glass fiber–reinforced composite'. *Biomaterials* 2002, **23**, 2221–9.
63. Bouillaguet S, Schutt A, Alander P, Vallittu PK, Schwaller P, Buerki G, Michler J, Cattani-Lorente M and Krejci I. 'Influence of hydrothermal and mechanical stress to interfacial bond strength glass fibers to polymer matrix'. *Journal of Biomedical Materials Research, Part B*, 2006, **76**, 98–105.
64. LeBell A-M, Tanner J, Lassila LVJ, Kangasniemi I and Vallittu PK. 'Bonding of composite resin luting cement to fibre-reinforced composite root canal post'. *Journal of Adhesive Dentistry* 2004, **6**, 319–25.
65. Vallittu PK, Ruyter IE and Ekstrand K. 'Effect of water storage on the flexural properties of E-glass and silica fiber acrylic resin composite'. *International Journal of Prosthodontics* 1998, **11**, 340–50.
66. Vallittu PK. 'Effect of 180 weeks water storage on the flexural properties of E-glass and silica fiber acrylic resin composite'. *International Journal of Prosthodontics* 2000, **13**, 334–9.
67. Krenchel H. *Fibre Reinforcement.* Thesis, Technical University of Denmark, Copenhagen, 1963.
68. Tezvergil A, Lassila LVJ and Vallittu PK. 'The effect of fiber orientation on the thermal expansion coefficients of the fiber reinforced composites'. *Dental Materials* 2003, **19**, 471–7.
69. Vallittu PK. 'The effect of glass fiber reinforcement on the fracture resistance of a provisional fixed partial denture'. *Journal of Prosthetic Dentistry* 1998, **79**, 125–30.
70. Alander P, Lassila LVJ and Vallittu PK. 'The span length and cross-sectional design affect values of strength'. *Dental Materials* 2005, **21**, 347–53.
71. Vallittu PK and Ruyter IE. 'The swelling phenomenon of acrylic polymer teeth and the interface with the denture base polymers'. *Journal of Prosthetic Dentistry* 1997, **78**, 194–9.
72. Vallittu PK and Ruyter IE. 'Swelling of polymethyl(methacrylate) resin at the repair joint'. *International Journal of Prosthodontics* 1997, **10**, 254–8.
73. Vallittu PK. 'Oxygen inhibition of autopolymerization of polymethylmethacrylate-glass fiber composite'. *Journal of Materials Science Materials in Medicine* 1997, **8**, 489–92.
74. Vallittu PK. 'Flexural properties of acrylic polymers reinforced with unidirectional and woven glass fibers'. *Journal of Prosthetic Dentistry* 1999, **81**, 318–26.

75. Narva K, Vallittu PK and Yli-Urpo A. 'Clinical survey of acrylic resin removable denture repairs with glass-fiber reinforcement'. *International Journal of Prosthodontics* 2001, **14**, 219–24.
76. Narva K. *Fibre-Reinforced Denture Base Polymers. Clinical Performance and Mechanical Properties.* Thesis, Annales Universitatis Turkuensis, University of Turku, 2004.
77. Narva KK, Lassila LVJ and Vallittu PK. 'The static strength and modulus of fiber reinforced denture base polymers'. *Dental Materials* 2005, **21**, 421–8.
78. Narva KK, Lassila LVJ and Vallittu PK. 'Flexural fatigue of denture base polymer with fiber-reinforced composite reinforcement'. *Composites, Part A* 2005, **36**, 1275–81.
79. Waltimo T, Luo G, Samaranayake LP and Vallittu PK. 'Glass fibre-reinforced composite laced with chlorhexidine digluconate and yeast adhesion'. *Journal of Materials Science Materials Medicine* 2004, **15**, 117–21.
80. Kangasniemi I, Vallittu PK, Meiers J, Dyer SR and Rosentritt M. 'Consensus statement on fiber-reinforced polymers: Current status, future directions, and how they can be used to enhance dental care'. *International Journal of Prosthodontics* 2003, **16**, 209.
81. Vallittu PK and Sevelius C. 'Resin-bonded, glass fiber reinforced composite fixed partial dentures–A clinical study'. *Journal of Prosthetic Dentistry* 2000, **84**, 413–18.
82. Behr M, Rosentritt M, Lang E, Chazot C and Handel G. 'Glass-fibre-reinforced composite fixed partial dentures on dental implants'. *Journal of Oral Rehabilitation* 2001, **28**, 895–902.
83. Bergendal T, Ekstrand K and Karlsson U. 'Evaluation of implant-supported carbon/graphite fiber-reinforced poly(methyl methacrylate) prostheses. A longitudinal multicenter study'. *Clinical Oral Implant Research* 1995, **6**, 246–53.
84. Ekstrand K, Ruyter IE and Wellendorf H. 'Carbon/graphite fiber reinforced polymethyl(methacrylate): properties under dry and wet conditions'. *Journal of Biomedical Materials Research* 1987, **21,** 1065–80.
85. Tezvergil A, Lassila LVJ and Vallittu PK. 'Strength of adhesive-bonded fiber-reinforced composites to enamel and dentine substrates'. *Journal of Adhesive Dentistry* 2003, **5**, 301–11.
86. Tezvergil A, Lassila LVJ and Vallittu PK. 'The shear bond strength of bidirectional and random-oriented fibre-reinforced composite to tooth structure'. *Journal of Dentistry* 2005, **33**, 509–16.
87. Nohrström TJ, Vallittu PK and Yli-Urpo A. 'The effect of position and quantity of glass fibers on the fracture resistance of provisional fixed partial denture'. *International Journal of Prosthodontics* 2000, **13**, 72–8.
88. Dyer SC, Lassila LVJ LVJ and Vallittu PK. 'The effect of internal fiber arrangement on the delamination failure in hybrid composite dental prostheses'. *Journal of Physical Mesomechanics* 2004, **7**, 119–22.
89. Dyer SR, Lassila LVJ, Jokinen M and Vallittu PK. 'Effect of fiber position and orientation on fracture load of fiber-reinforced composite'. *Dental Materials* 2004, **20**, 947–55.
90. Shinya A, Yokoyama D, Lassila LV, Shinya A and Vallittu PK. 'Three-dimensional finite element analysis of metal and FRC adhesive fixed dental prosthesis'. *Journal of Adhesive Dentistry* 2008, **10**(5), 365–71.

91. Dyer SR, Lassila LVJ, Alander P and Vallittu PK. 'Static strength of molar region direct technique glass-fibre-reinforced composite fixed partial denture'. *Journal of Oral Rehabilitation* 2005, **32**, 351–7.
92. Özcan M, Breuklander MH and Vallittu PK. 'Effect of slot preparation on the strength of glass fiber-reinforced composite inlay retained fixed partial dentures'. *Journal of Prosthetic Dentistry* 2005, **93**, 337–45.
93. Garoushi S, Lassila LVJ, Tezvergil A and Vallittu PK. 'Load bearing capacity of fibre-reinforced and particulate filler composite resin combination'. *Journal of Dentistry* 2006, **34**, 179–84.
94. Garoushi S, Lassila LVJ, Tezvergil A and Vallittu PK. 'Fiber-reinforced composite substructure: load bearing capacity of an onlay restoration and flexural properties of the material'. *Journal of Contemporary Dental Practice* 2006, **7**, 1–8.
95. Lastumäki T, Lassila L and Vallittu PK. 'Flexural properties of bulk fiber-reinforced composite DC-Tell used in fixed partial dentures'. *International Journal of Prosthodontics* 2001, **14**, 22–6.
96. Gegauff AG and Pryor HG. 'Fracture toughness of provisional resins for fixed prosthodontics'. *Journal of Prosthetic Dentistry* 1987, **58**, 23–9.
97. Osman YI and Owen CP. 'Flexural strength of provisional restorative materials'. *Journal of Prosthetic Dentistry* 1993, **70**, 94–6.
98. Chung KH, Ling T and Wang F. 'Flexural strength of a provisional resin material with fibre addition'. *Journal of Oral Rehabitation* 1998, **25**, 214–17.
99. Dixon DL, Fincher M, Breeding LC and Mueninghoff LA. 'Mechanical properties of a light polymerizing provisional restorative material with and without reinforcement fibers'. *Journal of Prosthetic Dentistry* 1995, **73**, 510–14.
100. Lahdenperä MS, Puska MA, Alander PM, Waltimo T and Vallittu PK. 'Release of chlorhexidine digluconate and flexural properties of glass fibre reinforced provisional fixed partial denture polymer'. *Journal of Materials Science Materials Medicine* 2004, **15**, 1349–53.
101. LeBell A-M, Lassila LVJ, Kangasniemi I and Vallittu PK. 'Bonding of fibre-reinforced composite post to root canal dentin'. *Journal of Dentistry* 2005, **33**, 533–9.
102. Le Bell-Rönnlöf AM, Lassila LV, Kangasniemi I and Vallittu PK. 'Load-bearing capacity of human incisor restored with various fiber-reinforced composite posts'. *Dental Materials* 2011, **27**, 107–15.
103. Nagase DY, Takemoto S, Hattori M, Yoshinari M, Kawada E and Oda Y. 'Influence of fabrication techniques on retention force of fiber-reinforced composite posts'. *Dental Materials Journal* 2005, **24**, 280–5.
104. Island G and White GE. 'Polyethylene ribbon fibers: a new alternative for restoring badly destroyed primary incisors'. *Journal of Clinical Pediatric Dentistry* 2005, **29**, 151–6.
105. Qualthrough AJ and Mannocci F. 'Tooth-colored post systems: a review'. *Operative Dentistry* 2003, **28**, 86–91.
106. Hatta M, Shinya A, Vallittu PK, Shinya A and Lassila LVJ. 'High volume individual fiber post versus low volume fiber post. The fracture load of the restored tooth'. *Journal of Dentistry* 2011, **39**, 65–71.
107. Butterworth C, Ellakwa AE and Shortall A. 'A fiber-reinforced composites in restorative dentistry'. *Dental Update* 2003, **30**, 300–6.

108. Van Dijken JWV and Sunnegård-Grönberg KS. 'Fiber-reinforced packable resin composite in class II cavities'. *Journal of Dentistry* 2006, **34**, 763–9.
109. Garoushi SK, Lassila LVJ and Vallittu PK. 'Short fiber reinforced composite: the effect of fiber length and volume fraction'. *Journal of Contemporary Dental Practice* 2006, **7**(5), 10–17.
110. Garoushi S, Vallittu PK and Lassila LVJ. 'Fracture resistance of short random oriented glass fiber reinforced composite premolar crown'. *Acta Biomaterials* 2007, **3**(5), 779–84.
111. Garoushi S, Lassila LVJ and Vallittu PK. 'Direct composite resin restoration of damaged incisors using short fiber-reinforced composite resin'. *Journal of Dentistry* 2007, **35**, 731–6.
112. Garoushi SK, Ballo AM, Lassila LVJ and Vallittu PK. 'Fracture resistance of fragmented incisal edges restored with fiber-reinforced composite'. *Journal of Adhesive Dentistry* 2006, **8**(2), 91–5.
113. Garoushi S, Lassila LVJ, Tezvergil A and Vallittu PK. 'Static and fatigue compression test for particulate filler composite resin with fiber-reinforced composite substructure'. *Dental Materials* 2007, **23**(1), 17–23.
114. Garoushi S, Lassila LVJ and Vallittu PK. 'Short glass fiber-reinforced composite with a semi-interpenetrating polymer network matrix for temporary crowns and bridges'. *Journal of Contemporary Dental Practice* 2008, **9**, 14–21.
115. Garoushi SK, Vallittu PK, Watts DC and Lassila LVJ. 'Polymerization shrinkage of experimental short glass fiber reinforced composite with semi-interpenetrating polymer network matrix'. *Dental Materials* 2008, **24**(2), 211–15.
116. Garoushi S, Vallittu PK and Lassila LVJ. 'Fracture toughness, compressive strength and load-bearing capacity of short glass fiber-reinforced composite resin'. *Chinese Journal of Dental Research* 2011, **14**, 1–5.
117. Garoushi S, Vallittu PK, Watts DC and Lassila LV. 'Effect of nanofiller fractions and temperature on polymerization shrinkage of glass fiber reinforced filling material'. *Dental Materials* 2008, **24**, 606–10.
118. Garoushi SK, Lassila LV and Vallittu PK. 'Direct composite resin restoration of an anterior tooth: Effect of fiber-reinforced composite substructure'. *European Journal of Prosthodontics and Restorative Dentistry* 2007, **15**(2), 61–6.
119. Garoushi S, Vallittu PK and Lassila LVJ. 'Depth of cure and surface microhardness of experimental short fiber-reinforced composite'. *Acta Odontologica Scandinavica* 2008, **66**, 38–42.
120. Peltola M, Vallittu PK, Vuorinen V, Aho A, Puntala A and Aitasalo K. 'Novel composite implant in craniofacial bone reconstruction'. *European Archives Otorinolaryngology* 2011, **269**, 623–8.
121. Hautamäki M, Meretoja VV, Mattila PH, Aho AJ and Vallittu PK. 'Osteoblast response to polymethylmethacrylate–bioactive glass composite'. *Journal of Materials Science Materials in Medicine* 2010, **21**, 1685–92.
122. Zhao DS, Moritz N, Laurila P, Mattila R, Lassila LVJ, Strandberg N, Mäntylä T, Vallittu PK and Aro HT. 'Development of a biomechanically optimized multi-component fiber-reinforced composite implant for load-sharing conditions'. *Medical Engineering and Physics* 2009, **31**, 461–9.
123. Shinya A, Ballo AM, Lassila LVJ, Shinya A, Närhi T and Vallittu PK. 'Stress and strain analysis of bone-implant interface: comparison of fiber reinforced

composite and titanium implants utilizing 3D finite element study'. *Journal of Oral Implantology* 2011, **37**, 133–40.
124. Ballo AM, Akca EA, Ozen T, Lassila LVJ, Vallittu PK and Närhi TO. 'Bone tissue responses to glass fiber-reinforced composite implants – a histomorphometric study'. *Clinical Oral Implants Research* 2009, **20**, 608–15.
125. Tuusa SM-R, Peltola MJ, Tirri T, Röyttä M, Aho H, Lassila LVJ and Vallittu PK. 'Reconstruction of critical size calvarial bone defects in rabbits with glass-fiber-reinforced composite with bioactive glass granule coating'. *Journal of Biomedical Materials Research, Part B* 2008, **84**(2), 510–19.

13
Luting cements for dental applications

MUTLU ÖZCAN, University of Zurich, Switzerland

DOI: 10.1533/9780857096432.3.375

Abstract: This chapter reviews the functions and working mechanisms of different cement types used in dentistry and discusses the clinical implications and effects of cement choice on the longevity of dental restorations, depending on the type of restoration and the clinical situation. The chapter then provides information on future trends and mentions clinical concerns in cement choice.

Key words: dental prostheses, dental tissues, glass ionomer cements, luting cements, resin-based cements, water-based cements.

13.1 Introduction

The longevity of indirect fixed dental prostheses (FDP) could be affected by multiple factors including the cementation mode that is basically the final stage of consecutive clinical procedures. At the beginning of the 20th century, luting cement selection was not of concern since there were no other options except zinc phosphate cements.[1] In fact, today we still have the longest experience of this cement. Yet, with the introduction of the acid etching technique described by Buonocore in 1955,[2] to promote adhesion to enamel, and the development of dimethacrylate monomers by Bowen,[3] adhesive materials and techniques have developed faster. Zinc polycarboxylate cement was the first chemically adhesive material marketed in the 1960s and glass ionomer cements and dentine bonding agents have become available from then.[4] Following an increase in awareness of tissue saving treatment options, after the implementation of resin-based materials in dentistry, clinical situations requiring minimally invasive treatment approaches have spurred the development of resin luting cements.

In general, the primary function of cementation, be it conventional or adhesive, is to establish reliable retention, a durable seal of the space between the tooth or implant abutment and the restoration, and to provide adequate optical properties especially for tooth-coloured ceramic or polymeric FDPs.[4] However, several features other than reliable retention during function became desirable for an optimally functioning cement, such as antibacterial efficacy, inhibition of plaque accumulation and caries formation, low solubility, low wear, hypersensitivity, adhesion, radiopacity, low film thickness, easy excess removal and providing adequate optical properties especially for tooth-coloured ceramic or polymeric FDPs.[1,5,6]

Currently, an increasing number of cements are available for dental use with a continuously expanding range of new products and applications. From the chemical point of view, the available cements could still be classified in two groups, namely water-based cements basically including zinc phosphate and glass ionomer cements (GIC) and resin-based or polymerizing cements consisting of resin modified glass ionomers (RMGI) and conventional composite and self-adhesive cements.[5]

13.2 Classification of cements

13.2.1 Water-based cements

Water-based cements have so far exhibited satisfying long-term clinical performance with cast metal inlays, onlays, partial crowns as well as single unit metal–ceramic and multiple unit FDPs with macroretentive preparation designs and adequate marginal fit.[5]

From water-based cements, zinc phosphate cement has been used for over a century to seal and retain metal, metal–ceramic and feldspathic porcelain jacket crowns successfully.[1] Zinc phosphate cement has served for decades as the universal cement for different applications in restorative dentistry relying on the retention and resistance form of the tooth preparation and an adequate marginal fit.[5] Because of its long history of successful clinical use with cast and metal–ceramic restorations, zinc phosphate cement is considered to be the 'reference' or 'gold standard'.[6]

The zinc phosphate cement sets by an acid–base reaction initiated on mixing a powder composed of 90% ZnO and 10% MgO with a liquid that consists of approximately 67% phosphoric acid buffered with aluminium and zinc.[7] The water content (33%) is significant because it controls the ionization of the acid, which in turn influences the rate of the setting reaction.[8] This is important for the clinician because an uncapped liquid bottle will permit loss of water resulting in a retarded set. Water evaporation should be suspected if the liquid appears cloudy on dispensing.[9] The setting reaction of a zinc phosphate cement is mainly due to the reaction between orthophosphoric acid and zinc oxide.[10] Aluminium phosphate delays the setting reaction of the cement and increases the hardness of the cement.[10]

This cement does not chemically bond to any substrate and provides only a mechanical retentive seal.[1,11] Thus, the taper, length and surface area of the tooth preparation are critical for its success.[7,8] Macromechanical retention is mainly determined by the geometrical configuration of the tooth preparation. The smaller the convergence angle, the larger the height and the larger the surface area of the prepared tooth, the higher the macromechanical retention will be. Retentive guiding grooves may also considerably increase the degree of retention. These characteristics are important to prevent the displacement of the crowns, affected by several factors such as hyperbalancing contacts during articulation, high occlusal forces and/or parafunctional habits and bruxism, and so on.[12]

Permanent luting cements should possess a maximum film thickness of 25 μm, a compressive strength of 68.7 MPa and maximum water solubility of 0.2% (ADA Specification No. 8). In general, when compared to other luting materials, zinc phosphate cement presents high compressive, low film thickness (18 μm), low tensile strength and is inexpensive per unit dose.[13] Being a rather stiff material, it might be an appropriate luting cement option for especially long-span FDPs. The compressive strengths of zinc phosphate cements range from 80–110 MPa and it has been reported that zinc phosphate cement exhibited no change in compressive strength over two years of ageing.[8,14]

The solubility and disintegration behaviour of luting cements that relate to the long-term loss of seal between the abutment and the prosthesis are important factors that determine the clinical longevity of FDPs and posts.[15] Zinc phosphate cements present continuous erosion in distilled water,[16] yet their solubility has been considered clinically acceptable.[13] However, when compared with GIC, RMGI and resin cements, zinc phosphate cement, under *in vivo* conditions has been demonstrated to disintegrate the most.[15,17]

In terms of temperature effects on pulp, zinc phosphate cement exhibits the highest temperature rise during setting reaction especially with an increasing powder or liquid ratio (10.92–13.80°C), whereas GIC exhibits the lowest rise (1.82–2.75°C).[7]

Zinc phosphate sets by an acid–base reaction and its physical properties are sensitive to several mixing variables such as the powder–liquid ratio, water content and mixing temperature.[1] The mixing technique is critical for an optimum outcome and should be completed on a cool slab, over a wide area, to incorporate small increments of powder into the liquid for approximately 1 min and 30 s.[1,7,8] When mixing a zinc phosphate cement, the powder and the liquid should be dispensed as recommended by the manufacturer, preferably on a cool but dry glass slab (frozen slab technique) to control the working and setting times and the powder should be incorporated slowly into the liquid over a large area of the slab for approximately 2 min. This procedure facilitates maximal powder incorporation while keeping the viscosity low enough for the material to flow sufficiently to allow the restoration to set fully. The cool slab technique also presents improved physical properties such as increased compressive strength, decreased solubility, controlled film thickness and decreased possibility of pulpal damage by maintaining low temperature changes in the cement as long as the powder–liquid ratio is adjusted to maintain a proper consistency.[18]

When the mixing ratio of the zinc phosphate cement is increased from 2.3–2.4 g ml^{-1}, the number of powder agglomerates formed increases, leading to a higher strength.[19] Reducing the powder–liquid ratio of a zinc phosphate cement adversely affects its physical properties, such as retention.[20,21] The initial set occurs about 5–9 min after mixing (ADA Specification No. 8) and the clinician should not hasten to remove excess cement for at least several minutes after the initial hardening to reduce the risk of saliva contact since the material is very soluble in the non-matured state.[1,18]

It is generally recommended that the smear layer should be left intact and it is advisable to apply two layers of copal varnish or resin sealer after tooth cleaning before cement application to help reduce the potential negative effect of low pH and high setting temperature on the vital pulp after mixing (pH = 2.14 after 2 min to pH = 5.5 after 24 h).[1,13,22]

Despite several disadvantages of zinc phosphate cement, conventional luting of metal-based restorations using this cement has been clinically proven.[23] In a retrospective clinical study, a total of 73 patients who were delivered 102 four-unit FDPs cemented with zinc phosphate were followed-up for up to 20 years, with a mean survival follow-up time of 11.4 years.[20] The survival rate was 68.3% at year 20 and the main reason for irreversible failure was caries (32%). In another previous clinical study over a period of 10 years, zinc phosphate and RMGI cements were used for luting 39 pairs of metal–ceramic and all-ceramic crowns on 20 patients in a split-mouth randomized design blind to the recipient.[24] Clinical data were scored according to Californian Dental Association Criteria, Sillness and Löe criteria, patient satisfaction and operator-driven general clinical criteria. The statistical analyses revealed that there were no significant differences between either cement types used to retain single crowns over a follow-up time of 102-months.[24] The clinical performance of zinc phosphate on retaining metal-based restorations over an 38-month observation period has also been found to be comparable to a self-adhesive resin cement.[25]

Glass ionomer cements (GIC) were introduced to the profession about 40 years ago and have been shown to be a very beneficial restorative agent for dentistry.[60] They were formulated in 1969 by Wilson and Kent, at the Laboratory of the Government Chemist in England and production of first high fluoride GIC followed in 1972, originally called alumino-silicate polyacrylic acid (ASPA) because it was formed by the combination of silicate cements and polycarboxylate cements.[60] GICs were marketed for use as luting agents in 1976 and by the late 1990s, they had become the most frequently used definitive luting agents worldwide.[26,28] The goal was to produce a hybrid material that released fluoride and at the same time adhered to both enamel and dentin.[27–31] Dentin is a water-containing tissue that commonly has a film of odontoblastic tubular fluid on the cut surface. Since GIC is water-based, this cement is compatible with dentin.[4] GIC cements offer good strength and optical properties with the potential for fluoride release or recharge. However, they are sensitive to moisture or dehydration at an early setting stage and take time to set fully.

GIC were first introduced as cavity-lining materials and thereafter used as luting agents, primarily indicated for luting metal and metal–ceramic restorations although they could be used with all-ceramic crowns with high-strength cores such as alumina or zirconia.[29,32] The setting reaction for the GIC is an acid–base reaction and the cement sets by a reaction initiated on mixing a powder with a liquid solution.[22] The setting time of GIC is approximately 7 min with a film thickness of 25 μm, a compressive strength of 86 MPa, a tensile strength of 7 MPa and a solubility of 1.25% which is higher in the first 24 h.[26,29]

The powder (base) is composed of calcium, strontium and fluoride-containing aluminosilicate glass and the aqueous solution (acid) consists of copolymers of relatively weak water-soluble polyalkenoic acids, including itaconic, maleic and tricarboxylic, to form a hydrogel matrix.[1,7,26,30,31] Water is the most essential component present in the cement liquid. When the components are mixed together, a setting reaction occurs involving neutralization of the acid groups by the powdered solid glass base.[29,30] The acid attacks the glass, resulting in surface degradation of the glass and release of metal ions (e.g. strontium, calcium, aluminium), fluoride ions and silicic acid. The metal ions react with the carboxyl (COO-) groups to form a poly-acid salt, which becomes the cement matrix and the surface of the glass becomes a silica hydrogel. The unreacted cores of the glass particles remain as fillers. Although the clinical setting is completed within a few minutes, a continuing 'maturation' phase occurs over the subsequent month.[4,29,30]

There are several types of poly(alkenoic) acids available that undergo this reaction and the glass powder may also vary.[22] Further improvements have been achieved by the inclusion of more reactive polyacids (e.g. copolymers of acrylic and maleic acid), through pretreatment of the glass surfaces and with modified glass compositions. Radiopaque cements have also become available by addition of elements like pigments, silver alloy, lanthanum or strontium to the glass formulation.[28,32]

A convenient classification of GICs is based on their clinical application. Although the chemistry is essentially the same for all categories, there are variations in the powder–liquid ratio and powder particle size to accommodate the desired function.[4,26,29] Type I GIC luting cement has a fine powder particle size and the main advantages for its use as a luting cement include its thixotropic flow properties and resultant fine ultimate film thickness. There is also a small but positive fluoride flow which may be an advantage in the presence of a high caries rate. It also has a low solubility and an acceptable wear rate.[22]

GICs possess certain unique properties that make them useful as both restorative and adhesive materials, including adhesive bonding to enamel and dentin, release of fluoride ions over a prolonged period of time, anti-cariogenic properties from the release of fluoride, thermal compatibility with enamel, low shrinkage and biocompatibility. Besides these advantages, conventional GICs suffer from disadvantages such as short working times and relatively long setting times, brittleness, inherent opacity, low fracture toughness, poor resistance to wear and sensitivity to moisture contamination or dehydration during the early stages of the setting reaction.[22,26,31,33] Their biological compatibility have been well proven[28] and they are often known as biomimetic materials, because of their similar mechanical properties to dentin.[30] Thus, they are useful in situations where they are not disadvantageous by their comparatively lower physical properties, such as where there is adequate remaining tooth structure to support the material and where they are not subjected to heavy occlusal loading.[28,30]

Depending on the manufacturer, usually1.5 g of GIC powder is mixed with 1 ml of liquid. The setting reaction is mildly exothermic. Moreover, exposure to saliva, blood or water should be avoided, ideally for 7 to 10 min after mixing to prevent loss of cement at the restoration margin.[1] The powder–liquid ratio is important and varies in different products. A reduction in the powder–liquid ratio might result in poor physical properties. One great disadvantage of GICs for this purpose is the difficulty of varying the working time. If the material is mixed on a chilled glass slab, the time may be extended by about 25% but this may still present difficulties when cementing a full-arch prosthesis.[22]

GICs are self-adhesive and only require removal of the smear layer by pretreatment with a solution of polyacrylic acid.[30] However, they can bond to dentin surfaces even without the removal of the smear layer.[29] The application of a 10% solution of polyacrylic acid for approximately 10 s dissolves the smear layer and other contaminants leaving the dentin tubules relatively closed, yet the remaining surface clean. This will also alter the surface energy of the tooth structure sufficiently to facilitate the adaptation of the cement and ensure optimum placement of the restoration.[22]

The protection of the crown margins from water loss and water uptake in the first 24 h after luting with a GIC is of crucial importance.[4] Various materials have been used, including copal varnish and photopolymerized bonding resins, to overcome this problem. However, this is often impossible in the interproximal areas.[23,31] The sealing capacity of zinc phosphate cement was categorized as most favourable when compared with a GIC in an *in vitro* study.[34] These findings are in compliance with the results of an *in vivo* study where a higher solubility of GIC was detected compared with a zinc phosphate cement. Moreover, the bond strength to dentin in water had been shown to decrease depending on the exposure time to water: 1.5 MPa after 15 min, 2.67 MPa after 1 h, 1.1 MPa after 24 h, 5.2 MPa after 7 days and 3.6 MPa after 56 days.[35]

The bonding mechanism of the conventional GIC is very complex, but consists of initially wetting of the tooth surface with free polyacrylic acid, followed by ionic bonding between the carboxyl group in the cement liquid and calcium ions in the tooth structure.[30] Simply, an ionic bond occurs between the carboxyl (COO–) ions in the cement acid and the calcium (Ca^{2+}) ions in enamel and dentin.[4] It is essential, however, that the acid–base reaction remains dominant since the powder becomes bound to the matrix and the matrix, in turn, adheres to the tooth structure underneath throughout this reaction.[22] This effective bonding was reported earlier after long observation periods of conventional GICs in non-carious cervical retention, in the order of 90% after ten years.[36]

The fluoride-releasing properties of GICs are probably one of their greatest assets. It is assumed that GICs have a caries-inhibitory effect owing to their long-term and sustained fluoride release. Nevertheless, the cement has the capacity to take up more fluoride from the ambient environment, depending on the concentration gradient.[31] GIC releases fluoride, at high rates initially, and then decreasing after a few days to a consistent low level for many years. Because of this characteristic, GICs have a low incidence of adjacent secondary caries and high potential for remineralization.[30,37] Fluoride ions form fluorapatite in or on the tooth surface which is more resistant to acid attack and therefore inhibits demineralization.[30,37] Fluoride release from conventional GICs and RMGIC cements was evaluated in an *in vitro* study and the results showed that higher amounts of fluoride were released during the first days after cementation and this process stabilized after ten days.[38] Fluoride incorporation to the enamel was greater in the superficial layers of this tissue while the fluoride release behaviour was similar for all ionomer-based materials.[38]

In another *in vitro* study, a conventional GIC (Fuji IX GP, Japan) was compared to a GIC that was the same except that it incorporated 8 %wt hydroxyapatite in the powder to increase the mechanical strength. The highest fluoride release was recorded during the first 24 h, gradually decreasing until the 91st day in both GIC materials.[39] Forsten studied the fluoride release ability of GICs after they had been exposed to running water for 18 months and after they were treated with a 50 ppm fluoride solution. It was observed that after this treatment the specimens released more than twice the amount of fluoride than before treatment.[37]

The constant release of fluoride is assumed to be quite low level. In order to maintain the effect of constant release it is desirable to use a fluoride-releasing material that can be 'recharged' from external fluoride sources and the long-term release was shown to remain on the same level during a study period exceeding eight years.[37] Topical applications will increase the ambient level for short periods and promote a satisfactory uptake into tooth surfaces.[22]

A negative aspect of GICs relates to the occurrence of tooth sensitivity. It is assumed to be associated with the low pH after mixing (pH = 2.33 after 2 min, to pH = 5.67 after 24 h).[21,35] In order to avoid post-delivery sensitivity, it is recommended that the substrate tooth be carefully cleaned to maintain the smear layer and the tooth surface be dry but not dehydrated.[1]

According to the type of restoration, the placement of fired ceramic inlays with water-based cements have been shown to increase the fracture rate more than twice, thus this cementation mode cannot be recommended for predictable long-term restorations.[5] On the other hand, the high flexural strength and fracture toughness as well as the better fit of new all-ceramic systems including high-strength core materials allow for the use of water-based cements if their retention is primarily based on macromechanical retention.[5] Also, their bond strength to oxide based ceramics (i.e. zirconia) compared to resin cements is very low.[40]

13.2.2 Resin-based cements

Resin-modified glass ionomer cements

Polymerizing cements are considered in general as better alternatives not only to bonded indirect FDPs but also for all types of restorations, as improved retention as well as a better seal of the margins can be established.

The adhesive bonding of restorations using a resin-based cement allowed new types of materials to be used for tooth-coloured and/or tooth-preserving restorations (i.e. all-ceramic veneers and crowns, resin composite inlays, onlays, surface-retained or inlay-retained resin-bonded FDPs). The bond strength between dentin and resin cement was reported to be significantly higher than water-based cements.[25] RMGI cements, conventional resin and self-adhesive resin cements have all been developed in parallel with the development of new generation ceramics and minimally invasive adhesive techniques.

Among resin-based cements, RMGI cements are hybrid, dual-phase materials with similar manipulative properties to GICs but they set quicker and are stronger.[1,6] Despite all the improvements, moisture sensitivity, low physical properties, particularly their early mechanical strength, and the lack of controlled polymerization period problems still remained for GICs. In order to eliminate these problems, attempts have been made to combine GI chemistry with the well-known chemistry of composite resins.[1,27,33] In the late 1980s and early 1990s several 'photopolymerized' GICs were released onto the market. This cement was designed to produce favourable physical properties similar to those of resin composites while maintaining the basic features of a conventional GIC.[26]

After mixing, two types of reactions occur: the resin phase polymerizes quickly either by chemical or photoinitiation and the glass ionomer phase proceeds slowly towards normal maturation via an acid–base reaction over an extended period of time. During the setting reaction, polyacrylic acid protons liberate metal ions and fluoride from the glass, forming a silica hydrogel around the glass surface. The rising aqueous phase pH causes polysalt precipitates to form from the migrating ions, which act as cross-links to the polyacrylic acid chains. Setting times approximate to several minutes, although further maturation occurs over extended times. Conversely, the resin reaction rate is much faster, although complex, photoinitiated polymerization eventually results in a diffusion-controlled, polymer chain propagation as the concentration and mobility of monomer decrease amid the formation of the cross-linked matrix network and the final degree of conversion is dependent upon monomer mobility and diffusion.[41]

RMGIC cements have some advantages over conventional GICs, namely longer working time, controlled setting on application of the relevant light source, aesthetics closer to resin-based materials and the tooth, better strength characteristics, improved bond strength, reduced superficial degradation and increased wear resistance. However, RMGI cements suffered from certain drawbacks such as setting shrinkage, limited depth of cure especially with more opaque lining cements, dimensional change owing to water uptake of the resin phase and surface porosity.[26,28]

The RMGI cements present a mean compressive strength of 105 MPa, tensile strength of 20 MPa, low solubility and 40 HN hardness.[35] The film thickness has been reported to be under 30 μm (~25 μm) 2 min after mixing which is similar to GICs and self-adhesive resin cements and clinically accepted according to ISO Standard 9917, with the reference value being 25 μm.[42] RMGI cements have been demonstrated to present similar marginal gaps (~75 μm) compared to zinc phosphate cement and conventional GIC after luting.[43] Because the RMGI cements are mechanically stronger than GICs, they can be used as cements for restorations with moderate occlusal load-bearing areas.[22]

The fundamental acid–base polymerization reaction in RMGI materials is supplemented by a second curing process, which is initiated by photo or chemical curing. These products are considered to be 'dual-polymerized'.[26]

RMGI cements are defined as hybrid materials that retain a significant acid–base reaction as part of their overall curing process, as well as a photo- and/or chemical-initiated free-radical resin polymerization reaction. The fundamental acid–base curing reaction takes place by a second polymerization reaction. This latter process may be initiated by light, as in the photo-polymerized RMGICs which have the ability to set without light activation, although more slowly.[31]

In general, the powder of RMGI cements is similar to that in GICs. Addition of a small quantity of a resin such as hydroxyethyl methacrylate (HEMA) or bisphenol A glycidyl methacrylate (bis-GMA) in the liquid, water and a polyacid with or without pendent methacrylate groups in the powder creates the difference. More complex materials have been developed by modifying the polyacid with side chains that can be polymerized by a light-curing mechanism. They remain GICs by their ability to set without light activation, although this reaction takes place more slowly than for the traditional cements.[26,30] However, they are subjected to water uptake to some extent as a result of HEMA present in the formula and the wear factor is likely to be a little higher. As noted above, it is not essential to seal the restoration because only then it is immediately resistant to water uptake.[22]

The presence of HEMA has been demonstrated to slow the acid–base reaction in resin-modified materials.[44] In practice, the polymerization of HEMA contributes significantly to the strength of the set material. However, HEMA has been shown to have the potential to be systemically distributed from its location in the mouth and to be the source of adverse effects such as contact dermatitis and other immunological responses in patients and dental personnel. Since HEMA is volatile, there also exists a risk of inhalation of HEMA vapour. The biocompatibility of RMGI cements in dentistry, therefore has been considered not really biocompatible to nearly the same extent as conventional GICs as the monomer HEMA is responsible for this lack of biocompatibility.[44] However, a long-term clinical study of 13 years with RMGI cement restorations, revealed that in spite of the existing information about post-operative sensitivity, this aspect does not seem to be a concern with RMGI cements, with their limited histopathology of the pulp.[30]

The fluoride release profile of RMGI cement has been shown to be comparable to GIC,[46] being higher in the initial 24 h and then decreasing to constant levels after 14 days.[38] A systematic review also revealed that RMGI cements were able to promote a great reduction in demineralization in adjacent hard tooth tissues.[45] This fluoride can be taken up easily or recharged and subsequently released very rapidly, similar to the GICs. This mechanism of fluoride release was also described in an earlier report and suggested to be due to the fluoride being present in a very soluble form that has little or no interaction with the matrix.[48] Once the glass ionomer has set, the fluoride released by the set cement may originate from: (i) the remaining and not yet attacked leachable fluoride glass; (ii) the silica gel phase resulting from the acid–base reaction and covering the glass particles; (iii) the polysalt matrix where fluoride ions can be bound in strong complexes with the metal ions, especially aluminium and (iv) the pore liquid in which the fluoride ions are only loosely bound and free to move.[41,46,47]

An *in vitro* study demonstrated that cast crowns cemented with RMGI and resin cements had lower microleakage scores than zinc phosphate cement.[43] Confirming these results, a clinical study where metal–ceramic and Procera crowns luted with a RMGI cement or a zinc phosphate cement were observed over a period of 10 years and a low risk of clinical failure was recorded.[24] A 13-year clinical study with RMGIC restorations, revealed that the retention for RMGI cements was generally good, with an annual failure rate reported as being under 3%.[49] However, this study also concluded that the RMGI cements exhibited some loss of anatomic form and surface wear, particularly in the mid- to long-term. These findings might reveal that RMGI cements might work better for cementation purposes while they present weak mechanical properties when they are exposed to the oral environment for direct restoratives. Although RMGI cements used for paediatric restorative dentistry seem to be a better option when prolonged use of deciduous teeth is essential for space reservation, their possible immunological response stemming from HEMA content should also be considered.

Conventional resin-based cements

Methyl methyacrylate-based conventional resin luting cements appeared in the early 1950s and were chemically comparable to direct the acrylic filling materials of the time. As such, they did not adhere to tooth structure, underwent considerable polymerization shrinkage, had a relatively high coefficient of thermal expansion and absorbed water that contributed to microleakage at the tooth-resin interface.[6] Modern resin cements are a huge part of today's dental product market owing to their versatility, high compressive and tensile strengths, low solubility and very favourable aesthetic qualities. Their major shortcomings are difficulty of excess removal, technique sensitivity, difficulty of removal of the restoration and their high costs.[5] Many manufacturers have added fluoride in order to claim anticariogenic properties and to be competitive with GICs. The value of added fluoride to resin has not been fully determined at this time and it has been suggested that when fluoride toothpaste is used, the anticariogenic potential of a luting agent to reduce secondary caries may not be relevant.[8]

Although many improvements have been made to the GIC, the chemistry is basically different from that of current resin-based composite direct filling materials where a silica or glass particle-filled polymer matrix improves retention of the restoration. If the tooth is etched and conditioned with an adhesive resin and the restoration is etched or air-abraded, retention becomes 'micromechanical' which guarantees high tensile strength of the resin cement.[50]

Resin luting agents are primarily indicated for clinical situations where restorations lack retention and resistance form (such as short or tapered crowns, resin-bonded FDPs) and post-cementation in endodontically treated teeth.[5] Resin cements are categorized in three groups based on their polymerization mechanism: (i) chemically polymerized, (ii) photo- and (iii) dual-polymerized. The dual-polymerized resin cements should be used cautiously for luting veneers because they may discolour with time owing to their aromatic amine content.[5]

All-ceramic crowns, inlays and onlays made of glassy matrix ceramics present increased flexural strength after they are etched with hydrofluoric acid, silanized and cemented with a resin cement. *In vitro* and clinical studies indicated that microcrack propagation in glass ceramics could be avoided when cemented adhesively by resin cements.[51] Excess removal of these types of cement is usually performed after 2–5 s of spot curing and restorations are further polymerized after initial clean-up. Care must be taken during the initial bulk removal of excess resin cement to insure that the resin cement is not pulled from under the restoration margin, creating a gap or void.

Adhesion of resin cements has two features, one affecting the dental tissues and the other affecting the restorative material. Both substrates need adequate surface conditioning. Therefore, the adhesive properties of resin cements are generally dictated by the adhesive systems used to condition the dental tissues.[52] Until recently, resin cements were divided into three sub-groups according to the adhesive system used to prepare the tooth prior to cementation. The so-called chemical- or photopolymerized conventional resin-based cements often utilize etch-and-rinse adhesive systems. In the other group, enamel and dentin are conditioned using self-etching primers (simplified resin cements). The third group does not require any conditioning of the tooth surface (self-adhesive resin cements). These materials were designed to simplify the cementation procedures while achieving some degree of adhesion.[53]

Resin cements, be they conventional or simplified, may perform differently depending on their adhesive systems, since the latter are primarily in contact with the dentin. Contemporary adhesive systems used in dentistry interact with the enamel/dentin substrate either by removing the smear layer (etch-and-rinse technique) or by partially dissolving the smear layer, penetrating through it, decalcifying underlying intertubular dentin and impregnating any remaining smear layer for bonding (self-etch technique).[52] While the etch-and-rinse bonding technique is initiated by a separate etching step using 35–37% phosphoric acid that is later rinsed away, the self-etch/primer agent containing acidic monomers is only air-dried, thus remaining within the modified smear layer. The self-etch approach could also be called as 'etch-and-dry' approach. Such adhesives make the application less technique-sensitive for clinicians. Besides micromechanical interlocking through hybridization, specific functional monomers of 'mild' or 'intermediate' two-step self-etching adhesives were shown to interact chemically with residual hydroxyapatite crystals that remain available in the submicrometre hybrid layer.[53] While some studies reported higher bond strengths to dentin with two-step self-etching adhesives compared to one-step ones, others reported comparable or lower bonding efficacy to dentin (see review by Carvalho *et al.*).[53] In fact, testing resin cements with their adhesives/primers after ageing would deliver more realistic results that are often neglected in *in vitro* studies.[52]

Self-adhesive cements

The complexity of specific conditioning methods required for both the tooth surface, be it dentin or enamel, and the restorative material, glass or oxide-based ceramic, metals or polymers, increases the technique sensitivity of the adhesive cementation procedures. For this reason, a new group of resin cements were introduced to the market, the so-called self-adhesive cements that do not require any conditioning of either substrates.

Acid-functionalized monomers such as (meth)acrylate monomers with either carboxylic acid groups, like 4-methacryloxyethyl trimellitic anhydride (4-META) and pyromellitic glycerol dimethacrylate (PMGDM), or phosphoric acid groups, like 2-methacryoxyethyl phenyl hydrogen phosphate (Phenyl-P), 10-methacryloxydecyl dihydrogen phosphate (MDP), bis(2-methacryloxyethyl) acid phosphate (BMP) and dipentaerythritol penta-acrylate monophosphate (Penta-P) are used to achieve demineralization and bonding to the tooth surface.[54] In addition to these monomers, new proprietary acidic monomers, primarily those based on phosphates and phosphonates that have been developed to demineralize enamel and dentin as well as to promote stable salt formation, mainly involving calcium. The selection of the acidic monomer structure is critically important as exemplified by the formation of a strong, aqueous insoluble salt complex between calcium and the relatively hydrophobic MDP, whereas 4-META and Phenyl-P produce a calcium complex with more limited stability to dissolution.[54] The concentration of the acidic monomers in these materials must be balanced low enough to avoid excessive hydrophilicity in the final polymer but high enough to achieve an acceptable degree of self-etching character and bonding to dentin and enamel. The acidic monomers, depending on the type and concentration of acid functionality as well as the moisture content, have a pH between 1.5 and 3 immediately after mixing the cement which is certainly acidic enough to demineralize the tooth surface. As the acid–base reaction proceeds, ionic cross-links that form between acid groups and calcium or aluminium ions cause the pH to rise.

Microleakage of all-ceramic crowns was reported to be higher (1.78–13.12%) depending on the product than that of one conventional resin cement (0.76%) on enamel surfaces.[54] Their diffusion levels into dentin and their hydrolytic stability were reported not to be optimal.[55] Also recently, the bonding efficacy of self-adhesive cements especially in deep dentin was found to be more challenging for self-adhesive cements owing to reduced area of solid intertubular dentin associated with the increased water content, compared to superficial dentin.[52] From a clinical point of view, the depth of dentin could not be controlled during tooth preparation. Therefore, clinically the cements that adhere well to both superficial and deep dentin were recommended.

Self-adhesive cements can be polymerized either in self-cure mode or in dual cure mode. The degree of conversion was found to be much higher in dual cure mode, yet remained less than conventional resin cements.[56] Nonetheless, early clinical studies have not reported inferior results so far.[57,58] However, clinical evaluations are few and short term, so drawing long-term conclusions about the overall effectiveness of these cements in dental practice is not yet possible. However, the handling properties of these materials appear to be excellent and therefore their acceptance by the profession is increasing. The most common dental cement types, classified by application, benefits and drawbacks are listed in Table 13.1.

13.3 Clinical implications of cement choice

Considering that there is no ideal luting material for all cementation purposes on the market, the above-mentioned properties of a cement are also associated with several confounding clinical factors (i.e. occlusion, preparation design, moisture control, type of build-up material, type of supporting tooth structure, surface roughness, margin location, tooth location, amount of tooth destruction and abutment mobility) that determine the selection of the cement. One of the determinants of the choice between water-based or polymerizing cements is concern about microleakage and eventually secondary caries on the dental tissues underneath the FDP. Water-based cements are more prone to solubility than resin-based cements. An ideal fit of the restoration should be one of the major tasks of the clinicians and the dental technicians, especially for restorations that are conventionally cemented. On the other hand, resin cements are formulated to offer strength, aesthetics, flexible working times and very low solubility yet they are also technique sensitive and not cost-effective. An inappropriate luting agent selection or improper manipulation might affect the longevity of an indirect restoration.

With the implementation of all-ceramics, aesthetic considerations also play an important role associated with the choice of cements. Conventional

Table 13.1 Most common dental cements classified by application, benefits and drawbacks modified according to Powers and Sakaguchi[59]

Cements	Application	Benefits	Drawbacks
Water-based glass-ionomer	Class V restorations Retention of conventional alloy-based restorations Retention of alumina- or zirconia-based all-ceramic restorations Retention of long-term provisional restorations	Bond to tooth tissues; Fluoride release; Relatively great resistance to disintegration; Relatively biocompatible.	Short working time; Slow maturing process; Crack development during dry conditions; Low elastic modulus; High *in vivo* solubility.
Zinc phosphate	Retention of conventional restorations; Retention of long-term provisional restorations.	Long-term experience; Universal cementation agent; Good handling characteristics; Proven longevity with well-designed and well-fitting restorations.	Pulp irritant; Lack of adhesive properties; No anticariogenic ingredients
Polymerizing cements; Composites and adhesive cements	Retention of conventional alloy-based restorations; Bonded all-ceramic crowns, bridges, veneers, inlays, and onlays; Bonded laboratory composite crowns, bridges, veneers, inlays and onlays; Bonded posts and cores cements.	Very low solubility; Excellent compressive strength; Superior long-term bond to enamel; Acceptable bond to dentin under certain limitations; High fracture toughness.	Difficult handling characteristics; Pulp irritant; Lack of anticariogenic properties.
Resin-modified glass ionomer	Class V restorations; Retention of conventional alloy-based restorations; Retention of alumina- or zirconia-based all-ceramic restorations; Retention of long-term provisional restorations.	Increased elastic modulus; Increased compressive strength; Low solubility.	Hydrophilic properties; Water uptake expansion.

resin-based cements offer a wide variety of colours with which to manipulate the end result of the restorations. This is particularly important for anterior ceramic veneers where high aesthetics are demanded.

Water-based cements, using for instance, GIC could be preferred if the patient is known to be allergic to any of the ingredients present in adhesive bonding agents, if sub-optimal periodontal conditions are present, or when the visibility of the working field is poor. The basic requirements for water-based cements are an adequate marginal fit (<100 mm), tooth preparations that exhibit only a slight taper of 4–10° as well as rather long clinical crowns (>3 mm) which provide a large rough contact surface to prevent the loss of retention.[5] The choice of conventional resin-based cements is obligatory for ceramic veneers, inlays and onlays to increase the fracture strength especially of silica-based ceramics. However, to avoid a higher incidence of microleakage, it is advantageous to confine the preparation margins within the enamel.

With the introduction of high-strength oxide ceramics, compulsory application of adhesive cementation diminished. Reinforced ceramics do not seem to require adhesive cementation for ceramic strengthening purposes unless of course, the fit of the restorations is ideal and there is enough retention. Furthermore, early reports on more user-friendly self-etching cements are promising despite some unfavourable data regarding their polymerization degree, dentin infiltration or microleakage, although clinical long-term data are not available to date.

In all aspects of adhesive cementation, appropriate surface conditioning both for the dental tissues and the cementation surface of the restorations should be performed. In adhesive applications, at best tooth–cement–material unity should be achieved. This issue is particularly important in minimally invasive applications since retention of the restoration does not rely on mechanical retention. The type of tooth substrate, enamel or dentin, seems to have an impact on the type of failure and therefore appropriate conditioning of each substrate is crucial.[50] Absolutely clean surfaces are also required although in indirect restorations the dentin or enamel surfaces are often contaminated with provisional cements, implying that the substrate surface is not always ideal for superb adhesion.

13.4 Conclusion and future trends

In conclusion, clinicians should consider all confounding factors when deciding between water-based or polymerizing cements. The selection of cement type and cementation mode is dictated by the restoration (i.e. restorative material properties, marginal fit, type of restoration, surface treatment), the properties of the cement (i.e. viscosity, biocompatibility, adhesive potential, solubility, water uptake, colour stability, wear resistance, working and setting characteristics, sealing ability, optical properties, radioopacity) as well as various clinical co-variables such as occlusion, preparation design (retentive or non-retentive), moisture control, type of build-up material, type of supporting abutment (natural tooth structure: enamel, dentin, cementum), or implant abutment (titanium or oxide ceramic), mobility of abutment, surface roughness, margin location (enamel, dentin or cementum), tooth location, and degree of tooth destruction (see review by Edelhoff and Özcan).[5]

In many applications of FDPs such as implants, resin-bonded, or metal–ceramic restorations, the dental literature lacks split-mouth randomized clinical trials. Future study designs should consider this missing information considering both mechanical and qualitative criteria. In particular, the clinical relevancy of the degradation of luting-cement–tooth interface needs closer attention. Simplification of the cementation, especially with the new acidic monomers, needs long-term clinical evaluation, considering that current *in vitro* data are not always favourable for such materials when physical and chemical properties are considered. Still, one-universal cement, for all clinical indications does not exist yet.

13.5 References

1. Hill EE and Lott J. 'A clinically focused discussion of luting materials'. *Aust Dent J* 2011, **56**, 67–76.
2. Buonocore MG. 'A simple method of increasing the adhesion of acrylic filling materials to enamel surfaces'. *J Dent Res* 1955, **34**, 849–53.
3. Bowen RL, Rupp NW, Eichmiller FC and Stanley HR. 'Clinical biocompatibility of an experimental dentine-enamel adhesive for composites'. *Int Dent J* 1989, **39**, 247–52.
4. Tyas MJ and Burrow MF. 'Adhesive restorative materials: A review'. *Aust Dent J* 2004, **49**, 112–21.
5. Edelhoff D and Özcan M. 'To what extent does the longevity of fixed dental prostheses depend on the function of the cement? Working Group 4 materials: cementation.' *Clin Oral Implants Res* 2007, **18**, 193–204.
6. De la Macorra JC and Pradies G. 'Conventional and adhesive luting cements'. *Clin Oral Investig* 2002, **6**, 198–204.
7. Diaz-Arnold AM, Vargas MA and Haselton DR. 'Current status of luting agents for fixed prosthodontics'. *J Prosthet Dent* 1999, **81**, 135–41.
8. Norman RD, Swartz ML, Phillips RW and Sears CR. 'Properties of cements mixed from liquids with altered water content'. *J Prosthet Dent* 1970, **24**, 410–18.
9. Shillingburg HT, Hobo S and Whitsett LD. *Fundamentals of Fixed Prosthodontics*. 2nd edn, Quintessence Publishing, Chicago, USA. 1981, 454 pp.
10. Jabri M, Mejdoubi E, El Gadi M and Hammouti B. 'Optimisation of hardness and setting time of dental zinc phosphate cement using a design of experiments'. *Arab J Chem* 2012, **5**, 347–51.
11. Liu Y and Yu HY. 'Does dental zinc phosphate cement really shrink in clinical applications?' *Med Hypotheses* 2009, **73**, 257–8.

12. Heintze SD. 'Crown pull-off test (crown retention test) to evaluate the bonding effectiveness of luting agents'. *Dent Mater* 2010, **26**, 193–206.
13. Phillips RW, Swartz ML, Norman RD, Schnell RJ and Niblack BF. 'Zinc oxide and eugenol cements for permanent cementation'. *J Prosthet Dent* 1968, **19**, 144–50.
14. Drummond JL, Lenke JW and Randolph RG. 'Compressive strength comparison and crystal morphology of dental cements'. *Dent Mater* 1988, **4**, 38–40.
15. Gemalmaz D, Pameijer CH, Latta M, Kuybulu F and Alcan T. '*In vivo* disintegration of four different luting agents'. *J Prosthet Dent* 2011, **12**, 1–6.
16. Dupuis V, Laviole O, Pautin-Gautier M, Castetbon A and Moya F. 'Solubility and disintegration of zinc phosphate cement'. *Biomaterials* 1992, **13**, 467–70.
17. Yanıkoğlu N and Duymuş Yeşil Z. 'Evaluation of the solubility of dental cements in artificial saliva of different pH values'. *Dent Mater* J 2007, **26**, 62–7.
18. Newman SM. 'Frozen-slab technique for mixing zinc phosphate cement for cast restorations'. *J Prosthet Dent* 1980, **43**, 46–9.
19. Fleming GJP, Shelton RM, Landini G and Marquis PM. 'The influence of mixing ratio on the toughening mechanisms of a hand-mixed zinc phosphate dental cement'. *Dent Mater* 2001, **17**, 14–20.
20. Wacker DR and Tjan AHL. 'Effect of variation in powder-to-liquid ratio of zinc phosphate cement on the retention of posts'. *J Prosthet Dent* 1988, **60**, 49–52.
21. Assif D, Azoulay S and Gorfil C. 'The degree of zinc phosphate cement coverage of complete crown preparations and its effect on crown retention'. *J Prosthet Dent* 1992, **68**, 275–8.
22. Mount GJ. 'Clinical performance of glass-ionomers'. *Biomaterials* 1998, **19**, 573–9.
23. De Backer H, Van Maele G, De Moor N and Van den Berghe L. 'An up to 20-year retrospective study of 4-unit fixed dental prostheses for the replacement of 2 missing adjacent teeth'. *Int J Prosthodont* 2008, **21**, 259–66.
24. Jokstad A. 'A split-mouth randomized clinical trial of single crowns retained with resin-modified glass-ionomer and zinc phosphate luting cements'. *Int J Prosthodont* 2004, **17**, 411–16.
25. Behr M, Rosentritt M, Wimmer J, Lang R, Kolbeck C, Bürgers R and Handel G. 'Self-adhesive resin cement versus zinc phosphate luting material: A prospective clinical trial begun 2003'. *Dent Mater* 2009, **25**, 601–4.
26. Nagaraja Upadhya P and Kishore G. Glass ionomer cement – the different generations'. *Trends Biomater Artif Organs* 2005, **18**, 158–65.
27. Peutzfeldt A, Sahafi A and Flury S. 'Bonding of restorative materials to dentin with various luting agents'. *Oper Dent* 2011, **36**, 266–73.
28. Francisconi LF, Scaffa PMC, Barros VR, Coutinho M and Francisconi PAS. 'Glass ionomer cements and their role in the restoration of non-carious cervical lesions'. *J Appli Oral Sci* 2009, **17**, 364–9.
29. Berg JH. 'Glass ionomer cements'. *Pediatric Dent* 2002, **24**, 430–8.
30. Tyas MJ. 'Clinical performance of glass-ionomer cements'. *J Appl Oral Sci* 2006, **14**, 10–13.
31. Sidhu SK. 'Glass-ionomer cement restorative materials: a sticky subject?' *Aust Dent J* 2011, **56**, 23–30.
32. Guggenberger R, May R and Stefan KP. 'New trends in glass-ionomer chemistry'. *Biomaterials* 1998, **19**, 479–83.

33. Smith DC. 'Development of glass-ionomer cement systems'. *Biomaterials* 1998, **19**, 467–78.
34. Utz KH, Grüner M and Vothknecht R. 'Cervical discrepancies and closeness of marginal fit of full cast crowns in correlation with the luting agent used'. *Dtsch Zahnarztl Z* 1989, **44**, 901–4.
35. Phillips RW, Swartz ML, Lund MS, Moore BK and Vickery J. '*In vivo* disintegration of luting cements'. *J Am Dent Assoc* 1987, **114**, 489–92.
36. Matis BA, Cochran M and Carlson T. 'Longevity of glass-ionomer restorative materials: results of a 10-year evaluation'. *Quintessence Int* 1996, **27**, 373–82.
37. Forsten L. 'Fluoride release and uptake by glass-ionomers and related materials and its clinical effect'. *Biomaterials* 1998, **19**, 503–8.
38. Basso GR, Della Bona A, Gobbi DL and Cecchetti D. 'Fluoride release from restorative materials'. *Braz Dent J* 2011, **22**, 355–8.
39. Lucas ME, Arita K and Nishino M. 'Toughness, bonding and fluoride-release properties of hydroxyapatite-added glass ionomer cement'. *Biomaterials* 2003, **24**, 3787–94.
40. Attia A. 'Bond strength of three luting agents to zirconia ceramic- influence of surface treatment and thermocycling'. *J Appl Oral Sci* 2011, **19**, 388–95.
41. Berzins DW, Abey S, Costache MC, Wilkie CA and Roberts HW. 'Resin-modified glass-ionomer setting reaction competition'. *J Dent Res* 2010, **89**, 82–6.
42. Kious AR, Roberts HW and Brackett WW. 'Film thicknesses of recently introduced luting cements'. *J Prosthet Dent* 2009, **101**, 189–92.
43. Rossetti PHO, Valle AL, Carvalho RM, Goes MF and Pegoraro LF. 'Correlation between margin fit and microleakage in complete crowns cemented with three luting agents'. *J Appl Oral Sci* 2008, **16**, 64–9.
44. Nicholson JW and Czarnecka B. 'The biocompatibility of resin-modified glass-ionomer cements for dentistry'. *Dent Mater* 2008, **24**, 1702–8.
45. Creugers NH, Käyser AF and van't Hof MA. 'A meta-analysis of durability data on conventional fixed bridges'. *Community Dent Oral Epidemiol* 1994, **22**, 448–52.
46. Paschoal MAB, Gurgel CV, Rios D, Magalhaes AC, Buzalaf MAR and Machado MAAM. 'Fluoride release profile of a nanofilled resin-modified glass ionomer cement'. *Braz Dent J* 2011, **22**, 275–9.
47. Mickenautsch S and Yengopal V. 'Demineralization of hard tooth tissue adjacent to resin-modified glass-ionomers and composite resins: a quantitative systematic review'. *J Oral Sci* 2010, **52**, 347–57.
48. Verbeeck RMH, De Maeyer EAP, Marks LAM, De Moor RJG, De Witte AMJC and Trimpeneers LM. 'Fluoride release process of (resin-modified) glass-ionomer cements versus (polyacid-modified) composite resins'. *Biomaterials* 1998, **19**, 509–19.
49. Sidhu SK. 'Clinical evaluations of resin-modified glass-ionomer restorations'. *Dent Mater* 2010, **26**, 7–12.
50. Özcan M, Nergiz I and Pfeiffer P. 'A brief history and current status of metal-and ceramic surface-conditioning concepts for resin bonding in dentistry'. *Quintessence Int* 1998, **29**, 713–74.
51. Burke FJ, Fleming GJ, Nathanson D and Marquis PM. 'Are adhesive technologies needed to support ceramics? An assessment of the current evidence'. *J Adhes Dent* 2002, **4**, 7–22.

52. Özcan M and Mese A. 'Adhesion of conventional and simplified resin-based luting cements to superficial and deep dentin'. *Clin Oral Investig.* 2012, **16**, 1081–8.
53. Carvalho RM, Manso AP, Geraldeli S, Tay FR and Pashley DH. 'Durability of bonds and clinical success of adhesive restorations'. *Dent Mater* 2012, **28**, 72–86.
54. Ferracane JL, Stansbury JW and Burke FJT. 'Self-adhesive resin cements – chemistry, properties and clinical considerations'. *J Oral Rehabil* 2011, **38**, 295–314.
55. Monticelli F, Osorio R, Mazzitelli C, Ferrari M and Toledano M. 'Limited decalcification/diffusion of self-adhesive cements into dentin'. *J Dent Res* 2008, **87**, 974–9.
56. Vrochari AD, Eliades G, Hellwig E and Wrbas KT. 'Curing efficiency of four self-etching, self-adhesive resin cements'. *Dent Mater* 2009, **25**, 1104–8.
57. Trajtenberg CP, Caram SJ and Kiat-amnuay S. 'Microleakage of all-ceramic crowns using self-etching resin luting agents'. *Oper Dent* 2008, **33**, 392–9.
58. Azevedo CG, De Goes MF, Ambrosano GM and Chan DC. '1-Year clinical study of indirect resin composite restorations luted with a self-adhesive resin cement: effect of enamel etching'. *Braz Dent J* 2012, **23**, 97–103.
59. Powers JM and Sakaguchi RJ. 'Cements'. In: *Craig's Restorative Dental Materials*, 12th edition, Powers JM and Sakaguchi RJ (eds), Mosby Elsevier, St Louis, 2006, 481.
60. Wilson AD and Kent BE, 'A new translucent cement for dentistry. The glass ionomer cement'. *Br Dent J* 1972, **132**, 133–5.

Index

Lightning Source UK Ltd.
Milton Keynes UK
UKOW030505270613

212847UK00001B/92/P

9 780857 092441